THE NEW MIDWIFERY

THE
NEW MIDWIFERY

EDITED BY
FARAH M. SHROFF

women's
PRESS

Canadian Cataloguing in Publication Data

Main entry under title:
The new midwifery: reflections on renaissance and regulation

Includes bibliographical references.
ISBN 0-88961-224-2

1. Midwifery — Canada. I. Shroff, Farah Mahrukh Coomi, 1965-

RG950.N49 1997   618.2'0233'0971   C97-932534-X

Cover art: Maxine Noel/ioyan mani
Cover design: Denise Maxwell
Editor: Leslie Thielen-Wilson
Copy editor: May Yee
Author photograph: Janice Pinto

This book was produced by the collective effort of Women's Press.
Women's Press gratefully acknowledges the support of the Ontario Arts Council and the
Canada Council for the Arts for our publishing program.

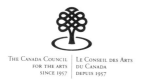

THE CANADA COUNCIL | LE CONSEIL DES ARTS
FOR THE ARTS | DU CANADA
SINCE 1957 | DEPUIS 1957

Published by Women's Press, Suite 302, 517 College Street,
Toronto, Ontario, Canada M6G 4A2.

Printed and bound in Canada.
1 2 3 4 5 2000 2001 1999 1998 1997

Contents

Acknowledgments... 9

Preface.. 11

Introduction: Midwifery — from Rebellion to Regulation
The Rebirth of An Ancient Calling
Farah M. Shroff *15*

SECTION I
Midwifery, Diversity and New Agreements with the State

A Path Towards Reclaiming Nishnawbe Birth Culture: Can the Midwifery
Exemption Clause for Aboriginal Midwives Make a Difference?
Carol Couchie and Herbert Nabigon *41*

Colonized Wombs
Sapna Patel and Iman Al-Jazairi *51*

Experiences of Mothers with Disabilities and Implications
for the Practice of Midwifery
Pat Israel *83*

Professionalizing Canadian Midwifery: Sociological Perspectives
Cecilia Benoit *93*

Midwives and Safe Motherhood: International Perspectives
Carol Hird and Brian Burtch......................................*115*

SECTION II
State Regulation of Midwifery Across Canada

Becoming Regulated: The Re-emergence of Midwifery in British Columbia
J. Alison Rice...*149*

Regulation: Changing The Face of Midwifery?
  Susan James *181*

Ontario Midwifery in Transition: An Exploration of Midwives' Perceptions
of the Impact of Midwifery Legislation in its First Year
  Mary Sharpe *201*

Prior Learning Assessment for Midwives and the TECMI-Coloured
Dreamcoat
  Farah M. Shroff,
  with Amy Hlaing and Betty Wu-Lawrence *245*

All Petals of the Flower: Celebrating the Diversity of Ontario's Birthing
Women within First-Year Midwifery Curriculum
  Farah M. Shroff *261*

Opinions of Certified and Lay Midwives About Midwifery in Quebec:
Perspectives for the Future of Their Profession
  Marie Hatem-Asmar and Régis Blais *311*

Midwifery in Atlantic Canada
  Charlene MacLellan *331*

Community Birthing Project: Northwest Territories
  Maureen Morewood-Northrop *343*

Closing Questions
  Farah M. Shroff *357*

Contributors *363*

Acknowledgments

Many people warned me that editing an anthology would be a very difficult experience. At the end of this journey, I feel enriched and inspired. It is impossible to name all the people who have nurtured this book's gestation, so to all of you whose names do not appear below, please accept a huge THANK YOU!!!!

Being pregnant for the first time as this book goes to print, I am excited about my continuing contact with midwives — this time as client.

Working with authors from all across the country was a very positive experience. The patience that you all exhibited for the slow process of publishing a book in difficult economic times, and more importantly, for the many drafts that I requested you to produce, has been a gift. Midwives Susan James and Mary Sharpe were authors who did more than just their own chapters. Amy Hlaing, Research Assistant, was helpful during some of the crucial phases of this book's creation. Ryerson Polytechnic University also supported this work.

Women's Press, particularly Martha Ayim, was a genuine delight to work with; I feel enlivened after our experience. Thank you Martha! — for being there in Calgary at the Learned Societies Conference — at the zygote stages of the book where some of the authors presented papers at a session I organized on state regulation of midwifery — and for being with me at every other stage. You midwifed this process like a truly compassionate and skilled companion.

My family/community was, as usual, a source of great love and compassion. Roozbeh, my beloved partner, Hoshang, my dad, Carole, my compañera, and others were great friends throughout this period: proofreading and gently criticizing the parts of the book I have authored. All the Bayanis/Mehrabadis (Yassi, Ladan, Behzad, Azar, and Kiwi my wag-tail walking/running/playing buddy), Milada Disman, Dale Edwards, Merwan Engineer, Elizabeth Flood, Noga Gayle, Toni Graeme, Dorothy Kidd, Janice Meilach, Fay Neuber, Manga, Rumi Shroff and family, Vee Shroff, Carole Yawney, and many others were encouraging and caring throughout this time. Although I did not come into this world with a midwife present, my mother and grandmothers fully compensated by ensuring that this baby was nurtured from infancy to adulthood. You continue to do this and I love you deeply.

Farah Mahrukh Coomi Shroff
Editor

Preface

Change is virtually always difficult. It brings forth the discomfort of those who have grown accustomed to and benefited from the status quo. It often creates anger, fear, resentment, jealousy and can also create or nurture excitement, joy and satisfaction.

This book is about change. Authors from all over Canada examine changes in the way that midwifery is positioned in relation to the state, hospitals, the legal system, and to birthing women, doctors, nurses, and other healthcare providers. The book's authors thus reflect on the burning issue in Canadian midwifery today: how is the experiment with state regulation going? (Or: what happens to the oldest women's profession when it goes to bed with the state?)

Midwifery is an ancient calling. The book's title, "The New Midwifery: Reflections on Renaissance and Regulation," and in particular the word "new," refers to the new agreements that midwives are making with the state. The term "renaissance" was inserted into the title to refer to the rebirth of this ancient calling and to recognize the French language as one of the patches of Canada's large and colourful linguistic quilt.

The book's authors are mostly midwives and social scientists (with a few exceptions) who live in various geographical locations of the country. Amongst the authors are some who have been consumers of midwifery services but the voice of midwifery consumers is not the strongest in the book. Journals that cover state regulation include *Mothering* magazine and *Birth Issues*. Hundreds of internet sites are devoted to midwifery issues; one that has discussed regulation from both consumer and practitioner perspectives is called "Midwifery Today." For Canadian literature on birthing women's perspectives on pregnancy (although it is unrelated to state regulation), readers may wish to turn to Daphne Morrison's *Being Pregnant*. Birthing women have been central to the success of state-supported and funded midwifery and several consumer groups around the country (e.g. "Midwifery Consumers of Alberta Network" and Saskatchewan's "Friends of Midwives") were formed with the express purpose of lobbying for midwifery's recognition and coverage. A wonderful addition to midwifery literature in Canada would be a book by women from diverse backgrounds who had given birth with the assistance of midwives, particularly if the publication examined issues of access to midwifery and had implications for state regulation.

Many other voices in this book could have been louder: those of lesbians, teen mothers, and many other women. The chapter on the midwifery needs of diverse women (by Farah M. Shroff) attempts to address some of these issues. Despite efforts, another voice that is not as strong in this collection is that of midwives who are against regulation and lost (or will lose) their livelihoods as a result of it. The introductory chapter (by Farah M. Shroff) thus outlines some of these issues.

One of the book's contributions is the foregrounding of First Nations midwifery issues as well as the inclusion of race and class analyses. The history of midwifery in Canada is usually written as colonial history and begins with European settlers' midwifery practices. For this book, each author was requested to acknowledge the presence of midwifery in their region before the arrival of non-Native peoples. In addition, Carol Couchie (a First Nations midwife) and Herbert Nabigon have written a chapter specifically on First Nations midwifery perspectives using the medicine wheel as a framework for their ideas.

A chapter by Iman Al-Jazairi and Sapna Patel documents and analyzes the views of some women of colour toward midwifery. Al-Jazairi and Patel spoke with dozens of racialized women about the status of midwifery in their home communities and in current-day Ontario. Their chapter scrutinizes colonization of the mind and body, interrogates racial dynamics in Ontario society, and provides an insightful perspective on women of colour's involvement — and lack thereof — in midwifery in this country. Another chapter scrutinizes a small project directed toward women of colour's involvement in midwifery assessment and certification (by Farah M. Shroff with Amy Hlaing and Betty Wu-Lawrence). This attention to racial and ethnic issues is also new in Canadian literature on midwifery.

Pat Israel's chapter on women with disabilities and midwifery is another of this anthology's highlights. Breaking through social notions that women with disabilities should not bear children, the author affirms the life-giving abilities of women with various disabilities. Israel discusses the place of midwifery in women with disabilities' pregnancies and births.

Canadian midwives have set themselves apart from other professional groups by trying very hard to be directed by the needs of their clients. Canadian midwifery clients are overwhelmingly satisfied with the work of midwives and have laboured alongside midwives for the recognition, financial coverage, and legitimization of this ancient women's vocation. In most parts of Canada their combined labour has borne fruit. This book examines the complex questions arising on this new leg of the midwifery journey.

Canada has already garnered attention from the rest of the world for the woman-centred midwifery legislation which is enshrined in Ontario, British Columbia, and other parts of the country. Canadian midwives and consumers worked very hard to learn from other countries about the benefits of various forms of legislation and were able to implement "a jewel" of such legislation in this country. This is unique because birthing women's needs, not those of midwifery practitioners, are the focus of midwives' work and this is mirrored in the legislation. Few professional groups have succeeded in turning their rhetoric into this kind of material reality; midwives are peerless in their dedicated attempts in this regard.

Ontario's Midwifery Education Program (based on a common curriculum at three universities — Laurentian, McMaster and Ryerson Polytechnic) was rated by a British and U.S. team of midwifery experts as the world's leading midwifery education program. Again, Canadians ought to know about this achievement, particularly as it is based on trying to push the boundaries of a didactic professionalized university education toward feminist knowledge bases and teaching methods.

This is Canada's first book exploring the complexities of state regulation of midwifery. As the years proceed there will be a need for regular analyses of these issues, for surely time will create new hurdles and new celebrations.

Farah M. Shroff

Introduction

Midwifery — from Rebellion to Regulation

The Rebirth of An Ancient Calling

Farah M. Shroff

do-di-seem	(Nishnawbe, Ojibway) "one who cuts the cord"
ikajurti	(Inuktituk) "the helper at birth"
m-kunga	(Swahili) "confidential advisor, especially an older friend who gives advice"
da.ii	(Hindi) "one who places/puts the baby"
porodni baba	(Czech) "birthing grandmother"
mid' wif	(Old English) "with woman"
ghabeleh	(Farsi) "a receiver" and "capable woman"
saavikaa	(Sanskrit) "one who assists in birth"
agbEbi	(Yoruba) "one who takes/accepts birth"
su.ii.n	(Marati) "one who assists someone else give birth"
sage-femme	(French) "wise woman"
jordmor	(Danish) "earth mother"
kyndik-sheshe	(Russian) "mother ligating the umbilical cord"
chu ch' an fu	(Mandarin) "a woman who helps to bear/give birth"[1]

In the rich linguistic and cultural heritage of Canada, midwifery has an ancient herstory. In First Nations cultures, as well as those of people who have arrived in the past few hundred years, midwives have played a vital and often highly respected role in social and health affairs, delivering most of the babies. (It is estimated that midwives deliver about 80% of the world's babies.)[2]

Non-native Canadians come from all over the world, and in most countries, midwifery is at least recognized if not respected. Despite this reality, midwifery is a term and concept unfamiliar to many Canadians. While it is practised in virtually every part of Canada, its practitioner base is very small. Regardless of its numbers, midwifery has only recently been legislated and regulated in many jurisdictions and the Ontario Midwifery Education

Programme has been rated by a U.S. and British evaluation team as a world leader in midwifery education.

This introductory chapter presents general social issues related to the practice of midwifery in order to lay the ground for the more detailed discussions in the book's following chapters. Included here are sections on Midwifery in Canadian Society, the Midwifery Model of Care, Debates about the State Regulation of Midwifery, Professionalization, Holistic Care, Caring, University Education, Diversity in Midwifery, and A Stork's Eye View of this Book. My knowledge of midwifery issues comes from my work as a Social Scientist with the Ontario Midwifery Education Programme.

MIDWIFERY IN CANADIAN SOCIETY

Lack of knowledge on the part of some Canadians regarding the world's oldest women's profession[3] is due to several factors, some of which are explored in the chapters of this book. Briefly, they include the medical take-over of reproductive health care, growing social and economic support for technological medicine, patriarchal domination of health care, colonial oppression which propped up Western medical practices, among many other factors.

The lack of societal knowledge about midwifery is a relatively recent phenomenon in this part of the world, as midwifery has thrived here in the heritage of the original peoples. Canada's oldest midwifery traditions stem from Aboriginal peoples. Midwives have been part of virtually every Aboriginal community and some midwives continue to practise today. English and French colonial oppression damaged many aspects of First Nations health culture, but resistance to this oppression has managed to maintain some of the ancient wisdom of midwifery. In Povungnituk, Northern Quebec, First Nations women have worked with midwives to revive natural childbirth, and the birthing centre in Povungnituk respects and incorporates some traditional Aboriginal midwifery practices. Mohawk midwife Katsi Cook is an active researcher and writer about traditional midwifery, cultural and ecological issues. There are other Aboriginal midwives who practice midwifery in other parts of Canada.

European traditions of midwifery — which are ancient too — were also brought here. European midwives were 'catching babies' for virtually as long as European societies have existed.[4] From the early days of colonialization in Canada, English and French midwives assisted women in childbirth.[5] Other immigrant communities — from the South and other countries of the North — which have long traditions of midwifery practice, brought midwifery with them as well.

Despite the presence of First Nations and immigrant traditions of midwifery in Canada for centuries, midwifery in Canada has been in limbo for over 100 years — with quasi-legal status.[6] Over this period, Western medical doctors and their supporters had wrestled control of childbirth from mid-wives. Midwifery practice in Canada declined.

By the early 1990s, midwives were practising in small numbers, under the threat of being charged with practising medicine without a license. Birth had gone from being a healthy, normal event to a highly medicalized one. Part of this medicalization was due to the fact that by the 1960s, fetal health became a high priority for families, physicians, and society in general. Birth rates had declined and couples were having fewer children. Improving pregnancy outcomes thus became more important. Also, infant mortality statistics became global indicators for a nation's well-being.

Most contemporary Canadians — across ethnoracial groups, cultures, geographical locations, social classes, ages and other categories — generally consider the best birth to be a high-tech(nology) birth, and labour and delivery best done in a setting where people are ill — the hospital. This situation has arisen out of a complex matrix of factors related to Western medicine's power in recent history and across continents. The result is that Western reductionist medical practices have compelled women to give birth in a position[7] and under circumstances that are convenient for medical staff but not necessarily conducive nor healthy for women.

Partly as a response to women's needs/demands for positive birthing experiences, midwifery is experiencing a rebirth. While midwifery is prac-tised by few women, and even fewer men, and is therefore accessible to only a few birthing mothers, these numbers appear to be growing. Consumers and midwives have worked within the women's movement to lobby governments to regulate midwifery. Many women have become disillusioned with obstet-rical birth. Public esteem for medicine and science has declined in the past few decades.[8] Greater scepticism about the efficacy of Western medicine has led some people to seek other types of care. Some birthing mothers have sought care which attends to their psycho-social needs and have gained more humanized hospital birthing practices. For other women, midwifery has been exceedingly successful at meeting psycho-social needs while continuing to maintain high standards of maternal and infant health. Holistic health care[9] in general is also experiencing a rebirth, and thus desire for 'natural child-birth' has grown, particularly amongst university educated and activist women who have thus far been largely middle-class women of European descent. Midwifery's resurgence converges with the evolution and growth of the environmental movement which, amongst other things, advocates 'natu-ral' living. Given the current efforts of the Canadian midwifery movement (and this very anthology!) to integrate Aboriginal and immigrant Southern communities and anti-racism perspectives, it will be most interesting to observe the challenging future of midwifery.

Further factors for the resurgence of midwifery include cost effectiveness imperatives of the Canadian state: midwifery may save tax-payers' money by, for example, reducing the use of hospital services. Even if midwifery care costs the same, through its perspective of birth as a natural, not pathological, process as well as its extended support for mothers, babies and families, the short and long term outcomes may be better.

Furthermore, midwives in Canada have successfully worked within the women's movement, using feminist concepts and organizational techniques to work with women in fulfilling their birth-related needs. Midwifery clients have worked alongside midwives to lobby for the recognition of this ancient women's calling. Midwives and their supporters have convinced the state and some members of the public that midwifery fills an important gap in women's health care. They have been successful at drawing upon clinical and social research to prove the efficacy and safety of their profession. Political timing, being in the right place at the right time, women Ministers of Health, and a number of other forces contributed to state collaboration with segments of the midwifery movement. In each region of the nation, differing factors led to midwifery's regulation, and many of these are discussed in the following chapters.

THE MIDWIFERY MODEL OF CARE

After years of working 'with woman,' midwives and their supporters have created a model of care that is genuinely concerned with meeting the needs of clients. This model has the potential for positively influencing the models of care that are entrenched in the mainstream health care system. Most medical models of care place the professional at the centre. The 'woman-centred' midwifery model, as espoused in Ontario and other Canadian regions, is composed of three main elements: informed choice, choice of birth place and continuity of care.

Informed Choice

The goal of informed choice ensures that midwives provide birthing women with comprehensive information about their care, so that *they* may be the primary decision makers during the course of their midwifery care. This may, for example, include information about ultrasound tests; midwives explain the results of research conducted on ultrasound technology and the most current ideas about its benefits and drawbacks. Birthing women may then decide whether or not to undergo testing.

This is in direct contrast to 'informed consent' which is, at least in practice, legal protection for physicians. 'Patients' are requested/required to sign legal consent and waiver forms before certain medical procedures are performed upon them. Unless 'patients' sign these forms, the procedure will not be carried out. In emergency situations when 'patients' are highly vulnerable, this kind of pressure may be viewed as coercive, particularly because physicians do not have a good track record for explaining procedures, based on the latest research, to ill people and their families.

Even the language of midwifery embraces egalitarian ideals. Midwives 'follow women clients'; they do not have 'compliant (or non-compliant) patients.' Obedience and subservience is not expected within the midwifery model. The power dynamic between midwife and client is ideally an egalitarian one and most midwifery clientele passionately agree that this is the case in practice.

Until now, most midwifery clients were a self-selecting group who generally chose to have as little intervention as possible. Most tried to eat healthily, get lots of exercise and sleep, and had enough middle-class privilege to have work they enjoy (and/or partners whose income was substantial) and therefore were able to support the lifestyle they chose. Informed choice for this group, most of whom have had some post-secondary education, has usually led to decisions which resonate with the values of most midwives. If and when the client base expands, it may be very difficult for midwives to accept clients' decisions in an informed choice process. Clients may choose, for example, to continue smoking during pregnancy, despite all the research-based evidence their midwives (and others) provide about smoking's damage to mothers and fetuses. Different midwives will likely feel differently about how to handle these situations. While some will respect their clients' right to smoke and make minimal mention of the issue after it has been fully discussed once, others will continually try to convince them to quit.

Midwifery clients may thus make informed choices that are not conducive to the health of themselves or their babies. While midwives must conform to legal codes which may apply in the case of, for instance, illicit drug use, few laws exist in the case of most lifestyle issues such as smoking. The same issues arise for women clients who may choose to have a wide variety of technological testing done despite the lack of research evidence to prove its worth. Strictly following the tenet of informed choice therefore, means that midwives work with their clients under a wide variety of circumstances and that midwives continue to provide woman-centred care to all their clients regardless of (informed) choices made by their clients.

Choice of Birth Place

Birthing women have the right to choose where they would like to labour and deliver their babies. Women who, after rigorous examination, are deemed to be at very low risk of having anything but normal and healthy deliveries, have the option of labouring and delivering in their homes, birthing centres, or hospitals. In most Canadian jurisdictions, midwives have privileges in all three options, though generally the choice is between home and hospital, as few birthing centres exist. Women whose health conditions deem their pregnancies to be potentially 'high risk' are either referred at the first visit, or transferred when a diagnosis is made, to the care of a physician. In exceptional circumstances, physicians and midwives may work together to care for women who specifically request midwifery care but also need the care of physicians.

A cornerstone of midwifery care is the right of birthing women to choose to give birth in their home environment with the hospital as a back-up option. To emphasize its importance home birth is discussed below in a separate section.

Birthing centres combine the advantages of hospitals' technological capabilities within an environment that is more home-like than hospital-like. Birthing women who are concerned about the potential for unexpected problems occurring during childbirth (or rural women who live far away from hospitals or those who are nervous about homebirth but like the idea of it) have expressed an interest in birthing centres. A few such centres exist in the country, but because governments view them as expensive, and not all careproviders believe that they are a good idea, the future for birthing centres does not appear to be strong.

Women may also choose to give birth in hospitals with the assistance of midwives;[10] midwives have or will likely gain privileges at hospitals throughout the country. In the case of a transfer of care, women may be admitted to hospital under the care of a physician and their midwives may still be involved in some aspects of her psychosocial needs — transmitting information about the progress of a Cesarean section to the partner, advocating for the birthing woman, etc.

Continuity of Care

Birthing women receive continuous care from two to four midwives during the course of their care. While they are pregnant, they may meet up to four midwives who practice together. In most midwifery practices, birthing women work with a primary midwife and a back-up midwife. The same midwives they have met during their pregnancies are present at their birth. In other midwifery practices, birthing women work with up to four midwives prenatally and could have any of them at the birth as well as for the six weeks of post-partum visits. This continuity allows women to develop rapport — and in some cases meaningful relationships — with their care providers. Close contact, mentally, emotionally and otherwise, with midwives, has catalyzed the 'midwife as friend' concept which has made midwifery so popular with women. Midwives often share their own lives with birthing women and this tends to foster the egalitarian model of care that midwives uphold, for it shows that midwives are not 'above' their clients and in fact may have much in common with them.

Women who have experienced medically-managed childbirth often complain that they met several care-providers who came and went during the course of their care; especially during labour and delivery, this fragmentation of care can be discombobulating, exhausting and even frightening. Having to repeat herself time after time, to the next person on shift or the new person involved in her care, can take away from the meaningfulness of the birth experience. Continuity of care is thus a critical component of midwifery.

Other aspects of midwifery care include appropriate technology, time with women, and home birth.

Appropriate Technology

Midwives regularly use and/or carry with them a variety of 'low' or relatively non-invasive technologies such as: blood pressure cuffs, stethoscopes, fetoscopes (which assist in hearing the baby's heartbeat), infant resuscitation bags and masks, maternal oxygen masks and sufficient oxygen for transport of mother and baby, suturing instruments, urinalysis supplies, urinary catheter, intravenous supplies, syringes, needles, oxytocic drugs, local anaesthetic, scissors for episiotomy and cord, baby scales, and a long list of other equipment. They also routinely recommend tests which require some form of technology such as laboratory blood and urine tests. In cases where it is required, midwives support the use of high technology interventions such as Caesarean births.

The midwifery model of care is thus not anti-technology. Midwives support the judicious use of technological intervention starting with an assumption that minimal technology may be required in the care of some women. When it is necessary, based on research evidence, that birthing women require technological intervention, midwives support it. Without sound reasoning to support the need for technological intervention, the midwifery model of care upholds the tenet of natural birth being best.

Time with Women

Women spend about forty-five minutes with their midwives at each appointment. Because counselling and education are central to assisting women to have self-confidence and knowledge, both of which are the foundation for healthy childbirth, time to discuss women's concerns is very important. For many women, childbirth can be a time of change and unknowns, so reassurance is also important. Medical doctors tend to spend less than ten minutes with their 'patients.' This lack of time is the source of much of the dissatisfaction with the care of physicians.[11]

Home Birth

As mentioned above, home birth is a critical component of midwifery care and sometimes, this principle is listed separately from the principle of choice of birthplace. Home birth has possibly been the most contentious aspect of midwifery care as many care providers argue that it is unsafe. They argue that unpredictable/unpredicted problems could arise in a split-second and these problems may be potentially fatal without the aid of technology. Those who argue for the safety of home birth cite research which shows that home birth outcomes are equally as safe as those of hospital births.[12]

The home, for most women, is the place where they have power, control, comfort and love. In familiar physical and social surroundings, women report that birthing is an infinitely less difficult process than being in unfamiliar, sometimes unfriendly, hospitals. At home, many women are accustomed to being in charge and having their wishes followed. Having competent caregivers who nurture and assist birthing women in having the most positive birthing experience possible is a joy for many mothers, especially those who have supportive partners, families and communities as well as sufficient economic and social resources (such as adequate income, paternity leave, and child care) to have a positive home birth. Home birth can only be a positive option for women for whom home is a positive environment. For women who face violence, abuse and other forms of oppression in their homes, hospital births may provide an alternative to the site of their abuse.

The College of Midwives' 1994 *Statement on Home Birth*[13] notes that most births occur in hospital and midwives must be capable of attending hospital births. It states that birth is more than a physical or medical event and that a number of expectant parents plan to have home births and that "normal birth at home must be encouraged and supported." The statement ends by discussing safety: "Available evidence does suggest that for low-risk women, a planned birth at home with trained attendants is a safe and viable option."

DEBATES ABOUT THE STATE REGULATION OF MIDWIFERY

Midwifery is moving, or has moved, from the margins to the centre. However, recent moves toward state regulation of midwifery in Canada have not been uniformly appraised. In this section, the 'pro' and 'con' sides of the regulation debate are sketched.

In a time of cutbacks and clawbacks, the inclusion of midwifery into state-regulated and financed health care may be considered a victory for birthing mothers. According to its proponents, state regulation of the world's oldest women's calling is a true celebration — a celebration of years of hard work by consumers, midwives and many others. They hope that midwifery's presence will influence other healthcare professionals' practices in a positive way. They note that Caesarean section rates, for example, have been known to decrease just by the presence of midwives in the healthcare system.

For those midwifery supporters who do not agree with the state regulation of midwifery, this is a time of concern that the woman-centred model has been coopted, colleagues have 'sold out,' and midwifery has become an elite profession. Those opposed to regulation are convinced that midwives will become part of 'the system' and lose a social justice focus and connections with their clients and the women's movement. Bureaucratic requirements, it is argued, may make it difficult for women/clients to remain the focus of midwifery as paperwork, 'accountability,' and keeping up with other health-care professionals will become more important. Critics also contend that midwifery practice will become more medicalized (e.g. more prenatal testing, "just in case") once midwives are part of the medical hierarchy and become accountable to doctors. They note that newly registered midwives may, through requirements to document and standardize their practices, comply with medically set standards for labour and delivery, even at home births. Some fear that home birth may be eliminated altogether or that midwives will be divided between those who specialize in home birth and those who specialize in hospital birth.

Perhaps most importantly, some opposition to state regulation centres on the lack of attention to the caring functions of midwifery; midwifery's bailiwick is the 85% of normal births. The clinical training of a midwife is a vital foundation for women's safety but the most celebrated aspect of mid-wifery care is its psycho-social face: midwives are often considered to be more like friends than detached professional medical staff.

These woman-centred elements of midwifery care have led to a high rate of client satisfaction. Critics argue that it is possible to legislate these principles and practices but that the caring, nurturing and friendship aspects of midwifery may get lost in the push for professional status. Supporters of state-regulated midwifery respond by stating that legislating the woman-cen-tred model is a huge step for birthing women and that following the model has almost always resulted in a friendly relationship between midwives and their clients. They also note that some clients are not necessarily seeking a friend in their midwife, as they may consider birth matters to be highly private or they are not the type of people who 'bare their souls' to others, especially professionals. These clients simply want a practitioner who is competent and can assist them to have a safe and positive birthing experience.

Women who were practising lay midwifery prior to the introduction of state-sanctioned/controlled midwifery are now legally barred from claiming the title 'midwife.' This group of lay midwives has lost their livelihood and is understandably upset. Ontario midwife Anne Maranta writes:

> I do not believe that the process that has gone on in this province in the last decade has been at all womyn-centred. I firmly believed that the process towards legalization was patriarchally-initiated and carried out. And that the process of becoming admitted to the Michener program[14] is a symptom of the whole male-dominated process. I firmly believe that womyn intuitively know among whom it is safe for them to birth and that given the opportunity they will seek those womyn out.... Paper certificates of competency say little. They may

indicate that a subject has been studied but they cannot be taken as an indication of knowledge or skill. They indicate that a specified amount of book learning has taken place, but not whether the womyn of the community this individual serves feel safe with this care provider. They say nothing about the soundness of judgment this practitioner may or may not hold.

We are still in the Burning Times ... the torture is different but we are still being asked to inform on our mothers, sisters, and daughters.... We are still considered a threat because we are able to empower by imparting information, supporting choice, respecting the decisions of individual womyn independent of their male counterparts.[15]

Some may feel that Maranta is absolutely correct, and that the process of legislating midwifery has not been favourable for women. Others may label the above sentiments as romanticization of pre-legislated midwifery, arguing that standards must be set for acceptable care and that some book learning does equate to knowledge or skill. They may also critique the above ideas as difficult to implement as it is not easy to support only those health practitioners favoured by the women of the local area.

Another Ontario midwife, Madeline Clin,[16] writes an open letter in 1993 to midwives (who at the time were in the process of the registration) asking them to help find a place for the midwives left out of the process. Clin appeals to registering midwives' sympathy by stating that upon the declaration of the legislation which regulates midwifery, women like her will not be able to continue their work. She declares that they may apply for admission into the university program but there are no designated spaces for them as there are for First Nations students and Francophones. Before the first group of students graduate, she points out, about 75 midwives are to be responsible for practice, clinical teaching and the College of Midwives. The only new midwives will be those who go through the Prior Learning Assessment (PLA) process and many of these "will be foreign-trained midwives, many of whom are nurses at present...[and] do not share the midwifery philosophy in Ontario that we share."[17] She continues, by asserting that yet others may choose to gain accreditation in other jurisdictions, which is very costly, and could lead to monetary factors determining who becomes a Registered Midwife.

In hindsight, Clin was correct about the difficulties inherent in a small number of midwives trying to keep together the entire profession; it was and continues to be extremely stressful for most midwives to keep up with the demands of practising midwifery and professional association and other unpaid midwifery work. They definitely could have used a few more hands to help with all the work. Her concluding point about financial factors determining who is registered as a legal midwife has also been borne out in many ways, including within the university program. Very few working-class students are admitted and even fewer are successfully moving through the program. However, during pre-legislation days, it was not necessarily cheaper to become a midwife; aspiring midwives travelled to other countries or worked for years as an apprentice, making very little money. Once they became fully trained midwives, most did not make more than $20,000 per annum, so they never became wealthy as a result of their private entrepreneurial midwifery practices.

Founding member and past president of the Association of Ontario Midwives, Ava Wheeler (currently a registered midwife practising in Northern Ontario), writes that legislation will bring a 'medical model' of midwifery where midwives become incorporated into the mainstream healthcare system. She notes that she would prefer to continue practising in the "very personal, intimate, creative, spiritual healing way that I've been practising in for the past fourteen years."[18] Her fear that midwifery will become medicalized represents the fears of most people who oppose state regulation of midwifery. Just as it is difficult to get into bed with someone and not get 'intimate,' critics argue, so is it difficult to become part of a dominant medical model without getting so close that you pick up some of its characteristics. On a personal level, Wheeler comments that she is not interested in a full-time midwifery career as being with her own children is important. She states that she would like to be able to continue to attend two to three births per month, for people with whom she feels very connected. In Northern Ontario, she mentions, the distances between settlements means that most of her clients are at least 30 to 60 minutes away from her and that it is too difficult to be on call for postpartum visits and other needs while trying to "do tons of births."[19]

The current regulations in Ontario allow midwives to work part-time, to a minimum of ten primary births per year (five of which must be home births and five of which must be hospital births), so midwives with similar lifestyle preferences ought to be able to balance their domestic lives with their midwifery responsibilities. Many midwifery students complain of the difficulties of coping with their families' needs and the exceedingly high demands of the profession. Wheeler is not alone in wanting to 'be there' for her own family while also being a midwife. The rigorous standards for midwives and the high expectations for participation in professional activities besides practice (such as being involved in the professional associations), make it very difficult to juggle home- and work-life for many midwives.

Regarding Wheeler's point about distances in the North, Northern midwives are currently provided with case-load variables and their needs are taken into account by the College of Midwives. Working with people to whom one feels connected would be a dream for most workers, but this kind of care could not be financially supported by tax payers in an equitable political system because the subjective choices of care-providers would inevitably mean that certain citizens would receive no service; for instance, would service providers feel connected to people who are very different from them with respect to sexual orientation, social class, ethno-racial identity, lifestyle choices and so forth?

Regulation has thus created divisions between midwives. Some would argue that midwives and consumers have also been divided by regulation. In many provinces, midwives and consumers joined together to form organizations designed to lobby for the recognition of midwifery. Once organizing efforts gathered steam, midwives formed their own professional bodies. This was largely in anticipation of regulation and self-regulation which would require midwives, as autonomous practitioners, to have their own professional association. Midwives argue that despite this separation, birthing women continue to set the midwifery agenda. Others argue that this separation during the 1970s and 1980s gave consumers less input into the direction in which midwifery was going. They feel that midwifery leadership used the support of consumers until they did not need it and then left consumers behind.

Differences of opinion regarding midwifery's regulation exist within other professional groups as well. Many nurses, nursing schools and associations fought to have midwifery become a sub-specialty of nursing and have remained bitter after their loss. Some labour and delivery nurses also lost the possibility of attending hospital births at which midwives are the primary caregivers; because two midwives must be present at every birth, the midwives displace the former role of the nurse (and doctor). This turf battle has also created rivalries between nurses and midwives. This is not, however, occuring on a large scale.

Physicians have remained the most powerful member of the healthcare hierarchy, and although the official organs of the profession may support midwifery in principal, many individuals and groups do not. For the first year of the Ontario university program for example, neither midwives nor midwifery students were granted privileges at one northern hospital. Practising midwives and students in various parts of Northern Ontario have experienced hostility and resistance from physicians and other members of the hospital hierarchy. Southern midwives and students do experience hostility but it tends to be less frequent and less audacious. An obstetrician is quoted in a Globe and Mail article (about the graduation of the first group of midwifery students) as saying "Good luck to the midwives. I don't want parity with them. I want to be recognized as far more experienced and trained than the midwives."[20] Midwives are trained for four years at university as specialists in birthing. Physicians' basic curricula usually do not include more than 14 weeks of obstetrical training.[21]

Physicians' scrutiny plays a major role in the ongoing development of the midwifery profession. Quebec and British Columbia midwives have especially experienced conflict with physicians. This being noted, a critical mass of physicians have supported midwifery. These physicians see their role as caregivers for women experiencing high-risk pregnancies and are willing to leave the rest of the 'labour' to midwives. Some physicians were relieved to have midwives taking over some births, as physicians' insurance rates were climbing. Yet others were indifferent to the entry of midwifery. It is never possible to make generalizations about an entire profession.

Professionalization
In order to gain state approval, midwives had to prove that they had a distinctive body of knowledge and sufficient willingness among members of the profession to become regulated. Critics contend that by conforming to state-approved standards, midwives will lose the ability to respond to individual women's needs, and that a professionalizing elite of midwives — a handful of women — orchestrated the move toward legislation.

Professionalization, according to sociological theory, is implicitly hierarchical and thus elitist and exclusionary. Sociologists on the left have oft quoted George Bernard Shaw's famous statement that professionalism is a conspiracy against the laity. Professionalism is partly about gaining elite status and having more power than nonprofessionals and having power over others. Professionals usually have codes of conduct that are set by their governing bodies and particular forms of language they use; some call this jargon. Professionals may try to mystify their knowledge base and practices so as to justify their high place in the social hierarchy and the concomitant salary that comes with it. (Simplifying knowledge and practices means that anybody could do it.) Maintaining a clearly defined epistemological and practice-based 'turf' is key to maintaining professional status. Cecilia Benoit's chapter explicates sociological theories of professionalization.

Practising within a medical system which is inherently inegalitarian, will midwives be able to maintain egalitarian relationships with their clients? Adherence to hospital policies and newly designed professional policies may hinder midwives' ability to respond to clients' needs. With state legitimization, particular forms of knowledge and clinical practice were approved. Those midwives who conformed to these standards, often because they had helped to set them in the first place, gained ascendancy within state-structured midwifery. Will the professionalizing elite represent the spectrum of midwives or their own interests?

Caring
Will registered midwives be able to place caring high on their agenda?[22] Within another state-regulated mostly female profession — nursing — caring has become compromised due to a number of cost and treatment issues. This is not to state that nurses in general do not provide compassionate care, because they do indeed, but simply to point out that other tasks are considered more important. When nurses have barely enough time to give out medica-

tions and attend to the basic necessities, it is virtually impossible to carry out
other functions. The 'extras,' such as spending time chatting with people, tend
to get left out.

University Education

In the early discussions about state regulation, some midwives argued for an
approximately two-year college program to train and educate future midwives. They believed that the required skills could be passed on in that time
period. Others argued that in the highly professionalized healthcare environment, midwives would surely gain even less respect from members of the
hospital hierarchy. This group also noted that a university education covers
more than just techniques; students gain broad-based knowledge and are
given a background to question, analyze and form educated ideas about
broader ideas and issues related to women's reproductive health. Pressure
from within and without thus created the agreement that midwives would be
educated in a university setting and earn a four-year Bachelor of Health
Sciences degree.

With regulation comes accountability to the state. Will accountability to
women be sacrificed? As part of this configuration of state regulation, the
university-based program, due to institutional rules, defines which knowledge
is legitimate and which is not, what kind of learning is legitimate and what
is not. The knowledge base of women who are self-educated or have learned
solely as apprentices are not generally validated within the confines of the
academy. Some women thus advocate a few different educational paths —
the university being just one. Midwives may have attained their skills as lay
midwives, traditional midwives, nurse-midwives or other. To some extent,
the Ontario Prior Learning Assessment (described in detail in the chapter by
Shroff with Hlaing and Wu-Lawrence) provides for this diversity of midwifery education and assessment.

Some critics of legislation note that university strictures will prohibit the
'essence' of midwifery from being passed on: "We are in danger of losing a
spirit which is caught, not taught and I believe it is caught by being self-mo-
tivated in one's learning, by being in apprenticeship with other midwives and
by being with women who are going through pregnancy and childbirth."[23]

The university style of education emphasizes academic performance.
However, in the Ontario model, which has already set the tone for the rest of
the country, students follow women from the beginning of their learning, thus
working in an apprenticeship-style with preceptors. Successful applicants
(especially those who were retained — some failed and a significant number
dropped out) to the Ontario university program have been made to go through
a rigorous and highly demanding academic program. Simultaneously, students are on call for births, thus requiring a vehicle, access to reliable child
care and solid financial resources. Students who are well prepared academi-

cally, who strongly desire to become midwives and who have the financial and social power to endure the university program are those chosen. Others have suffered.

Caring is not an explicit criteria for admission. In all fairness, it is virtually impossible to screen or test for 'caring' as it could be interpreted differently by various people. The admissions process is quite labour intensive for the assessors, as two people (independently) read each written submission and assign it a numerical score. If the two scores vary markedly, a third assessor is assigned to 'break the tie.' Those with the highest-scored written applications are invited to attend interviews. Of the approximately 500 applicants, about 30 students are admitted each year and this small number will only increase once the number of clinical preceptors grows.

Holistic Care

Currently, midwifery is becoming established as part of the dominant medical hierarchy. While some midwives use holistic healthcare techniques as part of their practice, holistic care has not been sanctioned by the state, except perfunctorily in British Columbia.

In Ontario's education program, midwifery students are introduced to some aspects of holistic care but no compulsory course exists for turning midwives into holistic healthcare practitioners. An elective course may be available to students, and this course was initiated at the same time that a new compulsory pharmacology course was introduced. While some midwifery faculty and preceptors consider their practices to be 'holistic,' virtually none of them are trained and certified in holistic healthcare modalities such as herbal medicine, naturopathy, traditional Chinese medicine, ayurveda and/or others. Other midwives are opposed to holistic health care because they believe there is no proof that it works. Pragmatically, they also know that midwifery has less chance of receiving state coverage if it is aligned to holistic health care in any way, as most forms of holistic health care are not regulated or supported. The latter group has been at the helm of the incorporation of midwifery and the development of the university curriculum.

Diversity within Midwifery

In most professional groups in Canada, as in most institutions, middle-/upper-class, heterosexual, able-bodied men of European descent hold the most powerful positions. This group does not represent the diversity of social class, sexual orientation, ability, ethno-racial or other categories of difference in this country. Activists have pushed socially conscious governments to try to make the workforce more representative of the Canadian population, and, in some cases, more diversity exists.

Diversity in the workforce is important for a number of reasons. Firstly, children are often influenced by role models. When young lesbians, for example, see older lesbians in 'important' positions, they get a sense that they too may be able to achieve this kind of status. Without this knowledge, young people may grow up feeling that they have no hope to become enfranchised and will always be fighting 'the system.' Some may wish to stay outside the system all their lives and argue that the system needs to change on a fundamental level before they want to be part of it. Others may wish desperately to be part of the status quo and may be inspired to know it is possible.

Diversity in the workforce is also important because the exclusion or devaluation of large numbers of qualified or potentially qualified people from the means of production may be bad for the economy. Incorporating immigrant midwives, doctors, nurses and other professionals may add to the gross domestic product. Additionally, because Canadian tax payers have not had to foot the bill for the education of immigrant professionals, net savings may be possible.

Diversity in the workforce is additionally important because lack thereof runs counter to the ideals of a just society. Oppressive beliefs and practices of classism, heterosexism, ableism, racism and sexism are hurtful to all parties involved — politically and socially.

Midwifery has been criticized for its lack of practitioner and client diversity all over the country, both in the provinces that have regulated midwifery and those that have not. Regulation of midwifery potentially opens the door for increased diversity within both the client base and the professional base.

Of Ontario, Erin Connell writes, "Ironically, midwifery was established to provide services to those women who have decreased access to traditional healthcare services, including: teenage mothers, immigrant women and women of colour. However, the majority of services are rendered to white, middle class, English speaking women."[24] Some midwives, in their defence, claim that their client base is diversifying, as more people hear about midwifery and learn that it is freely available, but that most of their clients continue to be middle-/upper-class, heterosexual, able-bodied women of European descent.

Amongst the practising group of midwives in Ontario (as of Spring 1997), a handful of the less than 100 are women of colour or First Nations women. Out of the first graduating class of 21 women from the Ontario Midwifery Education Programme in 1996, less than four were women of colour. The Ontario Midwifery Education Programme has a very low number of First Nations students and students of colour and does not adequately reflect the ethno-racial composition of the province.[25]

The few midwifery students of colour tend to be cognisant of their small numbers and have discussed their token status. They have noted that the handful of nonwhite students are so few that they do not begin to represent the diversity within the population at large. Some have complained that it is difficult for them to be motivated to come to class as they are constantly aware of their marginalized positions.

None of the leadership positions in the College of Midwives, Association of Ontario Midwives, and Ontario Midwifery Education Programme are held by women of colour or First Nations women. For the first four years of self/state regulation, one faculty member of colour was continually employed on the approximately ten-member faculty. The only other faculty of colour stayed for only one year.

Midwifery supporters have consistently advocated for setting better standards than their colleagues in other health professions. In the case of ethno-racial representation, midwifery thus far has failed. To date, more than three years into regulation, one of the biggest gaps in the midwifery model lies in its failure to be woman-centred to the full spectrum of women, in a country which is probably the most ethnically diverse in the world; Toronto, Ontario has been declared the world's most ethnically diverse city.

Some efforts are being made to address this issue, the most hopeful of which is the Prior Learning Assessment process (described in Shroff, with Hlaing and Wu-Lawrence's chapter). Within the Ontario Midwifery Education Programme, anti-racism and transcultural concepts are fundamental aspects of a compulsory first-year course (discussed in Shroff's chapter, "All Petals of the Flower: Celebrating the Diversity of Ontario's Birthing Women within First Year Midwifery Curriculum"). This may be the only compulsory anti-racism course in a Canadian university and has been written up in a book about innovative distance education courses in Ontario.[26] While there are plans to change this, there is currently minimal follow-up of this course's curriculum throughout the program.

Ontario midwifery students have become concerned with the lack of adequate ethno-racial representation of their peers and have formed an equity committee; part of the committee's work is to address the admissions process. To this end they have created an equity check-list which reminds interviewers of such things as not being deterred by an interviewee's accent if s/he is communicating clearly in the English language.

A STORK'S EYE VIEW OF THIS BOOK

Regulation of midwifery raises many issues which are of concern to nonlicensed midwives, licensed midwives, physicians, nurses, women clients and their families. *The New Midwifery* examines the tensions implicit in state regulation of midwifery. Covering all the regions of Canada, the chapters of this book examine state regulation of midwifery, exploring important questions: What happens to the oldest women's vocation when the state regulates it? What happens to midwife-client relations, midwife-nurse relations, midwife-doctor relations? Does midwifery clinical practice change? Will caring continue to be central to midwives' work? What is the potential social impact of these changes?

Clearly, this is an early attempt to grapple with these issues, for state regulation has only occurred in a few provinces — Ontario and Alberta in 1994, British Columbia in 1995, Quebec and Manitoba in 1997 at the time of this book's printing. As the authors of the book note, state regulation, even at this early date, appears to be a mixed success. Compromises to ideal midwifery care have already been made, particularly in places where governments are not willing to implement the woman-centred model of care. (Chapters about other regions present reports of progress so far.)

The chapters are generally organized in a geographical fashion, beginning with the West and moving East and North. Preceding these chapters is a conceptual section which frames the larger picture of midwifery in Canada. Most of these first chapters focus on midwifery and diversity. Each author also reflects on midwifery regulation and its implications.

Carol Couchie, an Ojibway midwife, begins with a co-authored chapter (with Herbert Nabigon) on traditional and modern First Nations midwives in socio-political perspective. They reflect on the rise and fall of midwifery within First Nations communities, and the possible outcomes of state regulation. Couchie and Nabigon provide a cultural and spiritual perspective to frame their work. The next chapter, by Iman Al-Jazairi and Sapna Patel, focuses on interviews of women of colour. The authors probe perceptions of midwifery, exploring why many women of colour may or may not choose midwifery care. Pat Israel then discusses midwifery needs of women with disabilities and critically analyzes Ontario midwifery legislation and its inability to meet the unique needs of women with disabilities.

Cecilia Benoit provides a theoretical perspective on sociological concepts of professionalization and regulation. Amongst other things, she examines the Swedish nurse-midwifery model, in which most births are conducted in hospitals and there is no continuity of care, but in which women may access woman-centred care for nonreproductive aspects of their lives (as opposed to just having access to midwifery during pregnancy, childbirth and six weeks postpartum, which appears to be the Canadian norm so far). Carol Hird and Brian Burtch offer an international perspective on maternal mortality and the need for state-supported midwifery to save women's lives.

In the second section, authors focus on different provinces/regions of the country. Alison Rice's chapter explores the breath-by-breath changes occurring in British Columbia. The summer 1996 re-election of the New Democratic Party in British Columbia appeared to promise the implementation of B.C. midwifery in a manner consistent with woman-centred care, but as of the Spring of 1997, the New Democratic Party has not been as supportive of midwifery as it could have been. Susan James poses many questions about state-sanctioned and state-controlled midwifery in Alberta, under a far-right government which is mostly concerned about cost issues and in 1997 made the decision to fund midwifery only in certain regions.

Moving to central Canada, three chapters are included in this volume about Ontario, since this is the first province to implement state-sponsored midwifery care. Mary Sharpe interviewed midwives a few months after state regulation and registration had been in effect. She analyzes their mixed responses. The primary research she conducted will potentially provide base-line data for future investigators of this topic. Farah M. Shroff, with Amy Hlaing, and Betty Wu-Lawrence report on a pilot project to support English as a Second Language applicants to become registered as midwives. Farah M. Shroff's chapter examines diversity issues as they are taken up in one course in the Ontario Midwifery Education Programme — recently rated as a world leader in midwifery education.

Marie Hatem-Asmar and Régis Blais expose the schisms in Quebec midwifery. Lay midwives' and nurse-midwives' disunity, coupled with unbridled skepticism on the part of physicians, has created a situation in which the state is testing midwifery through a series of pilot projects. Charlene MacLellan examines the history and renaissance of midwifery in the Atlantic provinces, telling her remarkable story as a practising midwife in the region. Maureen Morewood-Northrop describes a midwifery project in the Northwest Territories. A short chapter by Farah Shroff concludes the book.

Literature addressing the regulation of midwifery in Canada is not abundant. Brian Burtch's book, *Trials of Labour: The Re-emergence of Midwifery in Canada*, engages with many of the legal issues involved in state regulation, and Cecilia Benoit's book, *Midwives in Passage: The Modernization of Maternity Care* examines 'granny' midwifery in Newfoundland. Midwives have produced work in various places,[27] many unpublished, citing the pros and cons of the regulation of their vocation.

This book's contribution is that it brings midwives' and social scientists' (and a few others') writings together, to critically reflect upon regulation. One of its unique additions to the pool of literature in this area is that each chapter has at least some analysis of race, class and gender issues. Issues of diversity form a central role in the book. This will be one of the first such contributions to Canadian literature on midwifery. None of the authors, for example, cull out a colonial herstory of midwifery by neglecting the existence of First Nations midwifery.

While I as the editor was employed as the Social Scientist of the Ontario Midwifery Education Programme from 1993-97, my status as a nonmidwife excluded me from virtually all of the decision-making processes within the profession (rightly so). My current status, teaching part time through distance education media, and as a faculty member at the University of British Columbia, is that of an external observer with some internal experience. I thus have both an appreciative and critical view of regulation. I have tried to work within the midwifery education program to encourage diversity on the basis of class background, ethno-racial status, sexual orientation, ability and so forth. I have also focused on holistic health issues and health promotion. My goal in getting this book out is to bring people together to address the burning question: How is the Canadian experiment with state regulation going? This book has no conclusions because its purpose has been to raise questions and critically analyze them. There are no 'answers' to these questions, but we have collectively attempted to address the complexities of midwifery's legalization and regulation. Ideally, reflections on regulation should appear at regular intervals over the next many years. It may take generations for some changes to be felt, and I therefore welcome others to follow up with future analyses of state regulation of Canadian midwifery.

ENDNOTES

1. The *Tao Te Ching*, written 2500 years ago by Lao-tzu, describes the role of the midwife: You are a midwife: you are assisting at someone else's birth. Do good without show or fuss. Facilitate what is happening rather than what you think ought to be happening. If you must take the lead, lead so that the mother is helped, yet still free and in charge. When the baby is born, the mother will rightly say: "We did it ourselves!"

2. Anne Oakley and Susanne Houd, *Helpers in Childbirth*.

3. Popular mythology asserts that prostitution/sex-trade work is the oldest women's profession but others, including myself, claim that midwifery is the oldest women's profession.

4. European midwifery traditions have been the target of examination by European patriarchal knowledge systems for centuries. Under colonialism, these same patriarchal systems of knowledge targeted indigenous knowledge — including midwifery. Despite the parallel oppressive processes occuring to midwifery specifically and more generally by European women's knowledge systems (under patriarchy) and indigenous knowledge systems (under patriarchy and colonialism), few alliances between midwives from colonizing and colonized communities exist. It is thus not necessarily true that women of Euro-Canadian heritage, who wish to protect their own midwifery heritage, are interested in protecting that of First Nations or communities of the South. Addressing the survival of midwifery under state regulation, authors in this volume have tried to continually ask, which midwifery traditions and why? Without this interrogation, the tensions between Euro-Canadian midwives/women resisting colonialism/racism may be obscured. Will midwifery practised by women of European descent gain ascendancy in Canada in part because it is less 'upsetting' to the dominant Euro-Canadian patriarchal medical hierarchy? These questions point to the larger question facing the women's movement: are we, as women, always all on the same side of the power struggle?

5. The practice of medically based baby deliveries was also brought here by immigrants, not all of whom were on an equal footing. Differences in social class dictated their choices regarding childbirth care. Historically, the middle-class gentry leaned toward physician-managed birth and the peasantry, often due to lack of choices, had midwifery-assisted childbirths.

6. Lesley Biggs, "The Case of the Missing Midwives."

7. The lithotomy position, in which the woman lays on her back with legs apart, is still the most commonly used position for birth (Davis-Floyd, 1996), even though women find other positions more comfortable. The first time on record that a woman gave birth on her back was about 1728 when King Louis XVI wanted to observe the birth of his wife, Queen Maria, giving birth to her baby. French women in those days, like women all around the world, gave birth in a variety of positions, including occasionally lying partly on their backs, but this was not the norm. In order to satisfy the king's curiosity, his wife was asked to lie down and facilitate a clear view for him of the birth. The king actually stood behind a curtain for much of the labour, but his presence changed labour and delivery practices for centuries to come. Hence, the story goes, women in Europe (and later its colonies) came to give birth on their backs — defying gravity, and in most cases, common sense. By the 1770s European women were no longer labouring with a birth stool but were lying in bed on their backs. In the 1800s, a U.S. obstetrician began having birthing women bring their knees up while lying on their backs and this position later came to be known as the lithotomy position (Samuels and Samuels 1996).

8. Beth Rushing, "Ideology in the Reemergence of North American Midwifery."

9. Holistic health care is defined by Goldstein et al (1988) as: "an emphasis on the unity of body, mind and spirit; a view of health as a positive state, not merely the absence of disease; a concern for the individual's responsibility for her/his own health; an emphasis on self-care, health education and self-healing; a relationship between the provider and the client that is relatively open, equal and reciprocal; a concern with how the individual's health reflects familial, social and cultural environments; an openness toward using natural, 'low' technology and non-Western techniques."

10. This form of midwifery care may be viewed as very expensive because tax payers are funding both midwifery and medically-managed birthing. Instead of midwifery care in hospital, some see the need for doulas — birthing coaches who stay with the birthing woman throughout the course of her labour and delivery. Doulas have been proven to have a positive effect on virtually all the outcomes in pregnancy. Hodnett studied published and unpublished data of controlled trials that examined labour support during pregnancy and found that women who had the continuous presence of a trained support person had shorter labours and were less likely to have intrapartum analgesia/anaesthesia or an operative vaginal delivery. Doulas are trained for two weeks in some cases and for many months in other cases. Not having the same training as midwives, doulas are not substitutes for them. Critics note that this sets up a hierarchy of providers in which doulas are undervalued. Doulas generally work with women during childbirth and not before and after, although this may vary from place to place; doulas may function as midwives in some parts of the world where there are no midwives or midwives are not accessible to women.

11. Enid Balint and J.S. Norell, *Six Minutes with the Patient*.

12. Such research includes: Tyson (1991), Sullivan and Beeman (1983); Mehl and Whitt (1977); Campbell and MacFarlane (1986).

13. College of Midwives, *Statement of Home Birth*, Toronto, 1994.

14. The Michener Program was the pre-registration education and testing process for the first group of midwives who were regulated.

15. Anne Maranta, Editorial in the *Coalition of Ontario Midwifery and Birthing Schools Newsletter*, vol. 1, no. 2 (Spring, 1993): 5. Anne Maranta completed

her educational and assessment process in 1997 to become a Registered Midwife and now may have different sentiments than those expressed here.

16. Madeline Clin, Letter in *Coalition of Ontario Midwifery and Birthing Schools Newsletter*, vol. 1, no. 2 (Spring, 1993). Madeline Clin, in 1997, completed her education and assessment process to become a Registered Midwife.

17. Ibid., 25.

18. Ava Wheeler, "Reports from Ava Wheeler," *Coalition of Ontario Midwifery and Birthing Schools Newsletter*, vol. 1, no. 2 (Spring, 1993): 15.

19. Ibid.

20. Karen Unland, "Midwife Program Delivers 18 Graduates," *The Globe and Mail*, September 9, 1996, A6.

21. Graeme Duncan, Faculty of Medicine, University of British Columbia, personal communication, 1997.

22. While most midwifery consumers tout the caring aspects of midwifery as being vital to their childbirth experience, other consumers simply want a practitioner and are not concerned with the personalized friendship potentially offered by midwives.

23. Anne Smith, Letter in *Coalition of Ontario Midwifery and Birthing Schools Newsletter*, vol. 1, no. 2 (Spring 1993): 6.

24. Erin Connell, "Midwifery Education and Practice 3 Years Later," *McMaster Women's Health Office Newsletter* (April 1996): 5.

25. This would make the number of midwives who are currently registered and who are of First Nations background and of colour four, out of 92 registered midwives — this indicates only a 4% make-up, hardly representative of the First Nations and ethnic communities that exist in Ontario.

26. Norman McKinnon et al, *Technology and Learning: Innovative Projects* (Toronto: The Training Technology Monitor, 1996).

27. For example, Vicki Van Wagner, "Why Legislation?" (Mimiograph, 1994); Alison Rice, "For Safety's Sake, We Need Registered Midwives," *The Vancouver Sun*, June 9, 1995, A17; and Hilary Monk, "Ontario Midwifery in Western Historical Perspective" (Mimiograph, 1995).

REFERENCES

Balint, Enid, and J.S. Norell. *Six Minutes for the Patient*. UK: Tavistock, 1973.

Benoit, Cecilia. *Midwives in Passage: The Modernization of Maternity Care*. St. John's: Institute of Social and Economic Research, Memorial University, Newfoundland, 1991.

Biggs, Lesley. "The Case of the Missing Midwives: A History of Midwifery in Ontario from 1795-1900." In *Delivering Motherhood: Maternal Ideologies and Practices in the 19th and 20th Centuries*, K. Arnup et al, eds. New York: Routledge, 1990.

Burtch, Brian. *Trials of Labour: The Re-emergence of Midwifery*. Montreal: McGill-Queen's University Press, Montreal, 1994.

Campbell, R., and A. MacFarlane. "Place of Delivery: A Review," *British Journal of Obstetrics and Gynaecology*, vol. 93, no. 7 (1986): 675-683.

Clin, Madeline. Letter in *Coalition of Ontario Midwifery and Birthing Schools Newsletter*, vol. 1, no. 2 (Spring, 1993). Box 3924, Station C, Ottawa, Ontario.

College of Midwives. *Statement of Home Birth*. Toronto: 1994.

Connell, Erin. "Midwifery Education and Practice 3 Years Later," *McMaster's Women's Health Office Newsletter* (April 1996): 5. Hamilton: McMaster University.

Davis-Floyd, Robbie. "The Technocratic Model of Birth." In *Childbirth: Changing Ideas and Practices in Britain and America — 1600 to Present*, P. Wilson et al, eds. New York: Garland Publishing, 1996.

Duncan, Graeme. Faculty of Medicine, University of British Columbia, Vancouver, B.C. Personal communication, 1997.

Goldstein, Michael, et al. "Holistic Physicians and Family Practitioners: Similarities, Differences and Implications for Health Policy," *Social Science and Medicine*, vol. 26, no. 8 (1988): 853-861.

Hodnett, E.D. "Support from Caregivers during Childbirth." Cited in the Cochrane Library (1997) issue 3 [CD-ROM] Oxford: Oxford University Press, 1994.

Lao-tzu (500 BCE). *Tao Te Ching*, translation and commentary by Richard Wilhelm, translated into English by H.G. Ostwald. London: Arkana, 1985.

Maranta, Anne. Editorial in *Coalition of Ontario Midwifery and Birthing Schools Newsletter*, vol. 1, no. 2 (Spring, 1993). Box 3924, Station C, Ottawa, Ontario.

McKinnon, Norman, et al. *Technology and Learning: Innovative Projects.* Toronto: The Training Technology Monitor, 1996.

Mehl, L.E., G.H. Peterson, M. Whitt, W.E. Hawes. "Outcomes of Elective Home Births: A Series of 1,146 Cases," *Journal of Reproductive Medicine*, vol. 19, no. 5 (1977): 281-90.

Monk Hilary. "Ontario Midwifery in Western Historical Perspective: From Radicals to Reactionaries in Ten Short Years." Mimeograph, 1995.

National Institute of Child Health and Human Development Panel. "Facts About Cesarean Childbirth." Washington, D.C.: Office of Research Reporting at the National Institute of Child Health and Human Development, 1980. P.O. Box 29111, Washington, D.C., 20040, USA.

Oakley, Anne, and Susanne Houd. *Helpers in Childbirth: Midwifery Today.* New York: Hemisphere Publications Co., 1990.

Rice, Alison. "For Safety's Sake, We Need Registered Midwives," *The Vancouver Sun*, June 9, 1995, A17.

Rushing, Beth. "Ideology in the Reemergence of North American Midwifery," *Work and Occupations*, vol. 20, no. 1 (February 1993): 46-67.

Samuels, Mike, and Nancy Samuels. *The New Well Pregnancy Book*. USA: Fireside, 1996.

Smith, Anne. Letter in *Coalition of Ontario Midwifery and Birthing Schools Newsletter*, vol. 1, no. 2 (Spring, 1993). Box 3924, Station C, Ottawa, Ontario.

Sullivan, D., and R. Beeman. "Four Years' Experience with Home Birth by Licensed Midwives in Arizona," *American Journal of Public Health*, vol. 73, no. 6 (1983): 641-5.

Tyson, Holliday. "Outcomes of 1001 Midwife-attended Home Births in Toronto, 1983-1988," *Birth*, vol. 18, no. 1 (1991): 9-14.

Unland, Karen. "Midwife Program Delivers 18 Graduates," *The Globe and Mail*, September 9, 1996, A6.

Van Wagner, Vicki. "Why Legislation?" Mimeograph, 1994.

Wheeler, Ava. "Reports from Ava Wheeler," *Coalition of Ontario Midwifery and Birthing Schools Newsletter*, vol. 1, no. 2 (Spring, 1993). Box 3924, Station C, Ottawa, Ontario.

SECTION I

Midwifery, Diversity and New Agreements with the State

A Path Towards Reclaiming Nishnawbe Birth Culture:

Can the Midwifery Exemption Clause for Aboriginal Midwives Make a Difference?

Carol Couchie and Herbert Nabigon[*]

I have used the paradigm of the medicine wheel as an outline for this chapter. I wish to thank Herb Nabigan for his understanding of this healing tool. The medicine wheel is an ancient symbol that represents continuity over time. It provides our elders with a diagnostic tool and healing strategies at the individual and community level. It reminds us to consider all of creation in any of our endeavors and to integrate the mental, physical, emotional and spiritual aspects of our community.

PROLOGUE: WHO AM I AND WHERE HAVE I COME FROM?

Boozhoo! Nan-Doo-Geezik-kwe ndizhinikaz Nipissing endugnaba. My name is Carol Couchie (Healing Cedar Woman) and I am from Nipissing First Nation. I am just finishing my Bachelor of Health Science degree at Ryerson in the now four-year-old Midwifery Education Programme.

I am the oldest girl in a family of seven. My father was born at Nipissing in Garden Village and my mother was born in Bancroft, Ontario. Both were born at home with a midwife and both were fur trappers' kids. My mother was Scots and my father was Nishnawbe (Ojibway). We were raised with some strong traditional values. Our parents taught us to respect the bush, work hard and survive.

My mother was a tough woman and her early influence is largely responsible for who I am today. She often discussed our births with us as children. I knew what she was doing before she went into labour with me; I knew what day it was and the family reaction after I was born. I know she would have been proud and supportive of my decision to become a midwife.

---

[*]   As Carol Couchie is the primary author for this article, the first person has been used throughout; however, Herbert Nabigon's wisdom and insights have been integral to the shaping of this work, and is thus named as co-author.

I was not involved at all in the midwifery movement prior to legalization. However, I was busy learning, growing and healing within the Native community. I was intent on having a career in women's health. With this intention in mind I began developing a keen interest in feminist thought and theory. While attending the University of Toronto I was involved in the Aboriginal Health Professions program. I was asked to work as an elder's helper at a three-day workshop on traditional medicine and was assigned a traditional midwife, Katsi Cook, a Hotanoshoni woman, Aquwasasne. Meeting Katsi changed my life forever.

East

The first gift in the east is tobacco. Tobacco is used as an offering and it leads the way in all our sacred ceremonies. The sun rises in the east each day and it is a symbol of renewal. At the beginning of a new day, the sky turns reddish pink as darkness disappears. The colour in the east is red and it symbolizes Nishnawbe or red people. Our visions, animals, and feelings sit in the east. Our elders teach us that our feelings our sacred and if we understand our feelings we understand the language of the creator. Finally when searching for answers about life, we offer tobacco to an elder followed by questions.[1]

We, as First Nation's women, held onto our midwifery practice and skills longer then those women who later came and settled here.[2] In First Nation's communities many people of my parent's generation were born at home and remember midwives. This is generally not the case in third and fourth-generation Canadians, particularly in the more urban areas. Recently I visited two isolated First Nation's communities in the north. Midwives in these communities are still called upon in an emergency. These same midwives twenty years ago were attending the majority of women in their communities during childbirth.[3]

When Europeans began to come and live here at the height of the fur trade they brought no women with them. Many of these European men took Aboriginal women as wives. It was well known that survival was almost impossible without an Aboriginal woman's help. As time passed they began to have families and perhaps it is here that these men learned of our midwifery skills, as they have recounted them in their correspondence.[4]

Over the years, as these men began to adapt to the environment, they began to bring over their own women to live here and raise their families. Many of the skills and human resources that they borrowed from First Nations communities in Canada included midwives and midwifery skills. They knew and wrote about our midwifery expertise. They knew and wrote about the medicines we used for birth (for example, sqawvine or partridge berry).[5] In isolated areas Aboriginal healers and midwives were the only ones to call.[6]

My first question, and what I hope to begin to answer in this chapter is, what happened!? How did we as Aboriginal women go from experts in terms of midwifery knowledge and practice to having virtually no full-time practising traditional midwives left in Ontario?[7] Furthermore, why has our education level, traditional knowledge base and human resources in these fundamentally important areas fallen so far behind in such a short time span? Why are, our non-native sisters, largely belonging to the dominant culture, so far ahead of us in reclaiming this knowledge and practice for their own communities?

I would like to ask the question: will legislation help us and our communities gain back what we have lost? Does the exemption clause in the midwifery legislation begin to show respect to our traditional ways, practices and knowledge base — will it continue to marginalize us and create a two-tiered system of health care. Finally, how do we as Nishnawbe women define and revive our own birth culture and integrate past knowledge with modern obstetrics? In addition, how will we integrate a model of midwifery practised in Ontario, that has been reclaimed and developed by non-native women within their own birth culture?[8]

South

The sun moves from east to west each day, and at midday the sun faces the south. The sun is regarded by our ancestors as a symbol of time, patience, and relationship. The sun has a relationship with all the planets in our universe. It takes time to understand our teachings in the east. It also takes time to understand our relationship with the creator and spirit helpers. We also work to understand family, community and institutional relationships.

The sacred plant for the south is sage. Sage is woman's medicine. It is used for smudging and purification reasons. Sage tea, is also used for lactation suppression.[9]

As I begin to answer the first question, what changed? Why, when we as Aboriginal people were looked upon as knowledgeable resources for midwifery and obstetrical care, are we so far behind in developing and practising midwifery arts? I will be able to answer that question almost totally when I look at the relationship that First Nations people have had with Canadian society.[10]

Our past relationship with the newcomers became, and in many ways continues to be, one of colonization, oppression and suppression at every level — personal, political and institutional. Our relationships with Canadian society, particularly at the institutional level, became a twisted experience of lies and captivity.[11] My father, as well as his siblings, went to residential school.[12] I cannot recall any positive comments about Aboriginal people in my early education experience.

We went from a position of collegiality and sharing with the newcomers to one of mistrust, suppression, domination and dependence.[13] The attempted suppression of our language, culture and ceremonies has had a devastating effect on our traditional healing knowledge base, human resources and our ability to deliver our own services.

Colonization is the first cousin to patriarchy, and in many similar ways Canadian women have also been subjugated and dominated like Aboriginal people. The suppression of midwifery practice has been a part of that oppression. Although we, as First Nation's women, share in the same patriarchal oppression, we as a people have had many more struggles.

For example, many Caucasian women have greater access, have more resources, are better educated, and possess privilege far beyond many First Nation's men or women. They have the luxury of being able to fight sexism and develop feminist theory because many of their basic human rights have been intact for a longer period. For example, Canadian women have had the federal vote for some forty years before Aboriginal men or women were allowed to vote.

Aboriginal women have had to work hard to protect, define and strengthen cultural ideology that is often articulated on a much more universal theme. However, I am not saying that First Nation's women have not fought for their own rights. For example, in 1983, Bill C-31 was an amendment to the Indian Act that was fought for, and by, First Nation's women. The amendment allowed basic treaty rights around heredity, property, education access and health care for many women previously denied these rights. Despite oppression and patriarchy Aboriginal women have been picking up their medicine bundles.

In order to have a deeper understanding of the gap between Native and non-native women practicing midwifery, I will give an example. The example will attempt to explain some of the relationship issues that we as Aboriginal women are facing with Aboriginal men. I will also define what I mean when I discuss Nishnawbe birth culture.

With the development of modern industry, the opportunity for a hunting and gathering economy became extremely limited. Traditional knowledge and education for men, i.e. hunting, trapping, ceremonies, were replaced with an oppressive residential school education. Traditional spirituality, ceremonies and values that the men depended on for good health were suppressed, forced underground and became inaccessible to the majority of the people.

In contrast, the main role and ceremony for women involved childbirth and caring for the home and children. Although Nishnawbe women lost culture and language and were forced into the margins in the same way that Aboriginal men were, in many cases a large part of their identity regarding their work and traditional roles was still left intact.

It is for this reason that, as Nishnawbe people have been healing, we have focused more on the traditional ceremonies that belong to the men. Those ceremonies being the purification lodge, sun dance, and drumming. These ceremonies in the past were run and maintained by men. However, the main metaphor behind much of the ceremony is birth and rebirth.

In recent times ceremonies and culture have been revived by elders and traditional teachers. Both men and women have shared in the responsibilities of preparing for and maintaining these ceremonies. Together we have strengthened our cultural roots as indigenous people.

What we share as Aboriginal women with the rest of North American society is the patriarchal oppression seen in every aspect of modern society.[14] With all of these historical forms, like patriarchy and colonization, it is easy to see why Nishnawbe women lost control of their own ceremony, of childbirth. It is also clear why women must to continue to support the men in their work of healing.

While it is important to understand that a patriarchal medical model of childbirth took control away from Aboriginal women, in that traditional care-providers, like midwives, no longer attended First Nation's women, the actual physical ceremony has never and will never leave us — or we will cease to exist as a people. Children are born to women. They give us hope and purpose, and make us strong. So, where we need to reclaim our own ceremony as women is to have a better relationship and understanding of birth. Only then will we be able to articulate birth in a way that has cultural significance to us as Nishnawbe people.

West

The Thunderbird sits in the west door. She reminds us to go inward and heal our inner life. The Thunderbird brings us the sacred gift of water. When it rains. Water gets in our eyes, and we use our eyes to look twice at everything we do; hence the word *respect*, *re* — meaning again — and *spect*, meaning to look. Therefore, the word respect literally means to look again. All major decisions should be made by looking twice before we move toward solutions — this teaches us to look back at yesterday in order to heal ourselves today. If we use our minds in this way, our memories function as a way to build our knowledge base. When we exit from the darkness of our mother's womb, we enter the world on a river of water — that is why little babies are natural in water. The colour of the west door is black, that represents the Black Nation. They also teach us about respect.[15]

The sacred plant that sits on the west door is cedar. Cedar is another woman's medicine and is used in birth. It is offered to the sacred fire to help those spirits who exit from the west door as they journey to the land of the creator. Cedar also is used in the purification lodge to connect fire, which is male, and the lodge, which is female — the line is called the path of life.

As I mentioned earlier, compared to most of North America, midwifery in many Aboriginal communities has not been gone long and in some cases still exists in a limited capacity. We have a great advantage in that we do not have as far to go in beginning to regain this knowledge. However, we should not take the knowledge or the maintenance of it for granted. The many hands-on skills that are a part of midwifery only take one or two generations to be lost. Knowledge is synonymous with power. If we no longer have skills and understanding surrounding the birth process, we will continue to hand over the control of our most sacred ceremony, the birth of our children. After answering the question, what happened, we must continue to remind ourselves of the answer in order to correct and prevent further damage.

Nishnawbe women must look twice at where we have come from, namely an autonomous traditional society, with primary healthcare providers like traditional midwives. We must begin to learn once again about the physiology of birth. When we have relearned birth physiology to a level that it has once again become common knowledge, we will be able to articulate that knowledge in a way that reflects who we are as Nishnawbe people.

Children must also be educated. They need to have a sound understanding of how their bodies work. If we locate reproductive education within our culture we will educate ourselves on our own values, re-enforcing parenting skills and conveying respect to our children. Sound reproductive education gives young people a better understanding of themselves as human beings, strengthens the women, and in return empowers the community.[16]

Balance is also important for us to keep in mind with regards to what we have gone through in terms of colonization and our relationship to the medical model of practice.[17]

We are not the people we once were. Our communities are confronting a total health crisis that effects every First Nation's person in Canada. The effects are felt on all levels of the individual: the physical, mental, emotional, and spiritual. Although Western medicine is helpless on some levels in terms of healing our communities, they do have some expertise in specific areas from which we can benefit.[18]

For example, modern obstetrics has many monitoring devices that help monitor women with type II diabetes. On the other hand, many traditional herbal medicine could offer solutions in controlling glucose levels, where antihypoglycaemic agents such as Metformin HCl, used by type II diabetics, are contra-indicated. Balance is important in the healing process. We must look twice at what Western medicine has to offer and use it appropriately. Yet not undermine what our own traditional medicines have to offer.[19]

These recommendations have also come from research done by Carol Terry and Laura Calmwind in Nashnawbe-Aski territory. The territory is also known as the Sioux Lookout Zone of Northwestern Ontario. Elder traditional midwives when interviewed felt that traditional midwives, as well as younger people looking to become midwives, should be trained in both ways.[20]

Clearly our history dictates that, if healthcare providers in any of our communities are to be effective, they must be educated in both Nishnawbe culture and traditions, and Western medicine. Education in both areas of expertise must be accessible to present midwives and any of those who decide to learn and go into midwifery practice in the future.[21]

The Ontario government needs to think seriously about supporting self-government and promoting health by providing more then token acknowledgement of our traditional healing practices — like the midwifery exemption clause. They must support education programs and services for First Nation's women and their families.[22] Similar programs exist in the areas of social work and education. Native students should have access and priority to educational resources in areas that service a large Aboriginal population.

There has been some support through the provincial Aboriginal healing and wellness program. The Hotinashoni women at Six Nations have received support to train traditional midwives and build a birthing centre. The vision of the birthing centre is to provide the kind of holistic care that incorporates many aspects of the reproductive cycle, including education and health promotion.

The traditional birth attendants are being educated in midwifery skills within the present Ontario model and scope of practice. They are learning traditional skills that include clinical hands-on applications. In addition, important counselling skills that reflect the traditions, values and culture of their own community are also being learnt. These skills are being taught in an environment that is familiar and gives respect to the particular needs of Aboriginal students. The clients at the birthing centre are members of their own community. The atmosphere is very welcoming and home-like. The education at the birthing centre appears to be progressing very well and helps to eliminate some of the barriers that often exist for Aboriginal students in mainstream professional faculties.

WHERE AM I GOING?

North

The north door is a door of peace. The north wind blows cold air over our Mother in the winter. If you walk in the bush during the winter, the cold blanket of snow covering the ground is very peaceful. It is absolutely quiet and you can hear the trees cracking in the cold. It is time to journey inward. The Bear sits in the north and we regard her as a healer. The Bear represents protection and it functions as a spirit policewoman. When the wind blows hard in the winter, it teaches us to care — if we don't find a warm place we could freeze. Caring is an action step and a survival tool. Grandfather air moves everything around and will work to direct good movement to heal our community dysfunctions. White is the colour of the north. It represents the white nation. The medicine for the north is sweetgrass, it is a male medicine and represents unity and balance.[23]

It is clear that in order for the exemption clause to mean anything to Aboriginal people in Ontario we must be provided with the support to move forward in developing Nishnawbe birth culture.

The feminist movement in the larger Canadian society worked long and hard in Ontario to bring midwifery back into mainstream healthcare services. They consulted with Aboriginal women and together they created the exemption clause in the midwifery legislation for traditional midwives.[24] It is important that we, as Nishnawbe women and other First Nation women, define how we want midwifery to work within our own communities.

The present Ontario model of midwifery, for the most part, would suit some Aboriginal communities. But, it will be necessary for more Aboriginal women to access midwifery education. The present model is an excellent one that is flexible in suiting the needs of birthing women and their communities well. However, some communities may find they need to modify it to suit their own individual needs.

It is in gearing the present model of midwifery that I see the exemption clause as beneficial for the people. For example, many community health representatives (CHRs) have been training, to give breastfeeding support and education. In time it is my hope and desire to move back to my home community. I would hope that the CHRs and nurses employed by the band council would express a desire to be trained as traditional birth attendants and train as second attendants. Together we would attend the births of some of the women in our community.

It is important to consider the contribution Aboriginal midwives could make when we look to the future of self-government and band-controlled medical services through National Health and Welfare. Midwives could be involved in health promotion and health education. Midwives have many areas of expertise, that could include: prenatal education, nutrition counselling, early parenting, breastfeeding, well-woman care, sexuality and sex education, birth control counselling, postpartum support groups, and herbology.

I have a dream of attending a birth in my own community at Nipissing. I will go to a woman's home where her extended family is there for support. Perhaps even my own daughter will accompany me to help with younger children. Perhaps the woman's mother is there to help prepare food and greet the baby in the Nishnawbe language. The father will light a fire outside and offer tobacco. We will boil cedar for the postpartum bath.

Since I am a registered midwife in Ontario, if anything should fall outside of the normal, I am able to transport her to a hospital where I have privileges. The woman will be attended by someone in her community that she knows and trusts who will provide cultural interpretation in both directions. In the end she will have it explained to her why any intervention was done to her. She will be knowledgeable and capable of making decisions for herself and her family.

At present this is only a dream, but hopefully not for long. I hope to graduate in three months and begin to practise as a new registrant. I have received a lot of healing and personal growth from my midwifery education, and with the strength of my community behind me, I will hopefully live up to my name *Nan-Do Geezik-kwe*.

It was the realization of a dream for women in dominant Canadian society to legalize midwifery practice. It has brought about a higher degree of accessibility of both midwifery services and education to the public. Within that legislation is the recognition of Aboriginal midwifery as a distinct entity with particular and individual needs. However there is an enormous amount of work to be done with those communities that find themselves on the margins. I have outlined some of the barriers that we have faced in the past. I have also discussed some of the important relationship issues that are particular to colonized people.

Nishnawbe women are the guardians of their culture, families and communities. They will want to be a leading force in the future development of midwifery on their homelands. The professional practice of midwifery reflects their traditional values. That is the compassionate and respectful care of the newly emerging mother and baby. This is the very future of our Nations.

ENDNOTES

1. H. Nabigon and A.M. Mawhiney, *Aboriginal Theory: A Cree Medicine Wheel Guide for Healing First Nations* (Social Work Treatment).
2. J. Mason, "Midwifery in Canada," in *The Midwife Challenge*, ed. Sheila Kitzinger (London: Pandora Press, 1988).
3. A.R. Ford, "Aboriginal Women," in *An Equity Reader for Midwifery Students*, ed. Farah Shroff (Winter, 1993). L. Calm Wind and C. Terry, *Nishnawbe-Aski Nation Midwifery Practices* (Sioux Lookout, Ontario: Equy-wuk Woman's Group, 1993).
4. S. Van Kirk, "Many Tender Ties," in *Women in the Fur-Trade Society 1670-1870* (Watson and Dwyer, 1980). "Report of the Task Force On the Implementation of Midwifery In Ontario," Appendix 1, in *History of Midwifery in Canada* (1987).
5. I believe partridge berry is the translated Aboriginal reference to sqawvine which uses a derogatory name for native women.
6. "Report of the Task Force..." op. cit.
7. L. Calm Wind and C. Terry, op. cit.
8. A.R. Ford, op. cit. College of Ontario Midwives, Registrants Booklet, Exemption for Aboriginal Midwives, January 1994.
9. H. Nabigon and A.M. Mawhiney, op.cit.
10. G. York, *The Dispossessed: Life and Death in Native Canada* (Toronto: Little, Brown and Company Limited, 1990).
11. Ibid.; F. Fanon, *Toward the African Revolution: Political Essays* (New York: Grove Press Inc., 1967); *The Wretched of the Earth* (New York: Grove Press

Inc., 1963); A. Memmi, *The Colonizer and the Colonized* (New York: The Orion Press, 1965).

12. G. York, op. cit.

13. Ibid.; F. Fanon, *Toward the African Revolution...* op. cit.; *The Wretched of the Earth* op. cit.; A. Memmi, *The Colonizer and the Colonized ...* op. cit.

14. J.S. Frideres, *Native Peoples in Canada: Contemporary Conflicts* (Toronto: Prentice Hall Inc., 1988). S. Van Kirk, "Toward a Feminist Perspective in Native History" (University of Toronto, unpublished).

15. H. Nabigon and A.M. Mawhiney, op. cit.

16. L. Malloch, "Indian Medicine, Indian Health: A Study Between Red and White Medicine," *Canadian Woman Studies* (Summer/Fall 1989).

17. Ibid.

18. G. York, op. cit.; M. Boldt, *Surviving as Indians: The Challenge of Self-government* (Toronto: University of Toronto Press, 1993).

19. L. Calm Wind and C. Terry, op. cit.; *L. Malloch, op.cit.*

20. L. Calm Wind and C. Terry, op. cit.

21. Ibid.

22. Ibid.; College of Ontario Midwives, op. cit.

23. H. Nabigon and A.M. Mawhiney, op. cit.

24. College of Ontario Midwives, op. cit.

REFERENCES

Anderson, K. A. *Chain Her By One Foot: The Subjugation of Women in Seventeen-Century New France*. Routledge, 1991.

Boldt, M. *Surviving as Indians: The Challenge of Self-government*. Toronto: University of Toronto Press, 1993.

Calm Wind, L. and C. Terry. *Nishnawbe-Aski Nation Midwifery Practices*. Sioux Lookout, Ontario: Equy-wuk Woman's Group, 1993.

College of Ontario Midwives, Registrants Booklet, Exemption for Aboriginal Midwives, 1994.

Fanon, F. *The Wretched of the Earth*. New York: Grove Press Inc., 1963.

_____. *Toward the African Revolution: Political Essays*. New York: Grove Press Inc., 1967.

Ford, A.R. "Aboriginal Women." In *An Equity Reader for Midwifery Students*. Farah Shroff, ed., 1993.

Frideres, J.S. *Native Peoples in Canada: Contemporary Conflicts*. Toronto: Prentice Hall Inc., 1988.

Malloch, L. "Indian Medicine, Indian Health: A Study Between Red and White Medicine." *Canadian Woman Studies*. Summer/Fall 1989.

Mason, J. "Midwifery in Canada." In *The Midwife Challenge*. Sheila Kitzinger, ed. London: Pandora Press, 1988.

Memmi, A. *The Colonizer and the Colonized*. New York: The Orion Press, 1965.

Nabigon, H. and A.M. Mawhiney. *Aboriginal Theory: A Cree Medicine Wheel Guide for Healing First Nations*, Social Work Treatment.

"Report of the Task Force On the Implementation of Midwifery In Ontario, Appendix 1." In *History of Midwifery in Canada*, 1987.

Van Kirk, S. "Toward a Feminist Perspective in Native History." University of Toronto. Unpublished.

_____. "Many Tender Ties." In *Women in the Fur-Trade Society 1670-1870*. Watson and Dwyer, 1980.

York, G. *The Dispossessed: Life and Death in Native Canada*. Toronto: Little, Brown and Company Limited, 1990.

Colonized Wombs

Sapna Patel and Iman Al-Jazairi

IMAN

I was brought into this world by a midwife, *jeda* Bedor. I was born in Basrah, Iraq. When I was four years old, I climbed up to watch from a window as my aunt gave birth to her first child. *Jeda* Bedor and my grandmother were helping my aunt, while my mother was minding the children in the courtyard. My mother had four children including myself, with the assistance of *jeda* Bedor; she told me she always felt safe in the care of *jeda* Bedor. And she did not have to worry about her other children since we were close by and cared for by our aunts and grandmothers.

When I was much older, my mother delivered four more babies, all in hospital. During the latter deliveries, she always had many aches and pains, and often said she wished she could find a *jeda*. Until the hospital births, my mother had never been laid flat on her back on a hard bed while she delivered — nor had she ever been cut. I have always felt that if I ever had a baby, I would have a traditional midwife assist me.

SAPNA

Both myself and my sibling were born in hospital. I was born in Lusaka, Zambia. Mother died just over a year after I was born. I do not have access to her stories, except that she had a Caesarean section for at least one of us. When I was about a month old, my parents took us to India. I do not know if this visit was for the traditional 40-day postpartum period when a woman rests at her parents' home. (On a recent trip to India, I visited a woman who had a week-old infant; she was staying with her parents for 40 days. It seemed to be a peaceful time together for both mother and child.) My mother and her two sisters were all delivered at home with a *dai*. When she was recounting this story, my *masi* added, "That was in the old days, when we couldn't afford to go to the hospital."

When we began researching this chapter, I supported the option of a midwife-assisted birth. But I still wanted the reassurance of 'medical expertise.' I would go to a birthing centre, the 'middle ground' between hospital and home birth. However, the participants' stories, discussions with my co-researcher/writer, and my readings on lay midwifery dramatically shifted my perspective on the birth process.

> Behind [the] complex issues of midwifery and power, it may be the case that the idea of the midwife as 'being with woman' has nothing whatsoever to do with the modern notion of [midwifery]. It may be something else altogether — something much older, much more fundamental, much more challenging to the modern scientific world, obsessed as it is with the quantification of biological parameters of experience.[1]

Western medicine may be necessary when there are complications, but it becomes increasingly clear that the medical profession's methods are usually destructive to childbirth.

OUTLINE
We wanted to find out if women of colour would have midwife-assisted births now that midwifery is legalized and covered by the Ontario Health Insurance Plan (OHIP). It should be noted that this is only a first endeavour to collect and analyze the opinions of women of colour. It is representative of a few women, who themselves by no means entirely represent the vast category of 'women of colour.'[2]

After a discussion of the research process, we present our findings. Our research indicates that the overwhelming majority of women reject midwives as trustworthy birth attendants. In order to understand why this is so, we examined healthcare in 'the South.'[3] We found that the lack of faith in traditional midwifery is the result of imperialist (and later, neocolonialist) onslaught. An unconscionable alliance between the mysogynist medical establishment and racist, sexist development institutions means that traditional midwifery has been persecuted. The stereotype of the lay midwife as dirty and dangerous now comprises 'common knowledge.'

We give a historical analysis of the decline of lay midwifery in 'the South.' A separate section takes a close look at female genital mutilation (FGM). Finally, we outline factors that affect accessibility and conclude with questions for the direction of midwifery in Ontario.

METHODOLOGY

Outreach
We outreached to a diverse group of women. We placed notices on bulletin boards, passed around flyers, and phoned organizations. Women's groups, labour groups, ethno-specific organizations, and health centres, as well as community-based ESL (English as a Second Language) classes were contacted. We asked women we knew if they would participate.

Why Group Discussions?

In order to move away from the highly artificial construction of 'observer versus observed,' we held group discussions, which were less intimidating and encouraged story-sharing and openness. There was no formal set of questions, although the same or similar ones were usually asked of each group, and some questions only when it was comfortable (see Appendix 1).

Group Profile

Our sample comprises six ESL classes (including teachers) and two groups of women who are fluent in English. Thirty-seven women, of 46 in total, participated in the discussions.[4] All names used in this chapter are pseudonyms (see Appendix 2). There were women from China, Egypt, Iran, South Korea, Tunisia, Sudan, Sri Lanka, Pakistan and India. There are also women of Indian origin who were born and/or raised in the diaspora.

Barriers to Research

Obstacles to our research were: language; racism; ageism and marital status; and teacher/student and interviewer/interviewee power dynamics. Language was an obvious barrier to the detail of discussion in the ESL classes. Words are usually lost or changed when interpreted[5] into a different language. The emotional weight of the word is lost. We knew that women had much more to say.

In some classes, racism silenced women of colour. The numerous culturally-diverse women of colour sat on one side of the room, and did not have a chance to express themselves. The white women[6] crowded on the other side, and vocally dominated the discussions. One student even left her seat with the women of colour to squeeze in with the other white women.

In addition to cultural diversity in the classes, there were also differences in age and marital status. In the course of the discussions, it became apparent that students held several assumptions about each other's sexual experience. For instance, an older woman (Sarojini) silenced two younger women (Roshni and Geeta) when they hesitated to answer our questions. She seemed to feel obligated to protect "these children who are not even married. It's only when you're going to have a child that you can understand what to do and how. They can't know yet." Also, when another Indian woman did not participate, a classmate explained on her behalf that it was because she is unmarried.

Perception of authority was another obstacle. Even when a teacher uses elements of popular education to break down classroom hierarchy, adult students still relate to the teacher as an authority figure. Students often carefully gauge their teachers' attitudes and adapt their own responses accordingly. In addition, women were probably reserved because we were strangers asking them about very personal experiences, on record.

HISTORICAL CONTEXT

Ancient Knowledge

Holistic medicine, including midwifery, has been used extensively throughout the world.[7] Midwives have assisted childbirth since ancient times. Egyptian papyrus, dating as early as 1900 BC, demonstrates ample evidence of
the practice of midwifery.[8] Additional proof of this ancient female occupation
is found at Luxor: *bas reliefs* depict midwives attending to women of the
royal house with the use of birthing stools.

The Civilizing Mission

No aspect of life in the twentieth century can be dissociated from colonialism
and imperialism.[9] In the 15th century, Europe began its invasion of Africa,
Asia, the Americas and Australia. Despite evidence to the contrary, Europeans
claimed that our lands were "empty of people, 'vacant,' 'waste' and 'un-
used'.... [They] were thus able to describe their invasions as 'discoveries,'
piracy and theft as 'trade,' and extermination and enslavement as their
'civilizing mission.'"[10] Driven by their unquenchable thirst for profits, the
colonizers seized and sold people, gold, silver, spices, and other resources.
They succeeded in annihilating entire nations as well as many of our traditional social, economic, and political systems. Chinweizu concisely summarizes this movement:

> Enlightened, through their renaissance, by the learning of the ancient Mediter-
> ranean; armed with the gun, the making of whose powder they had learned from
> Chinese firecrackers; equipping their ships with lateen sails, astrolabes and
> nautical compasses, all invented by the Chinese and transmitted to them by
> Arabs; fortified in aggressive spirit by an arrogant, messianic Christianity of
> both the popish and Protestant varieties; and motivated by the lure of enriching
> plunder, white hordes...sallied forth from their western European homelands to
> explore, assault, loot, occupy, rule and exploit the rest of the world.[11]

It became the 'white man's burden' to salvage the 'ignorant natives' from
our 'backward' ways. Vandana Shiva cites *Encyclopaedia Britannica*'s description of indigenous people: "Man in Australia is an animal of prey. More
ferocious than the lynx, the leopard, or the hyena, he devours his own
people."[12] Not only is this a vicious dehumanization of people, it is an
inversion of the truth about cannibalism.[13]

Lord Cromer, British Consul General in Egypt from 1883 to 1906,
reasoned, "[We] govern them by sheer weight of character and without use
of force...[because we] possess in a very high degree the power of acquiring
the sympathy and confidence of any primitive races with which [we] are
brought into contact."[14] And Cromer's contemporary in India, Viceroy Lord
Curzon, declared, "In the Empire we have found not merely the key to glory

and wealth, but the call to duty, and the means of service to mankind."[15] By 1914, Europe held in its power approximately 85 percent of the earth, in some form or other.[16]

A Drastic Transformation

As with plant regeneration, where agriculture has moved from the Green Revolution technologies to biotechnology, so too with human reproduction, a parallel shift is taking place..., the relocation of knowledge and skills from the mother to the doctor, from women to men [is being] accentuated.[17]

In Europe, woman and nature had long been characterized as evil and base. The wise woman healer was persecuted "as witch..., the image of deceitful nature, enticing and fair without but filled with foul corruption underneath, dragging male consciousness down into the power of sin, death, and damnation."[18] Almost one million people, mostly women, were murdered in the Catholic Inquisition's witch hunts during the late 15th and early 16th centuries.

During the Renaissance, the rise of science and the humanities broke the Church's stranglehold on crucial facets of life such as health and healing, morality, and politics. As Ira Lapidus points out, "The cultivation of scientific and of humanistic mentalities relegated religion to a narrowed sphere of worship and communal activities."[19] The end result was a drastic transformation of the Western world view, from "the notion of an organic, living, and spiritual universe" to "that of the world as a machine, and the world-machine became the dominant metaphor of the modern era."[20]

Health care and childbirth were a necessary part of this change. Surgical and pharmaceutical developments, such as anaesthetic, forceps, and microsurgery, were actively applied to parturition and to the sphere of women's health in general. Hand-in-hand with rise of modern techno-medicine was the impetus to control women's bodies, especially those of working class and poor women. In 1809 when the first ovariectomy was performed, male gynaecologists were competing to find various ways in which to perform invasive surgery. Dr. David Gilliam affirmed the view that castrating women (removing part or all of the reproductive system) was effective. Cleansed of her cumbersome womb, the woman became docile, hardworking and easily managed.[21] Women were inherently inferior to men and incapable of taking care of themselves,

...as if menstruation, childbirth, defecation, etc. were too undignified for a lady to experience. Male doctors would have to take over the female body for women's own protection. The vagina, which had for too long sullied 'woman's sphere,' would have to be removed to the province of medical professionalism.[22]

If medicine were to progress at all, if women knew what was good for them, they should leave the care of their health in the competent hands of modern male doctors.

Using the same deterministic ideology, the imperialists sought to impose their new medical model on indigenous health systems worldwide:

> Recourse to state power to enforce sanitary and health measures (as in Victorian Britain) gave the medical profession uprecedented authority in public life and affairs of state, and this was quickly reflected in Europe's overseas possessions too. One of the characteristics of the period of imperial administration between 1880 and 1930 was the spate of laws, proclamations and decrees giving state sanction to health measures of various kinds.[23]

Legislative changes were introduced to prevent or curb traditional practices. As colonial governments considered any indigenous authority a threat to their own, the legitimacy of traditional healers (including that of midwives) was attacked — both by missionaries and medical practitioners.[24]

In India, for example, when the missionaries encountered gender segregation in the Hindu and Muslim upper and middle classes, they sent women proselytizers to Indian women. As they observed the domestic lives of Indian women, the white women concluded that Indian birthing — specifically the practices of the *dai* — endangered the lives of both mother and child. They depicted the *dai* as filthy, ignorant and superstitious. However, there is evidence to refute this prejudiced image. Ancient Sanskrit *samhitas* describe care during the prenatal, labour, delivery, and postnatal periods. Geraldine Forbes remarks, "It is clear that the professional in charge was the midwife.... [*Dais* are] experienced and courageous women of advanced age and with clean clothes, ...[and] who have cut their nails and who cheer [the birthing mother] with friendly words."[25] In addition, Dr. John Fryer, who went to India at the end of the 17th century, observed that both upper-class and peasant women had little problem during parturition. Birthing in India was no more dangerous than in England.[26] In the early 1900s, an urban middle-class Indian woman describes the *dai* as "having a kindly face, wearing a 'spotless white sari' and being very knowledgeable about her work."[27]

Yet the stereotype of the *dai* was pervasive among women missionaries, and later, the wives of the viceroys. These women imperialists[28] felt duty-bound to lobby both colonial and home governments to secure English women doctors, midwives and nurses, and to set up midwifery schools for Indian women. Later, Lady Harriet Dufferin (wife of Viceroy Lord Dufferin) also called for training of *dais* and "envisaged a time when it would be 'illegal' for Indian midwives to practise without a license."[29]

In addition to government lobbying, the women imperialists enlisted the help of the Indian upper classes and the new professional middle class, all enthusiastic modernizers. As Indian women from these ranks formed organizations, they not only wanted to fill the imperialist agenda, but also raise their own status as women in Indian society. In doing so, however, they were acting against their lower-class and lower-caste sisters, the *dais*. The 1931 All-India Women's Conference recommended that *dais* be licensed. Elite women and men, in India as in the rest of the colonized world, were advocating for the Western medical model to replace their own ancient indigenous traditions.

The imperialist agenda to suppress indigenous healthcare systems, while actively promoting their own, continues to this day. The enormous corporate power of wealthy pro-eugenics organizations, such as the Carnegie and Rockefeller Foundations, is manifest through their direct involvement in defining and implementing the goals and activities of international development bodies like the World Health Organization (WHO), the United States Agency for International Development (USAID), and the United Nations Fund for Population Activities (UNFPA). This coterie, which includes many other players, has been instrumental in enforcing drastic changes in healthcare services in 'the South.'[30]

Interior Spaces

The medical establishment has long fed on the bodies of women of colour. J. Marion Sims, who was praised by the *Journal of the American Medical Association* as the father of gynaecology, was lauded for his work "to relieve human suffering as much, if not more, than any man who has lived within this century."[31] This 19th-century doctor's rise to fame was because of a new surgical technique he developed by operating on African-American women slaves without anaesthetic. So great was his dedication to the cause of medical science that Sims inflicted his torture on a slave woman named Anarcha no less than 30 times.

People of colour everywhere have been targeted by European and U.S. governments, international bodies directed by affluent pro-eugenics corporations, and colonized puppet regimes around the world. These organizations execute their genocidal policies through state-sanctioned techno-medical and pharmaceutical industries. Eugenic sterilization,[32] also known as 'population control' and 'family planning,' has been aggressively aimed at Black women and men and Native women in the Americas, and at women throughout 'the South.'

"Black women are often afraid to permit any kind of necessary surgery because they know from bitter experience that they are more likely than not to come out without their insides,"[33] explains Frances M. Beal of the Student Nonviolent Coordinating Committee's Black Women's Liberation Committee. Stephen Trombley describes the experience of Ruth Cox, an 18-year-old Black woman who was coerced into a sterilization in 1965. She was assured the operation was reversible. It was not until 5 years later that she discovered she could never have children. "The doctors didn't respect me. They treated me like an animal that didn't have any brains.... When you're black and poor, you have to forget what you want and do what the rich, white people say. They want to stop the black population, that's what it is."[34]

During the 1970s, the U.S. government intensified its genocidal campaign against Black and Native peoples. By 1976, a quarter of all Native women in the U.S. had been sterilized by the Indian Health Service. "Our blood lines are being stopped," declared Choctaw doctor Connie Uri. "Our unborn will not be born.... This is genocidal to our people."[35] By 1982, 42% of Native women, 25% of Black women, and 35% of Puerto Rican women had had their ability to have children taken away.[36] Angela Davis reveals the massive cover-up by government agencies:

> At first the Department of Health, Education and Welfare claimed that approximately 16,000 women and 8,000 men had been sterilized in 1972 under the auspices of federal programs. Later, however... Carl Shultz, director of HEW's Population Affairs Office, estimated that between 100,000 and 200,000 sterilizations had actually been funded that year by the federal government. During Hitler's Germany, incidentally, 250,000 sterilizations were carried out under the Nazis' Hereditary Health Law. Is it possible that the record of Nazis, throughout the years of their reign, may have been almost equaled by U.S. government-funded sterilizations in the space of a single year?[37]

In 1993, two U.S. population agencies tested the sterilization drug quinacrine on 80,000 women in Bangladesh, Chile, Costa Rica, Croatia, Egypt, India, Indonesia, Iran, Pakistan, Venezuela, and Vietnam. In Vietnam alone, 30,000 women had their fertility removed.[38] This drug was not approved even by pro-sterilization bodies such as the WHO and the U.S. Food and Drug Administration.

If the early imperialists claimed to be morally compelled to remove vast amounts of land and riches from the inept hands of those whom they colonized, the multinational capitalists of the late 20th century clasp to their hearts and bank accounts the same stratagem. The 'white man's burden' has simply changed with the times. In a campaign that camaflouges the age-old drive to leech world resources for ever-increasing profits, the international corporate elite aim to control the reproductive lives of the same obstreperous peoples — particularly of women living in poverty. As Vandana Shiva remarks, "The land, the forests, the rivers, the oceans, the atmosphere have all been colonised, eroded and polluted.... [The] new colonies are... the interior spaces of the bodies of women."[39]

In Canada, racist abuse in the name of medicine is alive and well. Parvati told us that her sister had both her babies in Toronto, with a Caesarean section for the second child. The mother was sick for the first two days after surgery. And the baby weighed ten pounds, had heart palpitations, and was in an incubator. Parvati offers no information as to why the child was sick. She may not know the full story, and perhaps the mother was not given a proper explanation of what went wrong. Even when women communicate fluently in English, fear and awe of the medical establishment is so entrenched that we may not ask for information. Often when we ask, we do not receive a satisfactory explanation.

Sharmini tells us of a life-threatening experience she had at a suburban Toronto hospital three years ago. She was giving birth to her second child. The delivery was problem-free, but the afterbirth did not follow immediately. The nurse did not press on her stomach to induce artificial labour and ease the placenta out. Instead, she declared, "It's finished," and went off duty. Sharmini feels, "The nurse was not caring," and explains, "Afterwards, my whole body turned blue. The doctor told my husband that I had died, and transferred me to a room where dead bodies were kept." It was only at her husband's insistence that they re-examined Sharmini and revived her with a blood transfusion. She was also given a hysterectomy — without consent.

Sharmini tells us that now, although her child is healthy, she herself is very sick and in a lot of pain. She had previously been healthy. She and her husband feel the medical staff were racist. However, the couple did not lodge a complaint. Sharmini says her husband is happy her life was saved, and does not want to "create any more trouble." She does not express what she wants.

Given the deliberately uncaring behaviour of the hospital staff, the husband's refusal to pursue the institution or its employees for recompense is an understandable expression of his fear. Immigrants to Canada often do not know our rights. Or people of colour in general may not pursue our rights for fear of retribution. Given the context of racism in this society, such a reaction is understandable. As for the woman, not only is it her body that is subjected to such abuse, but she is also silenced by the patriarchal institutions both within her community and Canadian society at large, as well as by racism.

Some of the women speak about the lack of respect for our bodies as being different from white women's bodies, together with blatant disregard for our religious beliefs. Arvinder tells us of a woman doctor who exclaimed to her, "My, aren't you a hairy one!" Arvinder adds, "This is what Sikh women go through." She goes on to give further evidence of racism in Toronto hospitals. Her mother had requested that her pubic hair not be shaved before delivery. Yet the medical staff disregarded her request. It was the only time in her life Arvinder's mother had any hair removed. "For Sikhs, it's a big deal because in history, they have given their lives to not cut a single hair on any part of their bodies."

Referring to the involuntary sterilization of Native women in Canada, Arvinder does not trust doctors, adding, "They don't learn a lot about women's bodies. They treat our bodies like problems." She knows that birth is viewed as an operation where women are sometimes tied down during labour and delivery. Speaking about medical intervention, she says, "Everything is done to protect the doctors. Nothing is ever done in the interests of the woman."

New Imperialists

In segments of the middle class, there is increasing challenge to the medical interventionist hegemony. New Agers claim to provide alternatives to the establishment. Despite such assertions, the New Age movement is an integral part of corporacist culture. New Agers appropriate and patent the rich lore of cultural tradition of colonized societies all around the world — particularly of Aboriginal peoples — for the benefit and profit of a privileged few. Hema points out, "While the West is marketing its own medical model in South Asia, it is marketing yoga, Ayurveda, and other practices here." Shinnecock activist, Margo Thunderbird, describes the continuing genocide of Native Americans:

> They came for our land, for what grew or could be grown on it, for the resources in it, and for our clean air and pure water. They stole these things from us, and in the taking they also stole our free ways and the best of our leaders, killed in battle or assassinated. And now, after all that, they've come for the very last of our possessions; now they want our pride, our history, our spiritual traditions. They want to rewrite and remake these things, to claim for themselves. The lies and thefts just never end.[40]

The looting of people of colour's cultures is a continuation of genocidal policies around the world. The legacy of imperialism is the destruction of our cultures hand-in-hand with the disinheritance of people from our cultures.

A plethora of publications advertise the services of Eurocanadian and Euroamerican 'plastic medicine men' and women[41] purporting to be shamans and gurus selling 'exotic' formulas. These self-styled, self-named 'experts' create a melting pot of various cultural traditions ('ancient secrets'), with no regard for the sacred or for the context in which any set of beliefs must be placed. True to their own Western systems of the free market where everything has a price, their services exact a high fee, whereas traditional healers with integrity from within the respective cultures would be compensated on entirely different terms.

APPROPRIATION OF LAY MIDWIFERY

The early imperialists initiated the demonization of the traditional lay midwife. By portraying her as superstitious, barbarous, and repulsive, they formed a stereotype based on falsified information. In addition, her title has been changed. The lay midwife is referred to as the traditional birth attendant, (TBA) and not 'midwife' thus contributing to the decline of her status as a competent and reliable caregiver. Despite these efforts to eradicate the lay midwife, her services continue to be in demand in her community — and she prevails.[42]

Our discussions with the participants indicate that the following definition describes the traditional lay midwife (now known as the TBA) who is often knowledgeable about healing and/or spirituality:

> [She] is usually a mature woman who has given birth to live children. She is a member of the community she serves. Though often illiterate, she speaks the language and not only understands but is an integral part of the religious and cultural system. [Traditional lay midwives] are generally wise, intelligent women who have been chosen by the women in their family or village for their practical approach and experience. Many... have dynamic personalities and are accepted as figures of authority in the community. [They] are private practitioners who negotiate their own compensation with clients. Sometimes they receive payment in the form of cash or gifts; usually their compensation includes favoured status in the community.[43]

Some Tamil women,[44] as well as Nazneen, Hema, Zaynab, Sarojini and Arvinder, describe the knowledge and skills of the *mommah, marthuvichi* and *dai*. Nazneen believes that a *mommah* provides home remedies for morning sickness, backaches and swollen feet. She also offers advice on nutrition or exercise. Some of the Tamil women tell us the *marthuvichi* provides personal care unavailable in hospital. She comes to check on mother and infant every other day after the birth, and bathes the baby. She massages then lays the baby beside a window where the infant can safely absorb sunlight. The *marthuvichi* also advises the woman on nutrition, and recommends herbs for allergies. She provides emotional support when needed.

According to Zaynab, a *dai* does "everything," including giving the mother a massage and taking care of the other children. Sarojini concurs, adding that the *dai* helps with the fetus's position by massaging the woman's belly. She teaches the new mother how to breastfeed, how to hold the newborn, and generally how to take care of the infant.[45]

Hema was born in a village with a *dai*.[45] Her two younger sisters were born in a city, also in a home birth with a *dai* — under the supervision of a nurse. As to ancient Indian folk and medical traditions, Hema recalls that after her sisters gave birth, her mother prohibited bright lights, fans, loud noise or music around the newborns for at least a month. Certain foods were prohibited for the new mothers. Antiseptic herbs purified bath-water, while other herbs were burned outside the room as disinfectant, to help with healing after birth.

Arvinder is an exception. She and her siblings were brought up to firmly believe in homeopathy and yoga. Her family went to an allopathic doctor only in cases of emergency. She declares, "I'm very passionate about midwifery." Her mother had her first seven children under the care of a *dai* and her last two in hospital. Arvinder accompanied her older sister to prenatal yoga classes. She was also sent to family friends' homes to help care for newborns. She describes the Indian postpartum tradition in which the *dai* or an older female relative takes care of the mother and infant for 40 days. It is a restful time when the mother stays close to the newborn.

The medical establishment has been training the TBA with the aim of absorbing her into the allopathic model. Maydene speaks of the *tu tan se*, who she describes as a nurse midwife. The *tu tan se* provides legalized services in urban areas of China. Maydene also alludes to another kind of midwife, the *jib san po*, who cannot work legally. (*Jib san po* seems to be a different pronunciation of the term *chin shoon poa* used by another participant, Hulan.)[46] Hulan tells us that in mainland China, the *chin shoon poa* works in rural areas. The *chin shoon poa*'s services — which include family planning — are legal. She receives special training and is paid by the government.

Some of the Tamil women describe the *marthuvichi* as a nurse midwife. She visits the pregnant woman every month, and reports to the doctor. Laxshmi says the nurse midwife advises the expectant mother when to go to the hospital. The *marthuvichi* also distributes infant formula and gives vaccinations. Although many participants do not know about midwifery training in Sri Lanka, one says the *marthuvichi* is trained by the hospital for four to five years, and paid by the government.

Suha has no problems with recommending a *qabileh* to her daughters-in-law because the *qabileh* conjures up happy images, "She gives the mother happiness. The *qabileh* will try to relieve her pain and heal the mother as the baby comes through." When Suha mentions the use of surgical instruments, it becomes clear that the woman who attended her four home births was an obstetrician, not a midwife. Evidently, trust in this *qabileh* is easily won because she is a doctor. However, Suha knows that the traditional *qabileh* still practises in rural areas of Tunisia.

As is evident with the *qabileh, tu tan se, chin shoon poa*, and *marthuvichi*, the autonomy of the traditional midwife is increasingly taken away. Because of her tenacity, the medical establishment has developed training plans to phase out the TBA.[47] Part of TBA training is population control advocacy: "TBAs may be expected to promote family planning.... In areas with a functioning health centre, TBAs may also be taught to motivate clients to go to the health centre for injectable contraceptives, intrauterine devices, or *sterilization*. (emphasis ours)"[48] In the course of destroying traditional lay midwifery, racist patriarchal institutions are using the lay midwife to carry out their dirtiest deeds.

Even after she undergoes training, the TBA often does not have legal status.[49] In addition, midwifery schools produce a new breed of professional midwives who have been indoctrinated in the medical model. As informal apprenticeship is not a recognized form of education, these new midwives have higher status than the TBA.[50] They train and supervise the TBA and will probably fulfill the establishment's goal of eventually replacing her.[51]

FINDINGS ON ONTARIO MIDWIFERY

Thirty-five of the women with whom we spoke did not know about the status of midwifery in Ontario. The only participants who knew about practising midwives were Arvinder and Hema. These women were also involved in social change movements, and it is perhaps through this activism that they knew about midwives. None of the participants knew that midwifery services are now covered by OHIP.

When we explained the current status, there was a mixed reaction. Most women said if they had a midwife, it would be in a hospital or birthing centre. However, some women were more open to midwifery.

Home Birth

Some of the participants articulate the importance of the physical and psychological comfort of home birth.[52] Arvinder states she would choose to give birth alone in a garage rather than allow any doctor to touch her: "If I had a child, I would not go to the hospital. I would stay away. I'd rather take the risks than have them take my fertility away. Too many terrible things have happened that I've read and heard about."

Padma, whose aunt is a practising midwife in Sri Lanka, enthusiastically explains, "Back home, there are a lot of midwives. I think midwives are okay. A long time ago, they didn't have doctors, only midwives. Midwives are very important."

Zaynab was five months pregnant at the time of the discussion. She had her first baby with the assistance of a *dai* and the next three with her mother-in-law, as they could not get a midwife. She feels the experience with the *dai* was much better for her.

Nazneen feels, "There is something dreary, something cold" about being in a hospital. In addition, she would not want a male doctor examining her body. She mentions a Persian film, "A Bed for Three People," in which women in the family support a birthing mother as she delivers with the assistance of a *mommah*. Nazneen comments, "It seemed like a very inviting process. If I wanted to have a baby, I'd like to have it that way, with everyone around. I think having midwives and having them legalized is a very good thing."

In the all-Tamil women's group, it is pointed out that most women are here often without their mothers, grandmothers, or other older female relatives. Pregnancy and birthing can be frightening and lonely. "Back home, the mothers are there. They have experience. They can help the new mothers and tell them what to do," explains the teacher/interpreter. Their isolation may be broken by the comforting presence of a midwife.

Hema has had positive exposure to home birth in her family and articulates the importance of cultural similarity. "There are lots of words you can say in your own language. You can say you want this kind of food and the midwife will understand what you're saying. I didn't grow up here, so I'm more comfortable in my own language."

Ji-Eun also speaks about the comfort of home birth. She explains that a long time ago in Korea, hospital care was very expensive, therefore the *chu san wan* delivered the baby at home. She asserts, "I think she is better than a doctor because the whole family is together." She adds that older children feel "more love and respect when they see their mother's pain and mother's love" during birth. Her grandmother is a lay midwife, and she herself was born with the aid of a *chu san wan*. However, as both her children were breach babies, she delivered them in hospital.

Ji-Eun goes on to state, "I think that in Toronto, a midwife is very good because she gives good advice and has good control. The pregnant woman is going through many changes." She adds, "I think midwives are good," both in a birthing centre and at home. "Natural delivery with a midwife is good."

The remaining participants state they would accept the assistance of an Ontario midwife only in the presence of a doctor. Given the historical impact of imperialism on people of colour, their opinions are not surprising.

Internalized Medical Model
Imperialist and misogynist indoctrination have paid off: witness people of colour's abiding faith in the modern techno-medical machine.

> It is ironic that, at a time when 'natural childbirth,' upright delivery positions, the use of midwives, having babies at home and the avoidance of high technology are all becoming popular and receiving increasing scientific support in the United States and western Europe [and Canada], the Third World is bent on adopting high-technology obstetrics.[53]

Despite her mother's positive experience with home birth, Hema maintains, "As you grow up, you see the hospitals are the big thing. You lose that trust for *dais*." She adds, "I think it's just the way we are conditioned. In India, 20 years back, it was mainly [lay] midwifery and women having kids at home. These days, very few women are having normal births because they don't want to wait. They just want to cut it, have it, go home." As to whether she would seek the services of an Ontario midwife, Hema likes the reassurance of the medical model. Yet when the group explores intervention in hospital birth Hema remarks, "But it's such a natural thing, to give birth," adding, "It seems one loses all the power when one goes to hospital. It's like you have no control over your body, your child. The doctor decides what to do." In spite of her family's positive experience with home birth, Hema still wavers towards allopathy.

Although she "totally supports the idea of a nurturing birth," Samantha has fears about childbirth. She explains, "I'm really scared of having a kid, scared of pain. If anything goes wrong, I want to make sure I'm taken care of. That's a big part affecting how I or anyone else thinks about midwifery. There's sometimes a blind trust — that I don't think I'm immune to — in hospitals and doctors. I've questioned a lot of things my mother has done as a doctor. But I'm just basically a lay person questioning her. One of the privileges doctors have is all this knowledge. So if anyone ever questions them, [even] in a very light way, it's really hard to feel that you're taken seriously."

Reflecting a lack of confidence in traditional midwives, Hulan tells us, "We have a saying in China. If you're in labour, it's like having one foot in the coffin." And Maydene believes most young women in China these days prefer to go to the hospital. In an all-Tamil women's class, the teacher/interpreter summarizes that only rarely do women have a home birth, as "they are scared to have the baby at home." Sujata has heard of midwives, but does not know what they do since women of her generation in Bombay now only go to doctors. Kurshid feels that women in Iran cannot deliver without a doctor's assistance.

In Dilshad's community, middle-class women receive the care of a midwife only in a hospital. She explains, "In my community, which is closely associated with the British, midwifery was something I had heard about from my grandmother and read about in our stories. It was considered a very noble profession, with many of our ladies training in it. Our special hospital had a midwifery section."

Zahra's oldest sister had two babies with a *daya* at her parents' home, "It was easy, it was no problem for her." She herself had her first child in hospital. She wanted to have the second one at home but there were complications. The doctor told Zahra the baby would strangle on the cord, therefore she had a Caesarean section.

Even though Zahra concedes that *dayas* have experience and specialized knowledge, she nevertheless asks, "Why do you try to go back to the past?" as there are many female doctors available now. Zahra's comments reflect many women's greater comfort with a female doctor as well as her perception that women doctors provide better care than their male counterparts.

Hyung-Suk tells us she nearly died giving birth in a Seoul hospital. "I think, because it was my first experience, I thought I was going to die." After 28 hours of labour, she recounts, she was given a Caesarean section. Hyung-Suk tells us that *san pah* is Korean for midwife, but does not elaborate any further. Because of her experience, she prefers a doctor.

Ji-Eun, who is an enthusiastic advocate of midwifery, reflects on the possibility that some women may prefer allopathic birth because of popular trust in the supposed hygiene of modern hospitals. However, as Robert Mendelsohn, a well-established doctor of 30 years, points out:

> Despite their antiseptic appearance, [hospitals are] the most germ-laden places in town. Hospital patients contract so many germ-induced infections that doctors even have a word for them. We call them nosocomial infections, which enables us to discuss your new ailment in your presence without revealing that you wouldn't have it if you had stayed at home.... Hospitals harbor a variety of [germs] that could keep an army of bacteriologists busy for the rest of their lives.[54]

Mendelsohn discusses at length the hazards of hospital birth, citing numerous ways in which it is the obstetrician him/herself who puts the mother and baby at great risk. But this truth about the danger of hospitals is so well-camouflaged that even when women have positive experiences with lay midwives, they still promote hospital birth.

One would expect the older women we spoke with to support traditional midwifery, yet they advocate allopathic birth. Sarojini's husband's grandmother was a *dai*, and she herself was born at the hands of a *dai*. Sarojini had two *dai*-assisted home births, and a third child in hospital. She believes that midwifery is obsolete because "there have been small hospitals in the villages for 20 years now." Despite her strong family experience with *dai*-delivered births, Sarojini has nevertheless been firmly persuaded that hospital care is superior to that of a *dai*.

Another older woman, Dhanmati, tells us, "I was born at the hands of my grandmother," as no *dai* had been available at the time. Dhanmati had her first two babies with a *dai* in Afghanistan, and two in an Indian hospital. She states that the *dai*'s care was better ("It was very good") than that of the hospital. After the first trimester, the *dai* visited her at home every week, and after the second trimester, every day. The *dai* also cleaned the house, bathed both mother and infant, gave the baby a massage, and took care of the other children.

Given Dhanmati's positive experience, we expect her to advocate traditional midwifery. However, she is reluctant to do so, only saying, "It's one's own choice." Dhanmati's comments, like those of Hema and Sarojini, demonstrate how technological medicine imposes itself on tradition, persuading women to trust external, modern structures over their own body-knowledge.

Traditional midwifery is further rejected on classist grounds by middle and upper-class and caste women, in 'the South.' Lay midwives are perceived as being uneducated and from the lower classes and castes. Most women define *dai* as 'maid,' 'servant,' or 'nanny,' explaining that she goes to the new mother's house to take care of older children and to do housework. The services of lay midwives are predominantly used by working-class and poor urban women, as well as by rural women. Zahra explains there are many *dayas* in Egypt, especially in villages and poor parts of cities where hospital care is expensive. Also, some Tamil women tell us that when the hospital is too far, women go to the *marthuvichi* as a 'last ditch' option.

FEMALE GENITAL MUTILATION

Women's sexuality and women's lives have long been pathologized under the guise of medical necessity or tradition. Misogynistic beliefs and practices aim to remodel our bodies and our minds. Contrary to popular belief, FGM is not restricted to cultures of 'the South.' Physicians in England and the U.S. 'treated' hysteria, lesbianism, masturbation, and other so-called 'female deviance':

> There had been a brief fad of clitoridectomy (removal of the clitoris) in the [eighteen] sixties, following the introduction of the operation by the English physician Isaac Baker Brown. Although most doctors frowned on the practice of removing the clitoris, they tended to agree that it might be necessary in cases of nymphomania, intractable masturbation, or 'unnatural growth' of that organ.[55]

Barbara Ehrenreich and Deirdre English write, "The last clitoridectomy we know of in the United States was performed in 1948 on a child of five as a cure for masturbation."[56] And in recent years, an Ohio doctor is reported to have performed more than 4,000 clitoridectomies.[57] In 1996, a Toronto plastic surgeon was said to offer labia reductions.[58] In addition, vaginoplasty, a cosmetic surgery operation similar to episiotomy is reportedly being offered.[59] Needless to say, in the so-called democratic free world, both of these operations are offered for large sums of money.

In other parts of the world, FGM is "one of the [ancient] traditional rituals that prepare girls for womanhood,"[60] and practised in at least 27 African countries, as well as parts of Asia and the Americas.

There are three types of FGM.[61] Clitoridectomy (or *sunna* circumcision) could involve: pricking the clitoris; removing one third of the clitoris, specifically the most sexually sensitive part; or cutting away the entire clitoris. In excision, the entire clitoris is cut, together with all or part of the *labia minora*.

In order to remove part or all of the clitoris, a deep cut is made into a major vein. If the cut is not treated properly, it leads to excessive bleeding that may become life-threatening. Infections are very common and vary in degree. As the primary function of the clitoris is sexual, the circumcised woman loses her ability to feel sexual sensation.

Infibulation (or Pharaonic mutilation) is removal of the clitoris, the *labia minora*, and the *labia majora*. The remaining raw edges of the vulva are sewn together, leaving a small opening for urine and menstrual blood. In addition to the physical and sexual trauma experienced in excision, women develop scar tissue or benign tumors which cause intense pain and often burst open during childbirth. When the infibulated woman goes into labour, a second cut is made through the scar tissue all the way to the anus. The mother has to endure further pain after the delivery when she is reinfibulated, often to the same 'virginal tightness' as before marriage.

Female genital mutilation dates back two thousand years. It was practised by the Phoenicians, the Hittites, and the Egyptians. FGM is not advocated by any religion. Although FGM is often associated with Islam, it is also practised by Jews, Christians, and by people of other religions.

While the Torah does not mention FGM, Ethiopian Jews are known to practise FGM. As to Christianity, the Bible does not mention FGM. However, when the missionaries invaded African countries, the Catholic priests actively advocated the continuation of the practice as a means of preserving women's 'sexual purity.' In order to oppose the Catholic position, the Protestant church discouraged the practice amongst its new converts. After the end of colonization, many Africans created their own churches which actively support the practice of FGM. A woman cannot enter a church or participate in religious life if she is not mutilated for she is considered unclean.

Sunna circumcision is most often attributed to Islam. Many Muslim scholars believe that FGM is not an Islamic practice. There is no evidence in the Quran to support the practice of FGM.

The Daya

"When you ask me about the midwife, the daya — to me, she is scary. A dragon lady." (Latifa)

For the Sudanese women with whom we spoke, the *daya is* a frightening figure. *Dayas* are not only responsible for maternal and child care, they also traditionally perform FGM. Both women talk about the difficulties of childbirth.

Latifa tells us about a maternal relative's birth experience. The relative lives in a northern Sudanese village. Latifa describes the *daya* as "an old, old, old woman, maybe a hundred years old," and well-respected. When complications arose, the family wanted to take the labouring woman to hospital. But the midwife insisted on delivering the baby. Latifa explains that it is a question of pride. The woman remained in labour until she died three days later.

There is often mutual distrust between doctor and *daya*, and the pregnant woman often feels caught in the middle. Added to this is pressure from family members and neighbours to call a *daya*. Whether the woman gives birth at home with a *daya* or in hospital with a doctor, it is the *daya* who reinfibulates her. The two women say reinfibulation is a source of many problems for woman having babies in Sudan. Latifa believes that the *daya's* helpers are often people "who have no idea... how to deliver a baby, what kind of problems there are."

Latifa recalls that when her sister was in labour, her other sisters and eight aunts came to the expectant mother's house. Despite the pregnant woman's protests, the aunts insisted on a *daya*. When the *daya* arrived, she declared the baby would be delivered in two hours. However, the husband intervened and took his wife to the hospital. Latifa explains, the aunts and *daya* consequently tried to "make a scene" at the hospital.

Although the new mother has the choice of whether or not to be reinfibulated, both Huda and Latifa note that many women do not refuse. Usually the husband, mother, aunt, older sister or others force the woman to be reinfibulated to the extent she was before marriage. Two of Latifa's sisters were reinfibulated. However, one refused, and Latifa's mother was the only elder who knew about it.

Preferences

Huda initially prefers a doctor-assisted birth, but then favours a professional midwife over a male doctor. "I guess because she is a woman, she has more feeling, and she knows herself. She is with you from the beginning, so there is a relationship."

Latifa states that, for a woman who has been mutilated, "The most difficult thing in this world is to have a kid. So many things could happen, and I don't want to be at risk." She feels she could not trust a *daya*. She would prefer hospital birth "surrounded by people who know what's going on." Latifa believes doctors here know how to deal with FGM, and that there is no reinfibulation after birth. She feels, "The doctor shouldn't ask people if they want a midwife in a hospital. A hospital is for doctors and nurses. And the midwives can have their own centre."

Advocacy

The West has acted as though they... suddenly discovered a dangerous epidemic... creating a backlash of over-sensitivity in the concerned communities. They have portrayed it as irrefutable evidence of the barbarism and vulgarity of underdeveloped countries, a point of view they have always promoted. It became a conclusive validation [of] the view of the primitiveness of Arabs, Muslims and Africans all in one blow.[62]

FGM has been broached in a disrespectful way by both white feminists and feminists of colour. Women working against FGM have to not only educate their communities, but also defend their own people against the racism of the West. Although activists working to eliminate the practice are often accused of being co-opted by the West, they are in fact against direct intervention of Western powers in their countries.

FGM would be linked to women's economic development, human rights, health, family planning, child development, education, and religion. The work of indigenous activists, scholars, and sympathetic religious leaders, among others, could serve as an important source of valuable information. The common link among these efforts would be the extensive use of indigenous mass information, popular art and culture to create a multi-directional campaign. *Eradication efforts must be empathic, not alienating.* (emphasis ours)[63]

Women from outside the communities should look to activists for direction as to the kind of support they need. Financial support could take the form of donations to activist groups working to eradicate the practice. Political support can include pressuring governments to promote education against FGM.

There are increasingly larger numbers of women immigrating to Canada from FGM-practising countries. In order to care for those clients who have undergone FGM, midwives need to be aware of many issues.[64] For example a client might experience flashbacks when her genital area is touched during examination and delivery. Also, regular-sized speculums cause extreme pain because the vaginal opening may be unusually small.

An infibulated woman can have a vaginal birth, provided the midwife is knowledgeable about the risks involved as well as procedures such as dein-fibulation. The midwife provides information and counselling about physical changes after deinfibulation. And she advises as to whether it is better to have the deinfibulation procedure done before or during labour.

Because of social pressure from her family or community members, the client may request reinfibulation. It is important that midwives be able to refer the family to activist organizations or individuals from related communities. In addition, the new mother may request circumcision of newborn girls or of older girls in the family. Again, it is crucial that the midwife be able to dissuade and/or provide referrals for the family. It bears repeating that intervention should be done with utmost sensitivity and respect. Ontario midwives can consult organizations involved in eradicating FGM.[65]

CONCLUSION
Our research indicates that lack of information is one of the main barriers for women of colour in accessing midwives in Toronto. The majority of partici-pants did not know: that midwives are available here; that midwifery is legal; or that it is covered by OHIP.

Once we explained the status, there was excitement among many women about the prospect of a legal, affordable, midwife-assisted birth. Women expressed a need for a midwife of colour from within the respective culture, one who could provide the comfort of culturally-relevant care.

> To birthing... we bring our histories, our relationships, our rituals..., needs and values that relate to intimacy, sexuality, the quality and style of family life and community. [We bring] our deepest beliefs about life, birth and death.[66]

In addition, many women wanted to know how to contact midwives. Some women also enquired about the training program.

Midwifery organizations need to outreach to communities of colour. Information in various languages should be distributed to community agencies and disseminated in print and electronic media. Outreach should address not only midwifery as a service but also as a career option. When developing outreach programs, it is important to consider the medical establishment's historical campaign (which continues in 'the South') to undo popular faith in midwives' competence. Midwifery organizations need to use various forms of education to advocate nonmedicalized birth, in order to overcome women's internalized fear of birth. In addition, further research is needed on women of colour both as consumers and as practitioners of midwifery in Ontario. We stress that such research should be done in a respectful way, not in the framework of racist 'anthropology.'

The racist and sexist stereotypes placed on women of colour mean we are often treated differently in any context of life, including the workplace, educational institutions, and healthcare services. As birth is deeply related to all aspects of a woman's life, the care she receives during this time needs to be respectful and informed. Midwifery education must encompass cultural awareness training. Such training would not simply pay lip-service to anti-racism but would be designed and delivered with integrity. Although the following is specific to FGM, we believe it is equally applicable to midwifery training:

> The development of appropriate and discipline-specific education and training materials [must] be a joint venture between the different professional institutions and women from affected community.[67]

In conclusion, we offer some observations. Women's health as well as women's work are being made to fit themselves into the male-dominated, technology-dependent model of health and healing. Colonial education systems defined what was acceptable and valuable as women's work within colonial societies. In Ontario today, the professionalization of midwifery is redefining for us what is legitimate. The experience of midwives around the world confirms that socialization is a potent force — in spite of repeated assurance that midwives will remain autonomous from the techno-medical model:

Certified midwives now have something to lose: a salary, a title, respect. They are now devoid of any social movement and have become a part of the establishment. Previously when they were politicized, they had nothing to lose but their faith.... [The] capacity for professional collegial groups, in the long run, to resist bureaucracy is quite limited.[68]

Will midwives be able to make effective decisions in the interest of their clients? In addition, what is the impact of the proposed legislation of herbs and natural remedies on midwives' practice? As a legalized profession, will midwifery now be the new target for predatory pharmaceutical multinationals?

GLOSSARY

General

masi	maternal aunt
samhitas	Sanskrit collections or manuals
sunna	Prophet Muhammed's sayings and actions

Words for Midwife

Tamil	*marthuvichi*
Hindi	*dai*
	daya
	naun
Urdu	*dai*
	daya
Gujarati	*dai*
	dayan
Arabic	*daya*
	qabileh
	jeda (in classical Arabic, *jeda* means grandmother, but it is also colloquial Iraqi for midwife)
Farsi	*mommah*
Cantonese	*jib san po* or *chin shoon poa* (depending on pronunciation)
Mandarin	*tu tan se*
Korean	*chu san wan* or *san pah*

Note:
We transliterated the words from each language into English. As the definition of each word is subject to 'common knowledge' and the interpretation of each participant, we could not provide the etymological meaning for the word (e.g. in Old English, 'midwife' meant 'with the woman'). Such information could indicate more about the origins and traditional social context of midwifery within the culture and would be an interesting area of further study.

APPENDIX I

Sample of Questions Usually Asked
Not all of the questions directly pertained to the accessibility of midwifery for Ontario women of colour. Depending on the group, we asked some of the questions to stimulate thoughts or feelings about birth, so that we could move into a discussion of midwifery.

- What's the word for midwife in your language? What does she do? Are her services legal?
- Do you have children? Where did you give birth (hospital or home?) Who helped you?
- Can you tell us about your experience?
- Do you know that you can have a midwife for your birth here?
- (After explaining the status) Would you use a midwife? Would you advocate midwifery for pregnant women you know?

APPENDIX 2

Participants
A. *37 Participants Who Expressed Their Opinions*

no. of women	country of origin
2	China
2	South Korea
2	Iran
1	Tunisia
1	Egypt
2	Sudan
15	Sri Lanka (Tamil)
3	Pakistan
7	India
2	of Indian origin, in the diaspora

B. *24 Participants Quoted*

pseudonym	country of origin
Hulan	China
Maydene	China
Hyung-Suk	South Korea
Ji-Eun	South Korea
Kurshid	Iran
Nazneen	Iran
Suha	Tunisia
Zahra	Egypt
Huda	Sudan
Latifa	Sudan

Laxshmi	Sri Lanka (Tamil)
Padma	Sri Lanka (Tamil)
Parvati	Sri Lanka (Tamil)
Sharmini	Sri Lanka (Tamil)
Zaynab	Pakistan
Dhanmati	India
Dilshad	India
Geeta	India
Hema	India
Roshni	India
Sujata	India
Sarojini	India
Arvinder	of Indian origin, in the diaspora
Samantha	of Indian origin, in the diaspora

ENDNOTES

1. Ann Oakley and Susanne Houd, *Helpers in Childbirth: Midwifery Today* (New York: Hemisphere Publishing, 1990), 166.
2. Despite the reductionist implications of this term, we chose to use it because it is widely understood. Terminology has been problematized and discussed in depth. Vijay Agnew points out, "Power relations are embedded in terminology, and terminology reflects social and political realities, influences perception, and determines the material and social reality of individuals and groups. Women who are not part of the dominant white society are described as 'visible minority women,' 'women of colour,' 'black women,' 'racial minority women,' 'non-white women,' 'immigrant women,' and 'Third World women.'" VijayAgnew, *Resisting Discrimination: Women from Asia, Africa, and the Caribbean and the Women's Movement in Canada* (Toronto: University of Toronto Press, 1996), 106. See also Nahla Abdo's discussion of identity in "Race, Gender and Politics: The Struggle of Arab Women in Canada," in *And Still We Rise*, Linda Carty, ed. (Toronto: Women's Press, 1995), 73-98.
3. In contemporary discourse, 'the North' refers to Europe and North America, sometimes including Australia and New Zealand. This area is also alluded to as: 'the West,' 'developed countries,' and occasionally, 'the First World.' By contrast, 'the South' is variously referred to as: 'the Third World,' 'developing countries,' and 'under-developed countries.' These terms have their origins in the discourse of 'colonizer versus colonized.' As Chinweizu puts it in the title of his book, there is "the West and the rest of us." All of the above terminology is problematic. 'East/West,' a dichotomy used for so long that its usage has become commonplace, presupposes an imaginary line just east of Europe — a boundary more related to fiction than geography. 'North/South' does not address Aboriginal nations around the world or Asians north of the equator. Yet the North/South dichotomy encompasses more countries than do the other terms.
4. Because of relevance and redundancy, we quoted only 24 of the 37 participants.
5. By either of the researchers or the teacher.
6. European students from Romania, the former Yugoslavia, and Italy participated in the ESL group discussions. We have decided not to include their opinions

in this chapter, valuable as they may be. The aim is to give voice to women of colour, to express our views on midwifery.

7. It is difficult to discuss any form of health care and healing without using the dichotomous terminology of 'reductionist' versus 'holistic,' or 'dominant' versus 'alternative.' Even the word 'medicine' is problematic, as it applies not only to Western/scientific/rational/modern health care, but also to ancient systems around the world. See Herbert C. Northcott, "Alternative Health Care in Canada," in *Health, Illness, and Health Care in Canada*, B. Singh Bolaria and Harley D. Dickinson, eds. (Toronto: Harcourt Brace, 1994), 487-503.

8. Jean Towler and Joan Bramall, *Midwives in History & Society* (London: Croom Helm, 1986), 9.

9. We use 'imperialism' in the sense that Edward Said describes, to mean "the practice, the theory, and the attitudes of a dominating metropolitan center ruling a distant territory...." Colonialism, on the other hand, "which is almost always a consequence of imperialism, is the implanting of settlements on distant territory." Said goes on to quote Michael Doyle who explains, "Empire is a relationship, formal or informal, in which one state controls the effective political sovereignty of another political society. It can be achieved by force, by political collaboration, by economic, social, or cultural dependence. Imperialism is simply the process or policy of establishing or maintaining an empire." While historical colonialism has essentially ended, imperialism "lingers where it has always been, in a kind of general cultural sphere as well as in specific, political, ideological, economic, and social practices." Edward Said, *Culture and Imperialism* (New York: Vintage Books, 1993), 9.

10. Vandana Shiva, "The Seed and the Earth: Biotechnology and the Colonisation of Regeneration," in *Close to Home: Women Reconnect Ecology, Health and Development Worldwide*, Vandana Shiva, ed. (Philadelphia: New Society Publishers, 1994), 130.

11. Chinweizu, *The West & The Rest of Us* (New York: Random House, 1975), 3.

12. Shiva, 130.

13. Ward Churchill, *Indians Are Us? Culture and Genocide in Native North America* (Toronto: Between The Lines, 1994), 133-134.

14. Noam Chomsky, *Year 501: The Conquest Continues* (New York: Black Rose Books, 1993), 19.

15. Ibid.

16. Said, 8.

17. Shiva, 138.

18. Rosemary Radford Ruether, *Sexism & God Talk: Toward A Feminist Theology* (Boston: Beacon Press, 1983), 82.

19. Ira M. Lapidus, *A History of Islamic Societies* (Cambridge: Cambridge University Press, 1988), 554.

20. Fritjof Capra, *The Turning Point: Science, Society, and the Rising Culture* (New York: Bantam Books, 1982), 54.

21. Robert S. Mendelsohn, *Male Practice: How Doctors Manipulate Women* (Chicago: Contemporary Books, Inc., 1981), 30-31.

22. Barbara Ehrenreich and Deirdre English, *For Her Own Good: 150 Years of the Experts' Advice to Women* (New York: Anchor Books, 1978), 64.

23. David Arnold, "Introduction: disease, medicine and empire," in *Imperial Medicine and Indigenous Societies*, David Arnold, ed. (Manchester: Manchester University Press, 1988), 12.

24. David Arnold, "Public health and public power: medicine and hegemony in colonial India," in *Contesting Colonial Hegemony: State and Society in Africa and India*, Dagmar Engels and Shula Marks, eds. (London: British Academic Press, 1994), 131-151. See also Arnold, 1988.
25. Geraldine Forbes, "Managing midwifery in India," in Engels and Marks, eds., 154.
26. Ibid, 155.
27. Ibid, 169.
28. For a look at European (specifically British) women's role with regards to the oppression of colonized people, see Nupur Chaudhuri and Margaret Strobel, *Western Women and Imperialism: Complicity and Resistance* (Bloomington: Indiana University Press, 1992).
29. Forbes, 161.
30. For further information on eugenics and population control, see Stephen Trombley, *The Right to Reproduce: A History of Coercive Sterilization* (London: Weidenfield and Nicolson, 1988). For a study of imperialism and health, see Vicente Navarro, ed., *Imperialism, Health and Medicine* (New York: Baywood Publishing Co., 1974).
31. Mendelsohn, 33.
32. For a history of institutionalized sterilization, see J. David Smith and K. Ray Nelson, *The Sterilization of Carrie Buck* (New Jersey: New Horizon Press, 1989). For further reading on sterilization, see Loretta Ross, "Sterilization and 'de facto' sterilization," *The Amicus Journal,* Winter, vol. 15, no. 4 (1994): 29; and Monica Bahati Kuumba, "Perpetuating Neo-Colonialism through Population Control: South Africa and the United States," *Africa Today,* vol. 4O, no. 3 (1993): 79-85. Also see Alexander Cockburn, "Welfare, Norplant and the Nazis," *The Nation,* vol. 259, no. 3 (1994): 79-82.
33. Frances M. Beal, "Women in Black Liberation," in *Sisterhood is Powerful*, Robin Morgan, ed. (New York: Random House, 1970), 348-349.
34. Trombley, 188-189.
35. Angela Y. Davis, *Women, Race & Class* (New York: Vintage Books, 1981), 218.
36. Marlene Gerber Fried, *From Abortion to Reproductive Freedom: Transforming A Movement* (Boston: South End Press, 1990), 159.
37. Davis, Ibid.
38. Betsy Hartmann, *Reproductive Rights and Wrongs: The Global Politics of Population Control* (Boston: South End Press, 1995), 257.
39. Shiva, 129.
40. Quoted in Churchill, 216. See also Andy Smith, "For All Those Who Were Indian in a Former Life," *Sojourner: The Women's Forum,* (November 1990): 8-9.
41. *White Shamans and Plastic Medicine Men* (video), (Bozeman, MT: Native Voices Public Television, 1995).
42. Vaidya M. Radhika and A. V. Balasubramanian, eds., *Mother and Child Care in Traditional Medicine* (2 vols) (Madras: Lok Swaasthya Parampara Samvardhan Samithi, 1990). Both volumes give descriptions of the pregnancy, labour, delivery, and postpartum care provided by the *dai*. A group called Lok Swaasthya Parampara Samvardhan Samithi (LSPSS) is researching, funding, training and providing other support services to local health traditions. LSPSS fosters the revival and maintenance of folk, local and 'tribal' health practices in conjunction with formal medical systems such as Ayurveda, Unani and Siddha. Their goal is "to revitalise the traditional

self-reliant model of primary health care existing in... Indian Society."
LSPSS advocates the need for "a fresh outlook toward *dais* — the enormous
strength of the *dai* tradition needs to be understood and encouraged."

43. WHO, UNFPA, UNICEF, *Traditional Birth Attendants: A Joint
    WHO/UNFPA/UNICEF Statement* (Geneva: World Health Organization,
    1992), 5.
44. We say "some Tamil women" without specifying individuals because several
    women often talked at the same time and their comments were often
    interpreted as a group rather than individually.
45. Hema also offers another Hindi name for midwife, *naun*. She takes care of the
    expectant mother from the last week of pregnancy through postpartum, but
    does not do any housework. Although Hema describes the *naun* as "a
    midwife of the old style," we did not encounter further information in our
    research about the *naun*.
46. According to a Cantonese-speaking doctor of traditional Chinese medicine.
47. Forbes, 171-172.
48. WHO, UNFPA, UNICEF, 10-11.
49. A. Mangay-Maglacas, "Traditional Birth Attendants," in *Health Care of
    Women and Children in Developing Countries*, Helen M. Wallace and Kanti
    Giri, eds. (Oakland, CA: Third Party Publishing, 1990), 236.
50. WHO, UNFPA, UNICEF, 14.
51. Ibid, 16-17.
52. Regarding the safety of home birth, see: Houd and Oakley; Suzanne Arms,
    Immaculate Deception II: A Fresh Look at Childbirth (Berkeley: Celestial
    Arts, 1994); Brian Burtch, *Trials of Labour: The Re-emergence of Midwifery*
    (Montreal: McGill-Queen's University Press: 1994); Paul Thompson, "The
    Home Birth Alternative to the Medicalization of Childbirth: Safety and
    Ethical Responsibility," in *The Future of Human Reproduction*, Christine
    Overall, ed. (Toronto: Women's Press, 1989); Catherine Lusson, "Obstacles
    to Social Change: The Legalization of Midwifery in Ontario" (Master's
    Thesis, Trent University, 1994), 39-40; and Eleanor Barrington, *Midwifery is
    Catching* (Toronto: NC Press, 1985).
53. Brigitte Jordan, "High technology: the case of obstetrics," *World Health
    Forum,* vol. 8 (1987): 318.
54. Mendelsohn, 84.
55. Ehrenreich and English, 123.
56. Ibid.
57. Mendelsohn, 38.
58. Josey Vogel, "The Sex Files," *Flare Magazine* (September 1996): 141.
59. Sue Johanson, "Shape up sex life after pregnancy,"*The Toronto Star* (August
    22, 1996): B5.
60. Nahid Toubia, *Female Genital Mutilation: A Call for Global Action* (New
    York: Women Ink, 1993), 9.
61. Nawal El Saadawi, *The Hidden Face of Eve: Women in the Arab World*
    (London: Zed Books, 1980), 39; and Zainaba, "Lecture on Clitoridectomy to
    the Midwives of Touil, Mauritania," in *Opening the Gates: A Century of
    Arab Feminist Writing,* Margot Badran and Miriam Cooke, eds. (London:
    Virago Press, 1990), 67. Also see Toubia, 1993, 10. And Nahid Toubia,
    "Women and Health in the Sudan," in *Women of the Arab World,* Nahid
    Toubia, ed. (London: Zed Books, 1988), 101.
62. Toubia, (1988) 101.
63. Toubia (1993), 14.

64. For additional information, see Efua Dorkenoo, *Cutting the Rose: Female Genital Mutilation; The Practice and Its Prevention* (London: Minority Rights Publications, 1994); Asma El Dareer, *Women, Why Do You Weep?* (London: Zed Books, 1982); and Nawal El Saadawi (1980).
65. The following are some of the organizations in Toronto working to eradicate FGM at political and social levels, and can offer information on related health issues: Women's Health in Women's Hands, Canadian Centre for Victims of Torture, and Islamic Social Services and Resources Association.
66. Jane Pincus and Norma Senson, "Childbirth," in *The New Our Bodies, Ourselves: A Book By and for Women*, The Boston Women's Health Collective, ed. (New York: Simon & Schuster, 1991), 435.
67. Ontario Female Genital Prevention Task Force, *Report on Strategies for FGM Prevention/Eradication* (July 1995): 11.
68. Lusson, 73. For more on the question of professionalization, see: Barrington; Houd and Oakley; also Raymond DeVries, *Regulating Birth: Midwives, Medicine, and the Law* (Philadelphia: Temple University Press, 1985).

REFERENCES

Abdo, Nahla. "Race, Gender and Politics: The Struggle of Arab Women in Canada." In *And Still We Rise*. Linda Carty, ed. Toronto: Women's Press, 1995.

Agnew,Vijay. *Resisting Discrimination: Women from Asia, Africa, and the Caribbean and the Women's Movement in Canada.* Toronto: University of Toronto Press, 1996.

Arms, Suzanne. *Immaculate Deception II: A Fresh Look at Childbirth.* Berkeley: Celestial Arts, 1994.

Arnold, David. "Introduction: disease, medicine and empire." In *Imperial medicine and indigenous societies.* David Arnold, ed. Manchester: Manchester University Press, 1988.

Arnold, David. "Public health and public power: medicine and hegemony in colonial India." In *Contesting Colonial Hegemony: State and Society in Africa and India.* Dagmar Engels and Shula Marks, eds. London: British Academic Press, 1994.

Balasubramanian, A. V., and Vaidya M. Radhika, eds. *Mother and Child Care in Traditional Medicine.* (2 vols) Madras: Lok Swaasthya Parampara Samvardhan Samithi, 1990.

Barrington, Eleanor. *Midwifery is Catching.* Toronto: NC Press, 1985.

Beal, Frances M. "Women in Black Liberation." In *Sisterhood is Powerful.* Robin Morgan, ed. New York: Random House, 1970.

Burtch, Brian. *Trials of Labour: The Re-emergence of Midwifery.* Montreal: McGill-Queen's University Press: 1994.

Capra, Fritjof. *The Turning Point: Science, Society, and the Rising Culture.* New York: Bantam Books, 1982.

Chaudhuri, Nupur, and Margaret Strobel. *Western Women and Imperialism: Complicity and Resistance.* Bloomington: Indiana University Press, 1992.

Chinweizu. *The West & The Rest of Us.* New York: Random House, 1974.

Chomsky, Noam. *Year 501: The Conquest Continues.* Montreal: Black Rose Books, 1993.

Churchill, Ward. *Indians Are Us? Culture and Genocide in Native North America.* Toronto: Between The Lines, 1994.

Cockburn, Alexander. "Welfare, Norplant and the Nazis." *The Nation*, vol. 259, no. 3, (1994): 79-82.

Davis, Angela Y. *Women, Race & Class*. New York: Vintage Books, 1981.
DeVries, Raymond. *Regulating Birth: Midwives, Medicine, and the Law*.
    Philadelphia: Temple University Press, 1985.
Dorkenoo, Efua. *Cutting the Rose: Female Genital Mutilation; The Practice and
    Its Prevention*. London: Minority Rights Publications, 1994.
Ehrenreich, Barbara, and Deirdre English. *For Her Own Good: 150 Years of the
    Experts' Advice to Women*. New York: Anchor Books, 1978.
El Dareer, Asma. *Women, Why Do You Weep?* London: Zed Books, 1982.
El Saadawi, Nawal. *The Hidden Face of Eve: Women in the Arab World*. London:
    Zed Books, 1980.
Forbes, Geraldine. "Managing midwifery in India." In *Contesting Colonial
    Hegemony: State and Society in Africa and India*. Dagmar Engels and Shula
    Marks, eds. London: British Academic Press, 1994.
Gerber Fried, Marlene. *From Abortion to Reproductive Freedom: Transforming A
    Movement*. Boston: South End Press, 1990.
Hartmann, Betsy. *Reproductive Rights and Wrongs: The Global Politics of
    Population Control*. Boston: South End Press, 1995.
Houd, Susanne, and Ann Oakley. *Helpers in Childbirth: Midwifery Today*. New
    York: Hemisphere Publishing, 1990.
Johanson, Sue. "Shape up sex life after pregnancy." *The Toronto Star*, (August
    22, 1996): B5.
Jordan, Brigitte. "High technology: the case of obstetrics." *World Health Forum*,
    vol. 8, (1987): 312-319.
Kuumba, Monica Bahati. "Perpetuating Neo-Colonialism through Population
    Control: South Africa and the United States." *Africa Today*, vol. 40, no. 3,
    (1993): 79-85.
Lapidus, Ira M. *A History of Islamic Societies*. Cambridge: Cambridge University
    Press, 1988.
Lusson, Catherine. "Obstacles to Social Change: The Legalization of Midwifery
    in Ontario." Master's Thesis, Trent University, 1994.
Mangay-Maglacas, A. "Traditional Birth Attendants." In *Health Care of Women
    and Children in Developing Countries*. Helen M. Wallace, Kanti Giri, eds.
    Oakland: Third Party Publishing, 1990.
Mendelsohn, Robert S. *Male Practice: How Doctors Manipulate Women*.
    Chicago: Contemporary Books, Inc., 1981.
Native Voices Public Television. *White Shamans and Plastic Medicine Men*
    (video). Bozeman, MT: Native Voices Public Television, 1995.
Navarro, Vicente, ed. *Imperialism, Health and Medicine*. New York: Baywood
    Publishing Co., 1974.
Northcott, Herbert C. "Alternative Health Care in Canada." In *Health, Illness,
    and Health Care in Canada*. B. Singh Bolaria and Harley D. Dickinson, eds.
    Toronto: Harcourt Brace, 1994.
Ontario Female Genital Prevention Task Force. *Report on Strategies for FGM
    Prevention/Eradication*. July 1995.
Pincus, Jane, and Norma Senson. "Childbirth." In *The New Our Bodies,
    Ourselves: A Book By and for Women*. The Boston Women's Health
    Collective, ed. New York: Simon & Schuster, 1991.
Ross, Loretta. "Sterilization and 'de facto' sterilization." *The Amicus Journal*,
    vol. 15, no. 4, (1994): 29.
Ruether, Rosemary Radford. *Sexism & God Talk: Toward A Feminist Theology*.
    Boston: Beacon Press, 1983.
Said, Edward. *Culture and Imperialism*. New York: Vintage Books, 1993.

Shiva, Vandana, ed. *Close to Home: Women Reconnect Ecology, Health and Development Worldwide.* Philadelphia: New Society Publishers, 1994.

Smith, Andy. "For All Those Who Were Indian in a Former Life." *Sojourner: The Women's Forum,* (November 1990): 8-9.

Smith, J. David, and K. Ray Nelson. *The Sterilization of Carrie Buck.* New Jersey: New Horizon Press, 1989.

Thompson, Paul. "The Home Birth Alternative to the Medicalization of Childbirth: Safety and Ethical Responsibility." In *The Future of Human Reproduction.* Christine Overall, ed. Toronto: Women's Press, 1989.

Toubia, Nahid. *Female Genital Mutilation: A Call for Global Action.* New York: Women Ink, 1993.

Toubia, Nahid, ed. *Women of the Arab World.* London: Zed Books, 1988.

Towler, Jean, and Joan Bramall. *Midwives in History & Society.* London: Croom Helm, 1986.

Trombley, Stephen. *The Right to Reproduce: A History of Coercive Sterilization.* London: Weidenfield and Nicolson, 1988.

Vogel, Josey. "The Sex Files." *Flare Magazine.* (September 1996): 141.

WHO, UNFPA, UNICEF. *Traditional Birth Attendants: A Joint WHO/UNFPA/UNICEF Statement.* Geneva: World Health Organization, 1992.

Zainaba. "Lecture on Clitoridectomy to the Midwives of Touil, Mauritania." In *Opening the Gates: A Century of Arab Feminist Writing.* Margot Badran and Miriam Cooke, eds. London: Virago Press, 1990.

RECOMMENDED READING

Abdella, Raqiya. *Sisters in Affliction: Circumcision and Infibulation of Women in Africa.* London: Zed Books, 1982.

Ahmed, Leila. *Women and Gender in Islam.* New Haven: Yale University Press, 1992.

An Na'im, Abdullahi. *Toward an Islamic Reformation: Civil Liberties, Human Rights, and International Law.* New York: Syracuse University Press, 1990.

Arnold, David, ed. *Imperial medicine and indigenous societies.* Manchester: Manchester University Press, 1988.

Badran, Margot, and Miriam Cooke, eds. *Opening the Gates: A Century of Arab Feminist Writing.* London: Virago Press, 1990.

Bannerji, Himani, ed. *Returning The Gaze: Essays on Racism, Feminism and Politics.* Toronto: Sister Vision Press, 1993.

Churchill, Ward. *Struggle for the Land: Indigenous Resistance to Genocide, Ecocide and Expropriation in Contemporary North America.* Toronto: Between the Lines, 1992.

Doyle, Robert, and Livy Visano. *A Time for Action! Access to Health and Social Services for Members of Diverse Cultural and Racial Groups in Metro Toronto.* Toronto: Social Planning Council of Metropolitan Toronto, 1987.

Dua, Enakshi, Maureen FitzGerald, Linda Gardner, Darien Taylor, and Lisa Wyndels, eds. *On Women Healthsharing.* Toronto: Women's Press, 1994.

Frideres, J.S. "Racism and Health: Case of the Native People." In *Health, Illness, and Health Care in Canada.* B. Singh Bolaria and Harley D. Dickinson, eds. Toronto: Harcourt Brace, 1994.

Gupta, Nila, and Makeda Silvera, eds. *The Issue is 'Ism: Women of Colour Speak Out* (1983 reprint). Toronto: Sister Vision Press, 1989.

Kitzinger, Sheila, ed. *The Midwife Challenge.* London: Pandora Press, 1988.

Kumar, Radha. *The History of Doing: An Illustrated Account of Movements for Women's Rights and Feminism in India, 1800-1900.* New Delhi: Kali for Women, 1993.

Logan, Onnie Lee, as told to Katherine Clark. *Motherwit: An Albama Midwife's Story.* New York: Penguin Books, 1989.

Lorde, Audre. *Sister Outsider: Essays and Speeches.* New York: The Crossing Press, 1984.

McDonnell, Kathleen, ed. *Adverse Effects: Women and the Pharmaceutical Industry.* Toronto: Women's Press 1986.

Mendelsohn, Robert S. *Confessions of A Medical Heretic.* Chicago: Contemporary Books, 1979.

Moraga, Cherrie, and Gloria Anzaldua, eds. *This Bridge Called My Back: Writing by Radical Women of Color.* New York: Kitchen Table Women of Color Press, 1981.

Mukherjee, Arun, ed. *Sharing Our Experience.* Ottawa: Canadian Council on the Status of Women, 1993.

Overall, Christine, ed. *The Future of Human Reproduction.* Toronto: Women's Press, 1989.

Rafiq, Fauzia. *Developing an Antiracism Action Plan: A Handbook for Workers Working in Service Organizations of Metropolitan Toronto.* Toronto: Women Working with Immigrant Women, 1992.

Satzewich, Wotherspoon. *First Nations: Race, Class, and Gender Relations.* Scarborough: Nelson, 1993.

Sen, Gita, and Caren Grown. *Development, Crises, and Alternative Visions: Third World Women's Perspectives.* New York: Monthly Review Press, 1987.

Walters, Vivienne, Rhonda Lenton, and Marie McKeary. *Women's Health in the Context of Women's Lives.* Minister of Supply and Services Canada, 1995.

Experiences of Mothers with Disabilities
and Implications for the Practice of Midwifery[1]

Pat Israel

As a feminist with a physical disability, I have been involved in the issue of motherhood and disability for a number of years on behalf of DisAbled Women's Network (DAWN) Ontario. DAWN is a self-help organization of women with all types of disabilities. DAWN began in 1985 in response to the problems of exclusion experienced by many women with disabilities within the women's movement and the disability rights movement. The goals of DAWN include: to make women's services accessible; to act as a bridge between the disability consumer movement and the women's movement; to be role models for disabled girls; and to be a voice for women with disabilities.

Between 1993 and 1996, I had the privilege of serving as a public member on the College of Midwives. I was able to bring the issues of mothers with disabilities to the College and to the midwives I met there. I also had the chance to learn in far more detail what the issues of midwives are in providing care to all women.

At the age of five, my genetic disability began to show itself and I was introduced to the medical-model approach to disability which was the only option then. I have a rare disability which is Dopa Responsive Dystonia. The physicians were not able to diagnose my disability for most of my life, resulting in a lot of testing and different operations as a child and a teenager. I was 'enrolled' in a medical system over which I had no control at all.

Many disabled women have gone through that same process. They still go through it even today. It can make one very suspicious and wary of the medical system. However, now a person with a disability can connect with an Independent Living Centre or a self-help group and receive help around various options which may be nonmedical.

When you have a physical disability at a young age and are in a large urban centre, there is a good chance that you will go to a segregated public school and later to an integrated high school. You may have received very little information about sexuality. Sexuality education is often tied in with physical education classes and some disabled girls do not take the physical education classes.

HAVING CHILDREN

Having children is not a subject that is often discussed with girls with disabilities. Many parents assume that disabled girls will not have children. They would be shocked to find out that their daughter was even thinking about it. They do expect their nondisabled sons and daughters to be parents, but not their disabled ones.

A disabled woman that I talked to had told her father that she was pregnant. He asked her if she was going to keep the baby. Most parents would be happy if their daughter was pregnant. This is an unusual question to ask a woman who is in a committed relationship and is of childbearing age. She was asked simply because she has a disability.

Women with disabilities do have children even though they live in a society that actively discourages them from doing so. We face many barriers when we do become pregnant. These can include doctors who: do not have any knowledge about pregnancy and disability; have inaccessible offices and exam tables; or may even suggest that the disabled woman should have an abortion because they think that she could not be a good parent or the burden of having a child would be too great for her.

ATTITUDINAL BARRIERS

Many women with disabilities face anger from people if we are carrying a baby that might have the same genetic disability that we have. People with and without disabilities have expressed the belief that it is not right to knowingly bring a disabled child into this world. Others are in awe to see a woman using a wheelchair who is visibly pregnant. They wonder how it happened and may express concern over her parenting abilities. Or they may assume that the child will have to care for the mother with a disability when she/he is physically able to. People sometimes talk to children of disabled mothers when they should be talking directly to the mother.

ACCESSIBILITY

When mothers are ready to return to work, school, or to resume activities outside of their home, they quickly learn that many childcare centres are often not accessible. As well, information for pregnant women is not available in braille, large print or on tape. Information is not usually written in plain language, so that women with a developmental disability, low literacy levels or dyslexia can read it. Service providers who deal with pregnant women may not have a TTY in their office so that a deaf woman could phone them directly.

If the woman has chosen a hospital birth and she has a mobility disability, she may have to struggle with an inaccessible maternity floor. Accessible rooms with low beds and large washrooms with grab bars are often only on the rehabilitation floor. Hospital staff may not fully understand her specific needs for attendant care or that a woman with a disability may need a lot of help simply because she is in such an inaccessible environment. In her own home environment, she may not need any help at all or very little.

I believe women with disabilities could benefit from midwifery services in many ways. Women with disabilities could choose to have their baby at home which will probably be far more accessible than any hospital environment. Midwives will come to their client's home if necessary. With the lack of flexibility of para-transit systems and streamlining cutbacks, home visits may be the preference of a disabled woman. If the disabled woman does go to the midwife's office it is a lot easy for her to transfer to the couch in the examination room than to the typically high exam table in physicians' offices. At the midwifery office that I visited, an accessible washroom was available and there was a lot of space in the waiting room. Prenatal classes were also held in this same accessible office.

Midwives are excellent advocates for their clients, which could be quite beneficial for any woman with a disability who has to obtain services from an often large and impersonal bureaucratic system. Going to a midwife will give the disabled woman the opportunity for longer appointment times. She will have a greater opportunity to ask questions during a visit to a midwife rather than the short visits a physician offers. She can explore options for birthing positions that would be comfortable for her and her type of disability. If the midwife does not know the answers to her questions, she is more likely to try to find the correct resources and people who will know the answers. DAWN Ontario does receive calls from midwives when they have a disabled woman as a client. Finally, if there is a transfer of care to a physician for the birth, the midwife can still provide invaluable supportive care.

PERSONAL STORIES

The birthing stories of women with disabilities across Canada often have similar themes. One woman with a visual impairment spoke of her experience in the hospital when her husband was unable to be at the birth. Immediately after her baby was born, the nurses refused to let her hold her baby because they were afraid that she might drop the baby. As a result, the woman had to wait until her husband showed up a few hours later, at which time the nurses gave the baby to him to hold. He immediately gave the baby to his wife and she held her baby for the first time. As a woman with a disability hearing this story, this story both moved me and angered me. When this mom told me her story, she had tears in her eyes from the pain this situation caused her. It is hard to imagine having a baby and being denied the right to hold her or him right away simply because you have a disability. Healthcare professionals demonstrated utter disregard for the woman's ability to care for her baby and her right as mother to bond with it after giving birth.

Another example is of a disabled mother who had been born with a congenital disabilities. She used a prosthetic arm and her walking was affected. Prior to going into the hospital, she was confident in her abilities to be a good mother. She had taken all of the prenatal courses and had a very supportive partner. She was prepared and was looking forward to becoming a mother. After the birth of her son, a different nurse on every shift came in and said, "How can you possibly take care of a baby?" After hearing this several times from different nurses, the woman became quite upset and began to wonder herself what she would do when she got home with her newborn. However, when she did get home with her baby, she quickly moved into the role of being a mom and coped quite nicely with her new son.

BABIES ADAPTING TO THEIR MOTHER'S DISABILITY

Another aspect of parenting which is not often recognized is that often babies may be quite adept at adapting to their mother's disability, therefore making the job of mothering a bit easier. I have seen videos of disabled mothers picking up their babies or changing their diapers. The babies stayed still while being picked up or while their diaper was being changed. With mothers who were wheelchair users, when their babies were strong and agile enough to climb onto their mother's lap, they quickly did that when they wanted to be comforted and held. They knew that their mother could not easily pick them up but could comfort them when they climbed onto her lap.

ASSISTANCE AND RESOURCES

Despite all the problems and obstacles that women with disabilities face in the area of mothering, we still choose to have children. In fact, it seems that disabled women are even having a 'baby boom' judging from the increased calls that DAWN Ontario has been receiving. DAWN Ontario receives many calls from women who are pregnant and wanting information. They are looking for information on accessible cribs and other products that will help them care for their babies.

Disabled moms are also looking to link with other disabled moms who can talk to them and give them hints and advice. Women with disabilities are very isolated when they become pregnant and find it difficult to locate resources that are specific to disabled mothers. Many of the disability-specific service agencies have no information on disability and pregnancy. If the woman is lucky, the agency will have heard of DAWN Ontario and will refer her to us. Unfortunately, a lot of the time, she will be told, "Sorry, we do not have any information on this topic."

I am happy to say, however, that the situation is getting a little better for disabled Ontarions who live in or near Toronto. The Centre for Independent Living in Toronto (CILT) and the Canadian Paraplegic Association (CPA) have formed an alliance and are working on a project which will bring disabled parents together. Monthly meetings are held at the CILT office to allow parents with disabilities the opportunity to talk with each other. Ten thousand copies of the brochure which DAWN Ontario published on pregnancy and disability has been widely distributed and new requests come in every day.

HEALTH CARE FOR MOTHERS WITH DISABILITIES

When considering what constitutes adequate health care for mothers with disabilities, the following issues should be remembered:

Women with disabilities come from all backgrounds and have many different types of disabilities. These range from: mobility, visual, deaf and hard of hearing, developmental, non-visible (i.e. epilepsy, diabetes, chronic fatigue syndrome), learning, and psychiatric survivors. A lot of women will identify as having a disability, while others will consider it only a problem or inconvenience. Many deaf women do not feel they have a disability, as they identify as a cultural minority. Some women will have multiple disabilities.

We are from every ethnoracial community, including many Aboriginal communities. For many of us our first language may not be English. We may be confronted by a healthcare system which not only inadequately meets our physical access needs, but may not be linguistically or culturally appropriate or sensitive. We are bisexual, lesbian and heterosexual. Parenting for women who are lesbians or bisexual itself presents many challenges and is often steeped in misconceptions and stereotypes reflecting a heterosexist perspective.

Finally, the same care and sensitivity shown to nondisabled women who are survivors of violence must also be considered when working with women with disabilities, as many of us are also survivors of violence by spouses, family, members and caregivers.

SUGGESTIONS TO MIDWIVES

1. Midwives may have to deal with different service agencies that the disabled woman is associated with in order to get services for her. Often services are not well coordinated and may not collaborate efforts, so it can be confusing for the midwife when she first gets involved. While working at DAWN Ontario, I received a call from a midwife who was working with a disabled client. In addition to providing her midwifery care, she was also working to try to get the woman's motorized wheelchair repaired. I was impressed. This level of involvement reflected a

great deal about the level of commitment and care of the midwife. She understood the importance of her client having the proper wheelchair to get around, especially after she has the baby.

2. Healthcare providers will need to evaluate their office setting, as well as the level of access women have to services:
    *   Is it wheelchair accessible?
    *   Can a woman with a mobility disability get on your couch or examination table?
    *   Have you thought of different ways of examining her in case one way causes pain?
    *   Is the material that you give out to pregnant women available at least on tape for visually and print handicapped women?
    *   Is it written in plain language?
    *   Do you have a TTY so that your deaf clients can call you direct?

3. If a woman with a disability needs attendant care at her appointments, do not assume that she can bring the attendant from the project where she lives. Attendant services are not flexible and often not portable. When a disabled woman who uses attendant care in a project gets pregnant, all hell can break loose. The attendant care workers are not required to provide care for the woman and the baby — only for the woman. The project may even ask the woman to leave and find a new place to live. This puts her in a difficult situation since there are not many projects that will house a disabled mother and her family. So, when this woman becomes pregnant, she may need to make many quick changes within nine months.

    However, if a disabled woman is a self-manager — that is she receives funding from the government to pay for her own attendant care — then the situation will be different. She would be able to have an attendant come with her to appointments and would be able to have the attendants help her in caring for her child. This type of funding has allowed some women with disabilities the option of having children.

4. Compared to the varied services available to nondisabled moms across the province, there are few services specifically geared to the needs of disabled mothers — they are only located in the Toronto area. Currently, there are two programs which help parents with developmental disabilities to learn parenting skills. There is also a prenatal class taught by an instructor who is proficient in sign-language interpretation. There are some midwives who are skilled in sign-language interpretation as well. Midwives who have disabled women as clients will need to find out what resources are available. I strongly believe that

all midwives should know this information before they have a disabled woman as a client.

5. Read the books that are available on mothers with disabilities. They are invaluable resources. Call DAWN Ontario or the Centre for Independent Living in your area and find out if these organizations have names of disabled mothers willing to be contacted. They may also have information on accessible cribs and other products. Often, disabled moms are forced to get a regular crib adapted, as it is difficult to find accessible cribs readily available for purchase. However, this is very expensive and prices for an adapted crib can range from $1,200 to $3,000.

7. Remember that the disabled woman is the expert on her disability, but you will probably both learn together about how pregnancy will interact with her disability. If it is her second pregnancy, then the situation will be different and she will be able to inform you of her needs.

REGULATION OF MIDWIFERY

Originally, I believed that when midwifery became legal, women with disabilities could use midwifery care easily. This has not always been the case. Women with disabilities sometimes have to be under a doctor's care as well as a midwife. Because of funding rules, women are only allowed to be under a midwife's care or a doctor's care. This works fine for most nondisabled women, but because pregnancy can affect women with disabilities differently, we may also need to be under the care of a doctor in case of disability-specific problems.

The existing funding criteria will not allow any exemptions. I have received calls from disabled women at DAWN who were very disappointed that they could not use the services of a midwife because they needed to see a doctor during their entire pregnancy as well. Midwives themselves are frustrated by these rules and have tried to have them changed but have been unsuccessful. This has been a great disappointment, but we hope someday we can change this unfair ruling so that all disabled women who want midwifery care can get midwifery care.

Women within DAWN believe that there must be an exemption for women with disabilities and midwifery care should be allowed in conjunction with obstetric care. The issue of funded labour coaches has not been discussed by the members of DAWN, so it is not possible to give a policy statement from DAWN Ontario at this time. But if the government will not allow payment for a physician and a midwife, I think the government should at least fund physicians and labour coaches together.

Due to funding cuts, DAWN Ontario is struggling to stay alive. The local office of DAWN Toronto has closed its doors, but DAWN Ontario and several other local DAWN groups in Ontario are still open. DAWN Ontario has received vital funding from the Trillium Foundation to keep the office open and work on making the group strong and more financially viable. It would be disastrous to lose the resources and expertise developed by women with disabilities on mothers' issues. We will continue to struggle and to hope — to grow stronger.

Mothers with disabilities need a strong voice and strong representation. Given the right political climate and a sound funding base, DAWN can continue to expand and build upon the good work it has undertaken. Women with disabilities need healthcare providers to work with us to ensure our right to access quality healthcare services across Ontario.

ENDNOTE

1. I would like to extend my personal thanks to Fran Odette, who is also a disabled feminist for her help in editing this article and adding some sections which helped to clarify issues.

RESOURCES

Baby Tenda
123 S. Belmont Blvd.
Kansas City, Missouri, 64123
(816) 231-2300
Safety baby furniture which is adaptable to mothers with disabilities. Write or call company for brochure and name of Canadian distributor.

Childbearing and Parenting Program for Women with Disabilities/Chronic Illnesses
Elaine Carty, School of Nursing
University of British Columbia
206 — 2211 Wesbrooke Mall
Vancouver, B.C. V6T 2B5

Childbirth Education for Women with Disabilities and Their Partners
The Nisonger Center Publications
Ohio State University
1581 Dodd Drive
Columbus, OH 43210
A training manual for professionals. Cost is $65.00 U.S. funds, includes shipping and handling.

Disability, Pregnancy & Pregnancy International
Arrowhead Publications
1 Chiswick Staithe
London, W4 3TP England
A newsletter for professionals and parents to exchange information and experiences.

High Chairs & Children
by Sandie Waddell
Education Resource Centre
P.O. Box 1813 Whangarei, New Zealand
A book dealing with pregnancy, childbirth and aftercare for women with spinal cord injury. Cost is US $16.

"I want to be a mother. I have a disability: What are my choices?"
DisAbled Women's Network (DAWN) Ontario
P.O. Box 781, Station B
Sudbury, Ontario P3E 4S1
(705) 671-0825
web site: www3.sympatico.ca/odell/dawnpage.htm
A brochure on pregnancy and disability

Mother-to-Be: A Guide to Pregnancy and Birth for Women with Disabilities
by Judi Rogers and Molleen Matsumura
New York: Demos Publications, 1991
386 Park Ave. S. Ste. 201
New York, NY 10016

Parenting: An Accent Guide
Accent Special Publications
Cheever Publishing Inc., P.O. Box 700
Bloomington, IL 61702
Tips from parents (who happen to have a disability) on raising children.

The Baby Challenge: On Pregnancy for Women with a Physical Disability
by Mukti Jain Campion
New York: Tavistock/Routledge, 1990
Helpful information about how specific disabilities relate to pregnancy.

The Maternity Alliance
15 Britannia Street
London, WC1X9JP England

Through the Looking Glass
2198 Sixth St. # 100
Berkeley, California 94707
(510) 848-1112 and fax (510) 848-4445
e-mail: TLG@lookingglass.org
web site: www.lookingglass.org
A national research and training centre for families of adults with disabilities.
Publishes a newsletter.

Professionalizing Canadian Midwifery:
Sociological Perspectives

Cecilia Benoit

INTRODUCTION

Since the 1970s, midwives across Canada have established independent midwifery practices, forged loyal clientele, launched their own professional associations, established formal programs for training midwives, designed standards for practice, and altered their original knowledge claims in an attempt to gain legitimacy in the larger society. One clear indication of their success in the latter has been state legislation legitimizing midwifery services in Ontario, British Columbia, and Alberta, with many other provinces likely to follow suit in the near future. Another source of formal legitimation has been the four-year Baccalaureate Programme in direct-entry midwifery. Then, the Ministry of Health in Ontario agreed to fund an interim central agency, the Lebel Midwifery Care Organization (LMCO), governed by a voluntary board of directors, to manage the first midwifery programs in the province; midwives' salaries and expenses under the current funding scheme are fully-funded, thereby changing midwifery services from a consumer item to a public health service.[1]

These various trends in the Canadian midwifery movement, which are broadly captured by the sociological concept of 'professionalization,' have not been endorsed by midwives and clients without controversy. Internal conflict surrounding professionalization is not unique to midwifery nor peculiar to Canada. Sociologists in both the U.S. and Britain have made similar observations when studying other 'alternative occupations,' including chiropractors,[2] homoeopaths,[3] naturopaths,[4] and acupuncturists.[5] Sociologist Everett Hughes[6] some decades ago described the inner strain of Anglo-American professions in transition:

> The practitioners of many occupations — some new, some old — are self-consciously attempting to achieve recognition as professionals.... At first, the people who are recruited to the occupation come, of necessity, from other occupations. If they are women, many of them may have had no previous gainful occupation.

They will be of various social backgrounds, ages, and kinds of education. Some are more amateur than professional. In time, the question of training arises.... The development continues in the direction of standard terms of study, academic degrees.... These developments inevitably bring a campaign to separate the sheep from the goats, to set up categories of truly professional and less-than-professional people.

Advocates of the professionalization of midwifery in Canada, like their counterparts in other alternative healing arts, are apt to present a rather positive picture of their emerging profession, based upon a distinct body of midwifery knowledge, a quality training program, well-stated standards of practice, and dedication to clients. In Ontario, where the professionalization process is well underway, those in support of this development promise to also increase access to midwifery services for hitherto excluded groups of pregnant women. As Vicki Van Wagner[7] states:

> One of the main motivations to seek legislation came from the desire to make midwifery care accessible to a larger and more diverse group of women. The group of women served by midwives working outside the system tends to be white, middle-class and well-educated. In Ontario this stemmed from two problems: the lack of public funding for midwifery care and the lack of legal status and therefore credibility.... This meant that, for the most part, groups of women who often face barriers in accessing health care, such as immigrant women, native women and teens, did not have access to midwifery care.... To avoid regulation began to seem to many midwifery activists a form of elitism.

Some midwives and clients, however, disagree that professionalization will provide greater access to midwifery services.[8] They express fears shared with the North American consumer health advocates in general.[9] These include worry of midwives' co-optation by medicine, bureaucratization of reproductive services, emergence of a professional ideology of practice separating the midwife from those she serves, and lost of continuity of care.[10] In light of these threats, a more viable alternative is an independent source of legitimacy, outside of state institutions: "[t]hat is, they base their boundary claims on factors other than their relationship with the medical profession: a particular style of practice, commitment to family-centered or woman-centered birth, emphasis on personal responsibility for health, and safety of home birth."[11] Margaret Reid[12] understands the debate as one between "sisterhood" versus "professionalism":

> Sisterhood and professionalism are very different doctrines, stemming from different worlds and relating symbolically to different genders. The challenge that faces lay midwives is one familiar to those working within the radical feminist movement. Can midwives set up and achieve an alternative woman-centered occupation that lies outside the traditional sphere of professional

groups but is accepted by them and has access to professional resources and rewards? Or, in order to achieve those rewards, do midwives have to conform to the demands of (and be dominated by) professional authorities?

Jutta Mason[13] states the tension over midwives' professionalization in another way: "Whether legalization will give the midwife the security she needs to develop into a truly alternative worker or whether, instead, continued compromises with the obstetric establishment will turn her into the Trojan Horse of the alternative birth culture, remains to be seen."

This chapter has three main purposes: first, I discuss some of the main points of friction in the Canadian midwifery debate over professionalization. My aim here is to uncover the two models of midwifery that underlay the Canadian debate; secondly, I present a third model of midwifery found today in present-day Sweden; thirdly, I outline the main sociological theories of the service professions that offer conceptual tools for understanding the situation of women health professionals in the late 20th century. But first a brief sketch of my data and methods.

DATA & METHODS

This chapter draws on previous primary research I carried out in Newfoundland and Labrador (1989, 1991),[14] secondary research on Canadian and cross-national midwifery care arrangements (1992),[15] work on Aboriginal midwifery in British Columbia (1995),[16] and a recent two-country comparative study, "Envisioning Quality Reproductive Care: Stakeholders' Views in Canada and Sweden" (1996).[17] The first stage of the project (1993-94) was taken up with data collection from a variety of sources on the reproductive care system in Canada, including national and provincial government documents, academic publications, site observations, and semi-structured interviews with caregivers in British Columbia. The second stage of the project (1994-95) involved informal interviews in four additional Canadian provinces, and execution of a parallel study on the Swedish reproductive care system (January-May 1995). Site visits in three different Swedish counties, and semi-structured interviews with an assortment of stakeholders were conducted. Swedish government documents and related materials from research institutes were also collected, and informal interviews with academics and researchers carried out. All taped interviews have been transcribed and coded, and a number of academic papers are in the process of comparing the reproductive care systems of the two countries. Only a small portion of the data is considered here.

DEBATING MIDWIVES' PROFESSIONALIZATION

Close observation of the midwifery debate over professionalization in Canada indicates discord on a number of key issues. Here I will outline only three of the lines of disagreement: midwife's training, regulation of practice, and organization of work.

Becoming a midwife in Canada in the past few decades has involved a number of options: travel abroad to acquire foreign credentials, self-study, correspondence courses, apprenticeship with other midwives or a sympathetic physician, or simply 'learning by doing.' Apprenticeship with an experienced midwife proved to be especially attractive. Eleanor Barrington[18] notes, "As more of the practising midwives developed a comprehensive base of experience, apprenticeship became the increasingly popular route to training. It adapted to the needs of the community and the circumstances of the aspiring midwife."

Advocates of the recent academization of midwifery training point to some important limitations of the informal apprenticeship model, however:

> Ontario midwives hope that a government-funded education programme will address some of the weaknesses identified with apprenticeship. These include lack of any of the financial support usually available to students, lack of a peer group to facilitate academic learning and in some cases, lack of a structured curriculum. A recognized educational programme allows midwifery students exposure to the health care system and opportunities to work as colleagues with physicians and nurses, in a way that is not possible if midwives are outsiders.[19]

Advocates of the apprenticeship style of training rejoin by pointing to hidden dangers underlying formal academic education. On this point, Mary Neilans[20] writes:

> The standardization of formal training for midwives would mean that all currently practising midwives would have to prove themselves, often going back to school for several years.... The approved schools, as well as meetings of any governing councils, would require attendance in large urban centres, most likely in Toronto. This would be difficult for many midwives, particularly those in rural areas. Yet, if the midwifery degree were not attained and other routes of entry are deemed unacceptable, the midwife would risk criminal charges by continuing to practice as usual.... If the rural midwife is threatened, the women who need midwives most may lose them.

Regarding the second issue of contention — regulation of practice — advocates of the recent professionalization consider the best way forward is to institute a self-regulated College, analogous to the Canadian College of Physicians and Surgeons, with midwives themselves determining guidelines for safe practice and dealing with matters of discipline and potential malpractice.[21]

Not all Canadian midwives favour self-regulation under the control of an independent College of Midwives, however. Opponents focus on the likelihood of a 'new monopoly' emerging around pregnancy and childbirth, with but another 'professional stranger' deciding for pregnant women if they are 'at risk.' Opponents also fear a loss of continuity of care of the kind they now enjoy by virtue of having the choice of befriending a midwife who, in the woman's personal opinion, demonstrates the desired caring attitude and trust in the woman's own power to give birth to her baby:

> Part of our struggle has been to recognize that our support as women and as mothers, not particularly as experts, can help women in pregnancy and labour. [When I had my child], I didn't evaluate midwifery services — I found Mary, the woman who was willing to sit with me during the birth, through the advice of a trusted friend. No carefully-laid plans, no self-direction or prior information could have orchestrated this gift of strength and union.[22]

Finally, discord is observable regarding organization of midwifery practice. Proponents of the professionalization of Canadian midwifery maintain that there is an urgent need to improve the working conditions of midwives across the country. Many midwives in independent practice outside of Ontario live below the poverty line, while others support their 'midwifery habit' with a second or third part-time job in order to make ends meet. Independent midwives also tend to have little or no control over their timetables (around-the-clock, on-call duty is the norm), no work benefits, and inadequate medical backup; they are under continuous threat of being charged with criminal negligence. A secure income and improved working conditions are far more likely to occur with professionalization. At the same time, they contend, small autonomous midwifery group practices, combined with woman-centred framework of practice, focus on client choice of birthplace, and continuity of care by a like-minded team, would allow midwives to continue to follow the midwifery model of care. Without such change in working conditions, individual and occupational survival would be unlikely:

> Many midwives set out to become midwives and change their minds. The romantic allure of birthwork is rapidly offset by the exhausting hours and the emotional demands.... The midwife's personal and professional lives are more intertwined than most, with no time of day reserved for herself or her family. Clients' personal crises and unpredictable timed labours intrude on a 24-hour basis. Each woman [midwife] either copes with this or retires according to the limits of her stamina and her support systems.[23]

Yet midwives and clients opposing professionalization point to several drawbacks to the new forms of practice arrangements resulting from incorporation. They express particular concern about the development of mandatory professional standards of practice, negotiation for hospital attending privileges, and the funding arrangement for payment of services rendered. These changes mean, among other things, that midwives no longer practice according to what clients need and want; midwives must now also follow professional standards and hospital policies. Some feel that there is a exacting price to pay for guaranteed salary and widened scope of practice:

> Will there be a price to pay for that salary? Becoming an employee of the government legitimizes an expectation that midwives will work within the medical model... An emphasis on the medical model and its technologies may result in the deskilling of midwives, with a loss of traditional midwifery skills and knowledge.[24]

The Canadian midwifery debate over professionalization is ongoing. At this point I would like to put forward what I see as two distinct ideal-type models of midwife that are being contested and which find support in the second-wave feminist movements: the model of *lay attendant*, elements of which have been advocated by radical feminists;[25] the model of *autonomous professional*, which falls loosely within a liberal feminist framework.[26] Recent challenges by third-wave feminists have attempted to advance feminist theorizing on the diversity among women. Third-wave feminists have argued that second-wave feminist theories and their respective models of midwife and client tend to be constructed on the very real repressions of white, middle-class women who have been denied choice of provider and place of birth. Third-wave feminists note, however, that the struggles of second-wave feminists may not match the needs and concerns of women on the margins of Canadian society — rural women, visible minorities, Aboriginal women, teen mothers, poor women, women in nontraditional family arrangements.[27] If midwifery is to help meet the reproductive concerns of women from all parts of Canadian society, it must pay close attention to the multiple and integrated nature of the oppressions of race, class and gender.[28] Suggested here is the development of reproductive care arrangements that are founded on principles of equity, quality, and choice for clients, but which at the same time allow for diversity of backgrounds and family situations of midwives as workers.

Reproductive care arrangements in the Nordic countries offer interesting case examples in this regard.[29] Sweden in particular stands out in regard to its comprehensive model of reproductive care which attempts to strike a balance between the health concerns of Swedish women for quality reproductive care in their own communities, and the needs and interests of midwives as workers. The Swedish model of midwife approximates that of a *state professional*: midwives are public employees who work in public institutions (midwife centres, youth clinics, maternity wards, well-woman clinics) as frontline health workers taking care of most reproductive care concerns. This third model of midwifery finds tactical support from women's social mobilization referred to in Nordic countries as "state feminism," an umbrella term for a cluster of feminist groups and women's organizations joined together to solve social and economic problems that hinder gender equality.[30] State feminism diverges from second-wave feminism in key ways, particularly regarding the latter's largely negative views of the welfare state — as mainly serving the functions of the patriarchy and/or capitalism.[31] State feminists maintain that the overall evaluation of welfare states regarding health and social services for women as clients, as well as women's situation as professional workers, varies significantly across countries. The result is an open attitude towards the welfare state, especially in the Nordic countries where social democratic combined with grassroots feminism helps to create a more "woman-friendly" state.[32] What is needed, then, is close examination of particular social policies and worker models so that the benefits incurred are maximized for all involved, rather than promotion of the interests of some privileged actors over those on the margins of society. In brief, as Drude Dahlerup[33] states:

> Not all kinds of state intervention will improve women's position — far from that, as feminist theory of the state has shown. But from a [state] feminist perspective, certain types of intervention seem necessary.

State intervention in Sweden can be seen as advancing gender equality in many respects. The country has a long tradition in placing social and health concerns of citizens, including maternity care and women's other reproductive concerns, high on the national agenda. Public attention to structural variables of social class, geographical location, gender and parental statuses was given early on in the Swedish public debate about how to promote 'equality for all.' More recently, the disadvantaged circumstances of immigrant and refugee populations have been discussed and policies put forward to remedy their situation. It bears reminding in this regard that, as Christer Lundh and Rolf Ohlsson[34] point out, there are today "1.4 million people of foreign origin in Sweden. This means that Sweden is one of the most heavily immigrant-populated countries of Europe." At the same time, according to Kajsa Sundstrom-Feigenberg[35]

> Immigrants have access to the same public service as the Swedish population. They also participate to the same extent in antenatal care.... The favourable development of maternal and child health in connection with pregnancy and delivery in recent decades has to do with socioeconomic circumstances in Sweden — a relatively high and uniformly distributed standard of living and a generally high educational level.

Central to the public services available to Swedish people are reproductive care services organized by midwives. It is worth noting that the wide mandate to practice that Swedish midwives enjoy at present is legitimized by the state. Swedish midwives not only care for all pregnant women without medical complications, but they also impart information and advice on sexual matters and family planning, and perform an array of well-woman gynaecological services.[36] These include prescribing birth control pills, fitting diaphragms and IUDs, conducting pap smears and so forth— in fact, activities that are deemed 'medical events' in Canada and considered to be exclusively 'doctor's work.' Swedish physicians, by contrast, have a consultant role in reproductive care, checking the pregnant woman for signs of abnormality, and otherwise leaving the midwife to handle things.[37]

In brief, the organization of health and reproductive services within the Swedish state is far less patriarchal than what remains to a large extent the case in Canada. At the same time, the interests of women workers have received close attention in Swedish society, promoted by a variety of women's groups attempting to find realistic solutions to women's double work burden. The result has been the development of important social rights for women workers, including flexible work schedules, parental leaves, subsidized childcare, sick leaves, and pension benefits. What this means is that midwives can be both paid workers and mothers themselves, that they can have an opportunity to be both a 'caring' midwife and a 'caring' mother — an achievement, I would contend, that is far more difficult to realize for Canadian midwives, whether lay attendant or autonomous professional. Support for my position can be found in the sociological literature on the service professions, to which I now turn.

SOCIOLOGICAL PERSPECTIVES ON PROFESSIONALIZATION

Reflecting views of the public at large, North American sociologists have long been divided about the merit of service professions in meeting the needs of the public. The early schools of thought on the topic in Anglo-American sociology have followed two lines. One line of inquiry searches for specific *traits* that distinguished professions from other occupations; the other line of investigation involves analysis of the *functions* of the professions in the larger society.[38] The main purpose of either view is to establish the *diffentia specifica*, that is, the special attributes that distinguished the professions from other occupations.

Both the trait and functionalist approaches delineate professional workers in a largely praiseworthy light, demonstrating dedication to clients, and willingness to place the needs of those they serve above any personal desire for economic gain and societal prestige.[39]

Other scholars following in the tradition of sociologist Max Weber have gone to great length to challenge this laudable depiction of service professions. Much to the contrary of the trait and functionalist perspectives, neo-Weberian writers assert that professionals place the needs of clients far below the professionals' own yearnings for exclusive monopoly and professional powers.[40] Everett Hughes[41] put it this way:

Professions...claim a legal, moral and intellectual mandate. Not merely do the practitioners, by virtue of gaining admission to the charmed circle of colleagues, individually exercise the license to do things others do not do, but collectively they presume to tell society what is good and right for the individual and for society at large in some aspect of life. Indeed, they set the very terms in which people may think about this aspect of life. The medical profession, for instance, is not content merely to define the terms of medical practice. It also tries to define for all of us the very nature of health and disease.

According to this view, professionals and those they serve become increasingly separated into two communities: 1) professionals oriented towards technical achievements and ideals endorsed by their professional association; 2) consumers, dependent upon the professionals for major services, but short-changed in the process. The result has been the emergence of the "accountability movement": "[t]he public is asking whose interest the professionals are serving and who is benefiting most from those services — the professional or the client."[42]

Neo-Marxist scholars have entered into this debate about the capacity of service professions to benefit society, offering yet another perspective on the service professions. The argument here is that, like the public at large, service professionals are affected by cycles in the world capitalist system.[43] With the expansion of private healthcare services both North and South, professional workers are losing control to the corporate elite. The result is, on the one hand, polarization of health services in many countries between those who can pay for elite private health care and those who cannot, and at the same time, increasing power of owners of capital to dictate to managers and professionals how to organize their work to further corporate interests in profit realization above all else. Professionals, from this view, are internally divided, their circumstance dependent upon their market location. Sometimes professionals hold middle-class standing, practising relative work autonomy, opportunity to use their knowledge, and set the terms of their work; in other work situations professional workers become "deprofessionalized" or even "proletarianized."[44]

Feminist scholars have enlivened this theoretical debate concerning the situation of the service professions in society by placing the concept of gender at centre stage. Feminist scholars argue that until recently, theories of the professions have been gender blind and androcentric.[45] The perspectives outlined above give the reader the understanding of workers, including those claiming the professional label, of being male actors only. Once gender is brought to the foreground and investigated, then it becomes evident that men have sought to exclude women from a wide assortment of jobs and occupations, perhaps above all else, from entry into the service professions. Nevertheless, in the past few decades, women in Anglo-America and elsewhere have increasingly entered the paid workforce, and are found today among a variety of types of paid work, including the older professions, with law, clergy, medicine, and the academy as cases in point. These recent developments encourage a rethinking of existing conceptualizations of the medical and other service professions in Canada and elsewhere,[46] while at the same time keeping in mind that, at the larger societal level, women the world over have and continue to work for exploitative wages or for no monetary compensation at all.

In brief, medicine has been a prototypic example of *patriarchal* exclusionary closure,[47] whereby surface and hidden discrimination has inhibited the opportunities of all but a few token women. It is only since the 1960s and the pressures generated by the second-wave women's movement, that better representation is enjoyed by women in the medical and other health professions. Yet evidence suggests that patriarchal strategies continue to keep women near the bottom of the profession's internal hierarchy. As Pat Armstrong and Hugh Armstrong[48] argue:

> [E]ven when women are admitted, they do not often share the power and the glory... Women are more likely to be found in the least powerful fields where their work least matches the professional ideal. Similarly, women physicians are more likely than men to work in community health clinics or in group practice where they have less individual control over their work than they would in solo practice.

It is recognized by feminist scholars that women physicians and other women health workers share a similar fate. Female nurses, who comprise about two-thirds of the present-day health labour force in most developed societies and approximately ninety percent worldwide,[49] stand out in this regard. While gains have been made in regard to academic programs for training nurses, for example, the general portrait of nursing remains a "semi-profession" under patriarchal control.[50]

Feminist scholars point out that midwives share with their female physician and nursing counterparts low occupational status. Inadequate care of birthing women has been one result. The foremost view of pregnancy and delivery in Anglo-America is that these are ultimately 'high-risk milestones' necessitating prompt medical intervention. The not unexpected outcome is neglect of the birthing mother's psycho-social and physical concerns.[51] Patriarchal control is especially deep-rooted in North America where obstetrics remains largely under control of a white-male elite of physicians and hospital administrators, alienating midwives from properly caring for pregnant women, and at the same time depriving the latter of 'voice' about the birth of their child.[52] Robbie Davis-Floyd[53] uses the "technocratic model" of the body to conceptualize childbirth in America today:

Under the technocratic model the female body is viewed as an abnormal, unpredictable and inherently defective machine. During pregnancy and birth, the unusual demands placed on the female body-machine render it constantly at risk of serious malfunction or total breakdown.

Many writers sharing this viewpoint argue that midwives should adopt the radical alternative to patriarchal-medical control, that is, reject the professionalization model altogether, and in its place revive earlier forms of knowledge acquisition through informal apprenticeship and practice in clients' homes, keeping a distance from the entrenched medical establishment. They call for, in brief, midwives' embracement of a "holistic model of birth" in which "Self and Body are One, where Nature is best, and can be trusted, where intuition and inner knowledge are authoritative."[54]

Feminist scholars, however, do not all agree on this depiction of patriarchal dominance of female healers and the strategy of renunciation. Ann Witz[55] has recently engendered the Neo-Weberian approach mentioned above, to argue for a different perspective on female health professions. Witz suggests[56] that patriarchal control is maintained by denying women access to economically productive resources, but that women are not faceless and powerless, mere dupes of men, with the only viable path for them to exit from formal institutions altogether. Witz[57] notes that women employ "female professional strategies" in an attempt to be "mistresses of their own fates, rather than fatefully acquiescing to the role of handmaiden of male professionals." In examining the history of women health professionals in early 20th-century Britain, Witz describes how midwives developed their own "female professional project" which involved upgrading their credentials and campaigning to expand their mandate of practice, thereby challenging the patriarchal authority of medicine.

As mentioned earlier in this chapter, the radical and liberal feminist perspectives on midwives' professionalization have recently been challenged by third-wave feminists, who contest the very notion of the "grand narrative" of patriarchy. As Michele Barrett recently stated:[58]

Contemporary Western feminism, confident for several years about its 'sex-gender' distinction; analyses of 'patriarchy', or postulation of 'the male gaze' has found all these various categories radically undermined by the new 'deconstructive' emphasis on fluidity and contingency.

The conceptual turning point that feminists now face has caused anxiety for many of them, who increasingly find themselves faced with a range of uncertainties.[59] As bell hooks[60] puts it, "The overall impact of postmodernism is that many other groups now share with black folks a sense of deep alienation, despair, uncertainty, loss of a sense of grounding even if it is not informed by shared circumstances."

While acknowledging the uncertain circumstances at hand, Vijay Agnew[61] nevertheless views the recent turn in the feminist debate in Anglo-America as both positive and constructive:

> It has encouraged feminists to reconsider some of their initial rallying cries — for example, 'sisterhood,' 'the personal as political,' 'common oppressions,' 'men as the enemy,' and 'women as victims.' Feminists now see the need to question assumptions encoded in terms such as 'we' and 'woman,' which have tended to refer only to white, middle-class women. They see the need to re-examine the experiences from which their theories are derived and the practices that their theories recommend rather than to claim that their theories are unbiased, neutral, or universally applicable to all women.

The result has been an opening up of mainstream feminist associations to women of much more diverse backgrounds — First Nations, Asian, African, and Caribbean origin among them — than has hitherto been the case in Canada. At the same time, First Nations women, rural and minority women have launched their own community-based organizations. Despite notable limitations, these "services have empowered non-English speaking, working-class women to challenge the oppressions of race, class and gender biases."[62]

As I see it, the writings of Nordic feminists mentioned earlier also challenge second-wave feminist thought on 'the patriarchy,' arguing instead for a more open-minded perspective on the polity of capitalist societies, one that is based on empirical studies of actual state policies.[63] Harriet Silius[64] makes this point in a slightly different manner by calling for a new conception of power, one that portrays power as more nuanced and complicated than many writers on the service professions, second-wave feminists included, have hitherto conceived: "One possibility is to conceptualize power as *empowerment*, which focuses on *agency* and *resources*." The different processes embedded in the extension of welfare states in particular societies, Silius argues, have also empowered women in the public sphere. Nordic feminist scholars have successfully challenged the depiction of Anglo-American professions as the only type of professional service model, that is, one of monopoly of expert knowledge by independent practitioners operating on an open market for services.[65] Viewed from this perspective, midwives employed in midwife centres and other state institutions do not measure up to being 'real' professionals at all. John Holmwood and Janet Siltanen call this constricted view of the service professions into question, exposing it as a culturally-specific position that ultimately prevents development of fresh conceptual understanding of women professionals at work in state institutions, where market principles and mechanisms of patriarchal exclusion are more successfully challenged than in the private market. Imperative to "greater feminization of the professions," according to Holmwood and Siltanen,[66] is "greater feminization of the state."

SUMMARY AND CONCLUSION

The Canadian midwifery debate finds some support in the feminist literature on professions outlined above, although no direct comparison between the two is intended here. Some Canadian midwives and their supporters advocate a radical stance; theirs is the outsiders' view, based on a model of the 'lay midwife attendant' who learns her craft in an informal manner, whose art is practised ideally in the homes of birthing women, and who performs midwifery work because she is foremost concerned with helping other women.[67]

However, while serving the interests of a small category of empowered birthing clients,[68] the shortcomings of independent midwifery as it has recently been organized in Canada are readily apparent. For midwives, these include lack of stable income, burn-out due to long and unpredictable time schedules, work stress from fear (sometimes reality) of court battles, low public esteem, and intense conflict. For birthing women, lack of access to midwifery services tops the list, especially for women on the margins of Canadian society who fall through the cracks of existing informal midwifery networks.[69]

Advocates of midwives' professionalization in Ontario, as we have seen, are well aware of these shortcomings and have chosen to promote a very different model of midwifery — that of autonomous professional. The 'new midwife' in this model, aspires for equal footing with other autonomous professionals in Canada. She belongs to a self-governing profession separate from medicine and nursing. Brian Burtch[70] outlines the attributes that Canadian midwives need to possess in order to gain distinction as a profession: "control over their work, a self-regulating body to establish standards of care and 'disciplinary' measures, legal protection, and specialized research and education forums."

At the point of writing, gains towards female professionalization by professionally-oriented midwives have already been made in many Canadian provinces. The question remains, however, whether this particular model of midwife as autonomous professional will in the end cultivate the kind of midwifery service individual midwives and those they serve are looking for: that is, one based on a holistic model of reproductive care that avoids the pitfalls of the existing allopathic medical model, based on notions of 'technique,' 'risk' and 'intervention.'[71] As Ann Oakley and Susanne Houd[72] remind us:

> It is widely assumed that what is wrong with midwifery today is that its professional status is not as high as it ought to be— not as high as that of medicine, for example. Thus, the argument goes, to regain a central place in the control of childbirth, midwives must fight for further professionalization, tighter controls over practice, more specialized knowledge, and so on. At first sight, this argument appears sound, but it is seriously flawed. The problem is that the

consequences of professionalization may run counter to the reasons for defending the profession in the first place. Midwives, in short, may become more like doctors instead of more like midwives.

It can also be questioned whether the autonomous professional model will be sensitive to the needs and interests of midwives as workers. There is a very real danger that this model of midwife, with its weighty demand on midwives' time and energy, will result in a situation not unlike what seems to be happening to midwifery in Britain:

> [It has become] a divided workforce consisting of an elite core and casualized periphery based on the ability to give a full-time flexible commitment to work.... Providing continuity of care requires a radical change in the way that many midwives work at the moment in terms of increased flexibility and the impact of regular on-call work on midwives' personal lives.[73]

I have drawn on my Swedish research to offer food for thought concerning how both midwives' career interests and birthing women's health concerns are addressed in a third prototype of midwife — state professional. The vast majority of Swedish midwives fit this model of practice, enjoying high esteem as women's primary care attendants across their reproductive lives. There are, however, important shortcomings to this model — missing aspects which many Canadian midwives have struggled long to achieve. For one thing, during the short-term time frame of pregnancy-postpartum, the Swedish woman does not receive care from only a single midwife. On the other hand, it can be argued that Swedish women receive continuity of 'philosophy of midwifery care' from the team of antenatal, labour and delivery and postpartum midwives that attend the women's many needs and those of the families. Swedish midwives, moreover, provide the entire female population continuity of care across their reproductive life cycles (long-term continuity of care).[74] It can also be argued that the Swedish model of midwifery as state professional has no room for homebirth practice, which has had a major influence on the two models of midwifery discussed in reference to Canadian midwifery. It is worth noting, however, that home birth is neither illegal in Sweden nor popular with all but a small group of Swedish women; they seem less concerned about the actual place of birth than with early discharge from hospital, help with breastfeeding, parenting advice and the like.

Attacks on the welfare state in Sweden and subsequent restructuring of healthcare services in pockets of the country lead me to end this chapter on a cautious note. Midwives express uncertainty regarding their future. Their struggle is largely one of maintaining their privileged position in reproductive care. Close observation should also be given to the restructuring of health and reproductive care services in each province in our own country. The challenge here at home is to design a truly equitable reproductive care system that provides quality of care to different groups of women clients, yet at the same time recognizes the double-work burden that many midwives face. Bottom-up consultation with women from diverse locations in society is fundamental to this developmental process. Knowledge of the strengths and weaknesses of comparative reproductive care systems may also contribute important insights regarding the way forward.

ENDNOTES

1. Ivy Bougeault, *Delivering Midwifery: An Examination of the Process and Outcome of the Incorporation of Midwifery in Ontario* (Ph.D. diss., Graduate Department of Community Medicine, University of Toronto, 1996).
2. Lesley Biggs, "The Profession of Chiropractic in Canada: Its Current Struggles and Future Prospects," in *Sociology of Health Care in Canada*, ed. B. Singh Bolaria and Harley Dickinson (Toronto: Harcourt Brace Jovanovich Canada, 1989).
3. Sarah Cant and Ursula Sharma, "Demarcation and Transformation with Homoeopathic Knowledge: Strategy of Professionalization," *Social Science & Medicine* vol. 42, no. 4 (1996): 579-88.
5. Mike Saks, ed., *Alternative Medicine in Britain* (Oxford: Clarendon Press, 1992).
6. Everett Hughes, *Men and Their Work* (New York: Free Press, 1958): 133-5.
7. Vicki Van Wagner, "Why Legislation? The Regulation of Midwifery in Ontario from a Feminist Perspective," paper delivered at the CSAA Meetings, University of Calgary, 1994: 10-12.
8. Susan James, "Regulation: Changing the Face of Midwifery?" paper delivered at the CSAA Meetings, University of Calgary, Alberta, 1994.
9. Michail Betz and Lenahan O'Connell, "Changing Doctor-Patient Relationships and the Rise of Concern for Accountability," *Social Problems* vol. 31 (1983): 84-95.
10. Raymond DeVries, "A Cross-national View of the Status of Midwives," in *Gender, Work and Medicine* ed. Elianne Riska and Katarine Wegar (London: Sage, 1993).
11. Beth Rushing, "Ideology in the Reemergence of North American Midwifery," *Work and Occupations* vol. 20, no. 1 (1993): 50-1.
12. Margaret Reid, "Sisterhood and Professionalization: A Case Study of the American Lay Midwife," in *Women as Healers* ed. C. McClain (Rutgers: The State University Press, 1989): 238.
13. Jutta Mason, "Midwifery in Canada," in *The Midwife Challenge*, ed. Sheila Kitzinger (London: Pandora, 1988): 126.
14. Cecilia Benoit, "The Professional Socialization of Midwives: Balancing Art and Science," *Sociology of Health & Illness* vol. 11, no. 2 (1989a): 160-180; Cecilia Benoit, "Traditional Midwifery Practice: The Limits of Occupational Autonomy," *The Canadian Review of Sociology and Anthropology* vol 26, no. 4 (1989b): 633-649; Cecilia Benoit, *Midwives in Passage: The Modernization of Maternity Care* (Memorial University of Newfoundland: ISER Books, 1991).
15. Cecilia Benoit, "Midwives in Comparative Perspective," *Current Research on Occupations and Professions* vol. 7 (1992).

16. Cecilia Benoit with Dena Carroll, "Aboriginal Midwifery in British Columbia: A Narrative Still Untold," *Western Geographic Series* vol. 30 (1995): 221-46.
17. Cecilia Benoit, "Midwives in Canada and Sweden: Identities and Practices in Comparative Perspective," paper delivered at the Biannual International Conference on Professions in Comparative Perspective, Onati International Institute for the Sociology of Law, Onati, Spain, April 25-26, 1996.
18. Eleanor Barrington, *Midwifery is Catching* (Toronto: NC Press Limited, 1985): 44-5.
19. Van Wagner, 22.
20. Mary Neilans, "Midwifery: From Recognition to Regulation: The Perils of Government Intervention," in *On Women Healthsharing* ed. Enakshi Dua, Maureen FitzGerald, Linda Gardner, Darien Taylor and Lisa Wyndels (Toronto: Women's Press, 1994): 120.
21. Brian Burtch, *Trials of Labour: The Re-emergence of Midwifery* (Montreal and Kingston: McGill Queen's University Press, 1994).
22. Neilans, 122.
23. Barrington, 50.
24. James, 4.
25. Adrienne Rich, *Of Woman Born* (London: Virago, 1970); Susan Griffin, *Women and Nature: The Roaring Inside Her* (New York: Harper and Row, 1980).
26. Sheila Kitzinger, *The Midwife Challenge* (London: Pandora Press, 1988); Anne Witz, *Professions and Patriarchy* (London: Routledge, 1992).
27. Vijay Agnew, *Revisiting Discrimination: Women from Asia, Africa and the Caribbean, and the Women's Movement in Canada* (Toronto: University of Toronto Press, 1996).
28. Christina Lee, "Not Quite a Refuge: Refugee Women in Canada," *Healthsharing* vol. 9, no. 3 (1988): 14-16; Benoit and Carroll (1995); Sheryl Nestle, "'Other' Mothers: Race and Representation in Natural Childbirth Discourse," *Resources for Feminist Research* vol 23, no. 4 (1995): 15-9.
29. Cecilia Benoit, "Reforming Health Care Systems in Canada and Elsewhere: Prospects for Efficiency and Equity of Quality Care," presented to the Faculty of Nursing, University of Alberta, April 8, 1997.
30. Nina Cecilie Raaum, "Women in Local Democracy," in *Women in Nordic Politics: Closing the Gap*, ed. Lauri Karvonen and Per Selle (Aldershot, USA: Darmouth, 1995).
31. Barbara Ehrenreich and Dierdre English, *Witches, Midwives and Nurses: A History of Women Healers* (Oyster Bay, NY: Glass Mountain Pamphlets, 1973).
32. Arnlaug Leira, *Welfare States and Working Mothers: The Scandinavian Experience* (New York: University of Cambridge Press, 1992).
33. Drude Dahlerup, "Learning to Live with the State," *Women's Studies International Forum* vol. 17, nos. 2/3 (1994): 124.
34. Christer Lundh and Rolf Ohlsson, "Immigration and Economic Change," in *Population, Economy, and Welfare in Sweden*, ed. Tommy Bengtsson (Berlin: Springer-Verlag, 1994): 87.
35. Kajsa Sundstrom-Feigenberg, "Reproductive Health and Reproductive Freedom: Maternity Health Care and Family Planning in the Swedish Health System," *Women and Health* (1988): 44. The author notes that the surprising *lower* perinatal mortality among children of foreign women found in research on the topic could not be attributed to the distributions of mothers by age and

parity nor to children's degree of maturity. However, it should be noted that immigrants are screened along lines of education, skill, economic standing and so forth.

36. Ibid.
37. Anders Hakansson, "Antenatal Care in General Practice in Sweden," *Scandinavian Journal of Primary Health Care* vol. 6, no. 3 (1988): 143-48.
38. Talcott Parsons, "Professions," *International Encyclopedia of the Social Sciences* (1968): 536-47.
39. Bernard Barber, "Some Problems in the Sociology of Professions," *Daedalus* 92 (1983): 669-88.
40. Ivan Illich, *Medical Nemesis* (London: Calder & Boyars, 1975); Elliott Freidson, *The Profession of Medicine: A Study in the Sociology of Applied Knowledge* (New York: Harper & Row, 1970); Frank Parkin, *Marxism and Class Theory: The Bourgeois Critique* (London: Tavistock, 1979).
41. Everett Hughes, *Men and their Work* (New York: Free Press, 1958): 79.
42. Betz and O'Connell, 84.
43. Vincent Navarro, *Health and Medicine: A Social Critique* (London: Tavistock, 1986).
44. John McKinlay and John Stoeckle, "Corporatization and the Social Transformation of Doctoring," *International Journal of Health Services* vol. 18 (1988): 191-205.
45. Rosemary Crompton, "Gender, Status and Professionalism," *Sociology* vol. 21 (1987): 413-28.
46. Elianne Riska and Katarina Wegar, eds., *Gender, Work and Medicine* (London: Sage, 1993).
47. Witz, 1992.
48. Pat Armstrong and Hugh Armstrong, "Sex and the Professions in Canada," *Journal of Canadian Studies* vol. 37, no. 1 (1992): 118-35.
49. Helene Pizurki, Alfonso Mejia, Irene Butter and Leslie Ewart, *Women as Providers of Health Care* (Geneva: World Health Organization, 1987).
50. Jane Salvage, *The Politics of Nursing* (London: Heinemann, 1985); Mick Carpenter, "The New Managerialism and Professionalism in Nursing," in *Health and the Division of Labour* ed. Meg Stacey (London: Croom Helm, 1977).
51. Deborah Sullivan and Rose Weitz, *Labour Pains: Modern Midwives and Home Birth* (New Haven: Yale University Press, 1988).
52. Adrienne Rich, "The Theft of Childbirth," *The New York Review of Books* vol. 22 (1975): 25-30; Suzanne Arms, *Immaculate Deception: A New Look at Women and Childbirth in America* (San Francisco: San Francisco Book Inc., 1975).
53. Robbie Davis-Floyd, "The Technocratic Body: American Childbirth as Cultural Expression," *Social Science & Medicine* vol. 38, no. 8 (1994): 1127.
54. Ibid., 1136.
55. Witz, 1992.
56. Witz, 1990.
57. Ibid., 668.
58. Michele Barrett, "Words and Things: Materialism and Method in Contemporary Feminist Analysis," in *Destabilizing Theory*, ed. Michele Barrett and A. Phillips (Cambridge: Polity Press, 1992).
59. Nicholas Fox, *Postmodernism, Sociology and Health* (Toronto: University of Toronto Press, 1994).

60. bell hooks, *Yearning: Race, Gender and Cultural Studies* (London: Turnaround, 1991): 27.
61. Agnew, 49.
62. Ibid., 228.
63. Drude Dahlerup, "Learning to Live with the State," *Women's Studies International Forum* vol. 17, nos. 2/3 (1994): 117-27; Arnlaug Leira, *Welfare States and Working Mothers: The Scandinavian Experience* (New York: University of Cambridge Press, 1992).
64. Hariett Silius, "Gendering the Theories of Professions," paper delivered at the ISA Conference, Regulating Expertise: Professionalism in Comparative Perspective, Paris, April 14-15, 1994.
65. John Holmwood and Janet Siltanen, "Gender, the Professions, and Employment Citizenship," *International Journal of Sociology* vol. 24, no. 4 (1994): 43-66.
66. Ibid., 56.
67. Davis-Floyd; Mason.
68. Raymond DeVries, *Regulating Birth: Midwives, Medicine, & the Law* (Philadelphia: Temple University Press, 1985); Sullivan and Weitz.
69. Benoit with Carroll.
70. Brian Burtch, *The Sociology of Law: Critical Approaches to Social Control* (Toronto: Harcourt Brace Jovanovich Canada, 1992): 164.
71. DeVries, 1993.
72. Ann Oakley and Suzanne Houd, *Helpers in Childbirth: Midwifery Today* (Geneva: World Health Organization, 1990): 164.
73. Jane Sandall, "Choice, Continuity and Control: Changing Midwifery, Towards a Sociological Perspective," *Midwifery* vol. 11 (1995): 205.
74. Rudy Ray Seward, Jean Ann Seward and Vera Natoli, "Different Approaches to Childbirth and Their Consequences in Italy, Sweden and the United States," *International Journal of the Family* vol. 14 (1984): 1-16.

REFERENCES

Agnew, Vijay. *Resisting Discrimination: Women from Asia, Africa, and the Caribbean and the Women's Movement in Canada.* Toronto: University of Toronto Press, 1996.
Arms, Suzanne. *Immaculate Deception: A New Look at Women and Childbirth in America.* San Francisco: San Francisco Book Inc., 1975.
Armstrong, Pat, and Hugh Armstrong. "Sex and the Professions in Canada." *Journal of Canadian Studies,* vol 37, no. 1 (1992): 118-35.
Barber, Bernard. "Some Problems in the Sociology of Professions." *Daedalus* 92 (1983): 669-88.
Barrett, Michele. "Words and Things: Materialism and Method in Contemporary Feminist Analysis." In *Destabilizing Theory.* Michele Barrett & A. Phillips, eds. Cambridge: Polity Press, 1992.
Barrett, Michele, and A. Phillips, eds. *Destabilizing Theory.* Cambridge: Polity Press, 1992.
Barrington, Eleanor. *Midwifery is Catching.* Toronto: NC Press Limited, 1985.
Benoit, Cecilia. "Uneasy Partners: Midwives and Their Clients," *Canadian Journal of Sociology,* vol. 12, no. 3 (1987): 275-284.
-----. "The Professional Socialization of Midwives: Balancing Art and Science," *Sociology of Health & Illness,* vol. 11, no. 2 (1989a) : 160-180.

-----. "Traditional Midwifery Practice: The Limits of Occupational Autonomy," *The Canadian Review of Sociology and Anthropology*, vol 26, no. 4 (1989b): 633-649.

-----. *Midwives in Passage: The Modernization of Maternity Care.* Memorial University of Newfoundland: ISER Books, 1991.

-----. "Midwives in Comparative Perspective." *Current Research on Occupations and Professions*, vol. 7 (1992).

-----. "Paradigm Conflict in the Sociology of the Professions." *Canadian Journal of Sociology* vol. 19, no. 3 (1994): 303-329.

-----. "Aboriginal Midwifery in British Columbia: A Narrative Still Untold." *Western Geographic Series*, vol. 30 (1995): 221-46 (with Dena Carroll).

-----. "Midwives in Canada and Sweden: Identities and Practices in Comparative Perspective." Paper presented at *Biannual International Conference on Professions in Comparative Perspective*. Onati International Institute for the Sociology of Law, Onati, Spain, April 25-26, 1996.

-----. "Reforming Health Care Systems in Canada and Elsewhere: Prospects for Efficiency and Equity of Quality Care." Invited paper presented to the Faculty of Nursing, University of Alberta, April 8, 1997.

Betz, Michael, and Lenahan O'Connell. "Changing Doctor-Patient Relationships and the Rise of Concern for Accountability." *Social Problems*, vol. 31 (1983): 84-95.

Biggs, Lesley. "The Profession of Chiropractic In Canada: Its Current Struggles and Future Prospects." In *Sociology of Health Care in Canada*. B. Singh Bolaria and Harley Dickinson, eds. Toronto: Harcourt Brace Jovanovich Canada, 1989.

Bougeault, Ivy. *Delivering Midwifery: An Examination of the Process and Outcome of the Incorporation of Midwifery in Ontario*. Ph.D. Thesis, Graduate Department of Community Medicine, University of Toronto, 1996.

Burtch, Brian. *The Sociology of Law: Critical Approaches to Social Control.* Toronto: Harcourt Brace Jovanovich Canada, 1992.

-----. *Trials of Labour: The Re-emergence of Midwifery*. Montreal & Kingston: McGill Queen's University Press, 1994.

Butter, Irene, Eugenia Carpenter, Bonnie Kay and Ruth Simmons. "Gender Hierarchies in the Health Labour Force." *International Journal of Health Services*, vol. 17, no. 1 (1987): 133-49.

Cant, Sarah, and Ursula Sharma. "Demarcation and Transformation with Homoeopathic Knowledge: Strategy of Professionalization." *Social Science & Medicine*, vol. 42, no. 4 (1996): 579-88.

Carpenter, Mick. "The New Managerialism and Professionalism in Nursing." In *Health and the Division of Labour*. Meg Stacey, ed. London: Croom Helm, 1977.

Clarke, Juanne. *Health, Illness, and Medicine in Canada*. Second Edition. Toronto: Oxford University Press, 1996.

Crompton, Rosemary. "Gender, Status and Professionalism." *Sociology*, vol. 21 (1987): 413-28.

Dahlerup, Drude. "Learning to Live with the State." *Women's Studies International Forum*, vol. 17, nos. 2/3 (1994): 117-27.

Daly, Mary. *Pure Lust, Elemental Feminist Philosophy*. London: Women's Press, 1984.

Davis-Floyd, Robbie. "The Technocratic Body: American Childbirth as Cultural Expression." *Social Science & Medicine*, vol. 38, no. 8 (1994): 1125-40.

DeVries, Raymond. *Regulating Birth: Midwives, Medicine, & the Law.* Philadelphia: Temple University Press, 1985.

-----. "A Cross-national View of the Status of Midwives." In *Gender, Work and Medicine.* Elianne Riska and Katarine Wegar, eds. London: Sage, 1993.

Diderichsen, Finn. "Health and Social Inequities in Sweden." *Social Science and Medicine,* vol. 31, no. 3 (1990): 359-67.

Doyal, Lesley. "The Politics of Women's Health: Setting A Global Agenda." *International Journal of Health Services,* vol. 26, no. 1 (1996): 47-65.

Ehrenreich, Barbara, and Dierdre English. *Witches, Midwives and Nurses: A History of Women Healers.* Oyster Bay, NY: Glass Mountain Pamphlets, 1973.

Esping-Anderson, Gosta. *The Three Worlds of Welfare Capitalism.* Princeton: Princeton University Press, 1990.

Fox, Nicholas. *Postmodernism, Sociology and Health.* Toronto: University of Toronto Press, 1994.

Freidson, Elliott. *The Profession of Medicine: A Study in the Sociology of Applied Knowledge.* New York: Harper and Row, 1970.

Griffin, Susan. *Women and Nature: The Roaring Inside Her.* New York: Harper and Row, 1980.

Hakansson, Anders. "Antenatal Care in General Practice in Sweden." *Scandinavian Journal of Primary Health Care,* vol. 6, no. 3 (1988): 143-48.

Holmwood, John, and Janet Siltanen. "Gender, the Professions, and Employment Citizenship." *International Journal of Sociology,* vol. 24, no. 4 (1994): 43-66.

hooks, bell. *Yearning: Race, Gender and Cultural Studies.* London: Turnaround, 1991.

Hughes, Everett. *Men and Their Work.* New York: Free Press, 1958.

Illich, Ivan. *Medical Nemesis.* London: Calder & Boyars, 1975.

James, Susan. "Regulation: Changing the Face of Midwifery?" Paper presented at the CSAA Meetings, University of Calgary, Alberta, 1994.

Jonung, Christina, and Inga Persson. "Combining Market Work and Family." In *Population, Economy, and Welfare in Sweden.* Tommy Bengtsson, ed. Berlin: Springer-Verlag, 1994.

Jordan, Brigette. *Birth in Four Cultures.* London: Eden Press, 1983.

Katz-Rothman, Barbara. *In Labour: Women and Power in the Birthplace.* New York: W.W. Norton and Company, 1982.

Kitzinger, Sheila. *The Midwife Challenge.* London: Pandora, 1988.

Lee, Christina. "Not Quite a Refuge: Refugee Women in Canada." *Healthsharing,* vol 9, no. 3 (1988): 14-16.

Leira, Arnlaug. *Welfare States and Working Mothers: The Scandinavian Experience.* New York: University of Cambridge Press, 1992.

Lundh, Christer, and Rolf Ohlsson. "Immigration and Economic Change." In *Population, Economy, and Welfare in Sweden.* Tommy Bengtsson, ed. Berlin: Springer-Verlag, 1994.

Mason, Jutta. "Midwifery in Canada." In *The Midwife Challenge.* Sheila Kitzinger, ed. London: Pandora, 1988.

McKay, Susan. "Models of Care: Denmark, Sweden, and the Netherlands." *Journal of Nurse-Midwifery,* vol. 38, no. 20 (1993): 114-20.

McKinlay, John, and John Stoeckle. "Corporatization and the Social Transformation of Doctoring." *International Journal of Health Services,* vol. 18 (1988): 191-205.

Navarro, Vincente. *Health and Medicine: A Social Critique.* London: Tavistock, 1976.

Neilans, Mary. "Midwifery: From Recognition to Regulation: The Perils of Government Intervention." In *On Women Healthsharing*. Enakshi Dua, Maureen FitzGerald, Linda Gardner, Darien Taylor and Lisa Wyndels, eds. Toronto: Women's Press, 1994.

Nestle, Sheryl. "'Other' Mothers: Race and Representation in Natural Childbirth Discourse." *Resources for Feminist Research*, vol. 23, no. 4 (1995): 5-19.

Oakley, Ann, and Suzanne Houd. *Helpers in Childbirth: Midwifery Today*. WHO: Hemisphere, 1990.

Olsen, Gregg. "Locating the Canadian Welfare State: Family Policy and Health Care in Canada, Sweden, and the United States." *Canadian Journal of Sociology*, vol. 19, no. 1 (1994): 1-20.

Parkin, Frank. *Marxism and Class Theory: The Bourgeois Critique*. London: Tavistock, 1979.

Parsons, Talcott. "Professions." *International Encyclopedia of the Social Sciences* (1968): 536-47.

Pizurki, Helene, Alfonso Mejia, Irene Butter and Leslie Ewart. *Women as Providers of Health Care*. Geneva: World Health Organization, 1987.

Raaum, Nina Cecilie. "Women in Local Democracy." In *Women in Nordic Politics: Closing the Gap*. Lauri Karvonen and Per Selle, eds. Aldershot, USA: Darmouth, 1995.

Reid, Margaret. "Sisterhood and Professionalization: A Case Study of the American Lay Midwife." In *Women as Healers*. C. McClain, ed. Rutgers: The State University Press, 1989.

Rich, Adrienne. *Of Woman Born*. London: Virago, 1970.

-----. "The Theft of Childbirth," *The New York Review of Books*, vol. 22 (1975): 25-30.

Riska, Elianne, and Katarina Wegar, eds. *Gender, Work and Medicine*. London: Sage, 1993.

Rushing, Beth. "Ideology in the Reemergence of North American Midwifery." *Work and Occupations*, vol. 20, no. 1 (1993): 46-67.

Saks, Mike, ed. *Alternative Medicine in Britain*. Oxford: Clarendon Press, 1992.

Saltman, Richard. "Competition and Reform in the Swedish Health System." *The Milbank Quarterly*, vol. 68, no 4 (1992): 597-618.

Saltman, Richard, and Casten von Otter. *Planned Markets and Public Competition: Strategic Reformin Northern European Health Systems*. London: Open University Press, 1992.

Sandall, Jane. "Choice, Continuity and Control: Changing Midwifery, Towards a Sociological Perspective." *Midwifery* , vol. 11 (1995): 201-9.

Salvage, Jane. *The Politics of Nursing*. London: Heinemann, 1985.

Seward, Rudy Ray, Jean Ann Seward and Vera Natoli. "Different Approaches to Childbirth and Their Consequences in Italy, Sweden and the United States." *International Journal of the Family*, vol. 14 (1984): 1-16.

Silius, Hariett. "Gendering the Theories of Professions." Paper presented at the ISA Conference, *Regulating Expertise: Professionalism in Comparative Perspective*. Paris, April 14-15, 1994.

Sullivan, Deborah, and Rose Weitz. *Labour Pains: Modern Midwives and Home Birth*. New Haven: Yale University Press, 1988.

Sundstrom-Feigenberg, Kajsa. "Reproductive Health and Reproductive Freedom: Maternity Health Care and Family Planning in the Swedish Health System." *Women and Health* (1988): 35-55.

Van Wagner, Vicki. "Why Legislation? The Regulation of Midwifery in Ontario from a Feminist Perspective." Paper presented at the CSAA Meetings,

University of Calgary, 1994.Walby, Sylvia. *Theorizing Patriarchy*. Oxford: Basil Blackwell, 1990.

Witz, Anne. "Patriarchy and Professions: The Gendered Politics of Occupational Closure." *Sociology*, vol. 24, no 1 (1990): 675-90.

-----. *Professions and Patriarchy*. London: Routledge, 1992.

Midwives and Safe Motherhood:
International Perspectives

Carol Hird and Brian Burtch

INTRODUCTION

> How childbirth is managed has important implications for society as a whole; for its view of reproduction, for the position of women, for family relationships.[1]

It is estimated that at least half a million women die each year of childbirth-related causes. This means that over 1370 women die every day, one almost every minute. Most of these deaths are completely preventable.[2] Ninety-nine percent of these deaths are in the nations of the South. There is also extensive injury associated with many births in both developed and underdeveloped countries. Midwives can reverse these shameful figures, but only within a context of social, political, and economic change. In this essay, we look at causes of maternal deaths globally, and consider how Safe Motherhood Programs (SMPs) may be fostered locally through appropriate state support and regulation. We reconsider some concerns raised about state interference in women's reproductive choices, suggesting that state *involvement* in supporting women's rights and resources may reverse maternal deaths and increase women's status globally.

> The root causes of a woman's death can begin before her birth and are perpetuated during childhood and adolescence and continue later in her life. She generally has less access to food and education. Her childhood days are taken by the endless search for water, food and fuel. During adolescence, she is often subject to rejection, violence, prostitution, or early marriage.[3]

The health of women has a direct impact on *family* health. The number of children dying following the death of their mother is significant. Poor health as a result of childbearing thus affects the income, nutrition, and general well-being of women and their families.

Efforts to decrease maternal deaths have met with varying degrees of success. Reducing maternal deaths by 50 percent by the year 2000 will need " ...additional efforts regarding women's health, the care of pregnant women, and access to appropriate and adequate health services during pregnancy and delivery."[4] Each country has individual barriers to the implementation of Safe Motherhood Programs (SMPs). Leaders in health care admit "[we] have failed to exercise our full creative capacity and to commit our energies and resources to the health and development needs of women."[5]

The toll of lives lost during pregnancy, childbirth, and the postpartum period is well-documented in the medical literature. Ironically, maternal deaths are nearly invisible in feminist writing. Further, birth — and especially maternal deaths — is often ignored in accounts of discrimination against women. For example, the Human Rights Watch *Global Report*[6] says nothing about maternal deaths in its chapter on reproduction, sexuality, and human rights violations. This raises questions of alliances between western and third-world feminists in resisting medicalization of health, redefining women's needs, and empowering midwives and women globally.

What are often called 'developed' and 'underdeveloped' countries seem worlds apart in their experiences of maternal deaths. We use problematic terms such as 'developed' and 'underdeveloped' because these terms are often used by the midwives Carol surveyed, whose ideas we give voice to, and because the concept of underdevelopment through colonialism and capitalism is critical to understanding limited health care in much of the South. We recognize the ongoing debate about the appropriateness of these terms in various political and academic settings in North America, and use "the South" to refer to countries commonly referred to as 'underdeveloped.'

In Carol's survey, and in much of the literature on maternal mortality, poverty and inadequate health care are mentioned time and again. A midwife from Tanzania described a recent maternal death from haemorrhage: "The woman started bleeding after delivery in the village. She did not get transportation early. She managed to reach the hospital after two days of bleeding. Although blood transfusion was given the woman died after [a] few minutes in the hospital."

The maternal death described here is far less common in a developed country such as Canada. Yet there is common ground when we consider the status of women in Canada and other societies: their educational levels, access to health care, availability of contraception and abortion services, and exposure to violence. Specific concern is warranted for First Nations women, for example, and other women who are economically disadvantaged and who may be subject to racist treatment. Culhane-Speck[7] and Carol Reid,[8] among others, document patterns of increased health risks, and inferior, sometimes racist, health services for the First Nations in Canada. There is increasing awareness of how dominant medical approaches feed on cultural stereotypes and direct blame toward the First Nations in Canada[9] and the United States.[10]

In this essay, we trace how much of the maternal mortality literature reflects such a *medical* worldview. This means that social, economic, and political factors linked with globalization and underdevelopment are downplayed or absent, while the solution to maternal mortality is limited to an extension of the medical model to pregnancy and childbirth. This narrow focus draws attention away from the legacy of colonialism, and barriers to women's health, economic, political, and social status in underdeveloped countries.

We favour a *midwifery* model of care that goes beyond this medicalized approach to childbearing, and incorporates structural changes to the status of women. We draw on feminist theory and the political economy of health as key approaches to maternal mortality worldwide. We review programs sponsored by nongovernmental organizations (NGOs), departments of health, and other organizations working within a framework of improving maternal and infant care. A woman-centred approach must address which women are included in transforming political, economic, and social relations. Later in this essay we consider how the dangers of imposing a specifically western women's outlook on women in the underdeveloped world can be offset through a process of alliances and empowerment.

We review patterns of maternal mortality, with special attention to North America and the South. Next, we discuss several examples of Safe Motherhood Programs in the underdeveloped world. Specifically, we discuss services used to reduce maternal deaths, and barriers facing workers who provide these services. The next section looks at implications of safe motherhood policies for women at risk. We focus on barriers many women face in obtaining income, education, and in exercising more choice in reproductive decisions including pregnancy and birth. We underscore the importance of state sponsorship of health programs and literacy.

MATERNAL DEATHS WORLDWIDE

Maternal mortality is an important index of a community's commitment to women's health care. Maternal-related deaths are among the leading causes of death for women aged 15-44 in poor countries. It is the leading or second-leading cause of death in one-third of these countries. Adequate prenatal and birth care could prevent most of those deaths resulting from toxaemia, haemorrhage, sepsis, anaemia, obstructed labour and other complications. Teenage women having too many babies too quickly, who are inadequately nourished and rested, face an unacceptable high risk of death in childbirth...[11]

In the ten years since *Women in the World* was published, little has changed. As we set out below, women of colour, who are the *majority* of women in underdeveloped countries, and the majority of women worldwide, often experience health risks such as maternal mortality. Seager and Olson are correct to link poverty and higher mortality rates, and their focus on links between racism, global economics, and the political economy of health. In many countries, women continue to die in unacceptably high numbers. The implementation of Safe Motherhood Programs has not dramatically reduced maternal deaths in the South. Maternal death is defined as "...the death of a woman while pregnant or within 42 days of termination of pregnancy, irrespective of the duration and the site of the pregnancy, from any cause related to or aggravated by the pregnancy or its management, but not from accidental or incidental causes."[12]

Maternal deaths have only recently attracted systematic research and prevention activities on a global scale. Margaret Peters observed that: "It was not until the end of the decade dedicated to women [1976-85] that some emphasis was given to the unnecessary waste of women's lives."[13] International, national, and regional health agencies and sponsors of international health projects discussed maternal death issues at the first Safe Motherhood Conference in Kenya in 1987. Kwast notes that: "The Safe Motherhood Initiative's target was, and is to reduce maternal mortality by at least half by the year 2000."[14] Following the call for action, SMPs have been initiated worldwide.

In the North, maternal mortality is considered by some to be at an irreducible level. In Canada, for example, there were 10 maternal deaths in 1990. This meant that for every 100,000 live births, two Canadian women died of pregnancy-related factors.[15] In North America and most of the countries of the North, women dying of pregnancy-related causes are seen as tragic anomalies that are often unpreventable. Complications of anaesthesia, or unforeseen death through aneurysm are two examples of maternal mortality. In the South, however, maternal mortality is often 100-200 times higher than it is in Europe and North America.[16] As set out in Table 1, Africa has the highest rate of maternal deaths, followed by Asia, South America, the Caribbean, North America, and northern Europe.[17]

Table 1:
Estimated Lifetime Risk of Maternal Death for an Average Woman, by Geographic Region: 1975-1984

REGION	RISK (Ratio of deaths to live births)
Africa	1 in 21
Asia	1 in 54
South America	1 in 73
Caribbean	1 in 140
North America	1 in 6,366
Northern Europe	1 in 9,850

Safe motherhood affects all childbearing women and those who care for women. Using a feminist paradigm of equality of access to health education, equal pay, and political power we recognise that inequities in women's resources exist in all countries. In countries with the highest levels of maternal mortality the commonest causes of death are identified as haemorrhage, sepsis, abortion, infection, eclampsia and obstructed labour.[18] Social, economic and health policy initiatives have addressed these causes in many parts of the North. State involvement can serve as a fulcrum for efforts in support of women. For example, state support of midwives in Sweden since 1751 has been recognised as the main cause in the decline in maternal deaths. Sweden was the first European country to implement sweeping public health measures based on hygenic (aseptic) practices. Early regulation and state education of midwives helped to establish these measures. By the beginning of this century maternal deaths in North America were much higher than in Sweden.[19]

It is tempting to dismiss maternal death in Canada as rare and unavoidable. But midwives often care for disadvantaged women who may be at greater risk, even in relatively affluent societies: adolescents, poor women, illiterate women, and women of colour.[20] For women at risk, midwifery offers an important resource, balancing skilled care with intimacy with the woman and her family. But the question remains, how can lack of equal access to midwifery care affect women's lives in affluent societies? Access to midwifery care is not universal in North America. Midwives in western countries have historically often worked with poor women and high-risk populations. Our experience in contemporary Canada is that midwives have veered away from such outreach work, often working with a middle-class clientele, in part because midwifery services in many provinces are not covered by medical insurance plans. The point here is that midwifery services are now unreachable for many women in Canada, especially poor women who might benefit most from midwifery skills prenatally, during labour and birth, and postpartum.

Midwifery care has been linked with improved obstetrical outcomes for both women and newborns.[21] This lack of access to midwives for high-risk women can generate unsafe care and higher rates of death and injury. In the United States, for example, researchers concluded that "the racial gap continues" with women of colour 3.4 times more likely to experience maternal death than white women between 1974-1978. The same authors confirm that between 1979-1986, the risk of maternal death remained approximately three times higher for women of colour in America.[22]

Global statistics on maternal deaths are almost certainly underestimates. In most surveys, data are collected from official sources, primarily hospitals in urban settings. In underdeveloped countries with a predominantly rural population, thousands of maternal deaths are unrecorded. Another difficulty is the *lack of uniformity* in the data collection. Data are collected differently from country to country, and different time-frames are used to measure maternal mortality such that researchers must compare deaths in one country between the early and mid-1970s, and another country in the 1980s.

In the medical model, maternal deaths are often blamed on lack of medical resources and skills, something that can be remedied by medical personnel and clinical settings to educate expectant mothers and manage births. We believe that wider definitions are more helpful, since not all women die from 'medical' causes. Many are killed or injured from traumatic causes. Belying the image of protectiveness and respect extended to pregnant women, researchers have documented previously hidden rates of assault, sometimes fatal, against expectant women.[23] Researchers studied 95 maternal deaths in Cook County, Illinois. The largest category of maternal death was not medical complications (18.9%) or other, indirect health-related complications (12.6%), but *traumatic death* (46.3% of deaths studied).

> Maternal deaths from traumatic causes were attributed to homicide in 57% of cases and suicide in 9% of cases. The mechanism of injury in traumatic maternal deaths included gunshot wounds (22.7%), motor vehicle crashes (20.5%), stab wounds (13.6%), strangulation (13.6%), blunt head injuries (9.1%), burns (6.8%), falls (4.5%), toxic exposure (4.5%), drowning (2.3%), and iatrogenic [physician-caused] injury (2.3%)[24]

Researchers exploring violence against expectant mothers report great difficulty obtaining data on this subject. Official information on maternal mortality is difficult to find in U.S. jurisdictions. Atrash et al lament the end of maternal mortality review committees in many American states.[25] Routine reports on maternal death *underestimate* the numbers of maternal deaths. Some researchers recommend augmenting statistical analyses of maternal deaths and injuries through "personal histories" and "home-based records" to draw out the women's perspectives on health. Such research can offer important insights into women's experiences of violence and state control, using "standpoint feminism" as a key approach.[26] In terms of women's health, "The call for improved information on women's health by international and national agencies should be made in unison with the call for action [for Safe Motherhood]."[27]

Contributing causes to maternal death are easily identified in the literature. Unequal access to family-planning assistance and contraception condemns women to illegal, unsafe abortion facilities. It has been estimated that up to 50 per cent of maternal deaths in some Latin American countries are caused by complications of unsafe abortion.[28] Safer abortion practices have contributed to the decline in deaths from abortion-related causes in countries with liberal abortion laws and respect for women's reproductive choices. Even when the number of abortions rises, the number of deaths attributed to abortion falls rapidly.[29] It is estimated that maternal mortality would fall by 25 per cent if women were able to have the number of children they wished.[30]

Provision of family-planning counselling and family-planning devices is often beyond the means of many underdeveloped countries, and issues of political will and redistribution of resources need to be understood.[31] In countries with a large rural population, distribution of contraceptives is sometimes limited by cost, distance, and lack of personnel. The training of personnel relevant to the woman's community is sometimes negated by language barriers. In many countries, although an official language is stated, many rural women and their birth attendants do not communicate in that language. Females may also be barred from, or discouraged in continuing formal education, leading to their exclusion from midwifery training on the ground of 'illiteracy.' Such exclusions can reinforce women's oppression by blocking women from attending births, and subordinating specific dialects and languages to a dominant language. For midwives, it can mean the loss of traditional birth customs, as Western birth practices and technology eclipse traditional birth practices. Again, this is not specific to the South, as First Nations communities in Canada have protested systematic efforts, often successful, to stigmatize and extinguish their languages, and to impose Eurocentric norms not only on birth rituals, but all aspects of First Nations culture, economics, and politics.

Poverty and failure of family planning initiatives in some countries have been linked with high levels of infant mortality.[32] Lack of family planning contributes to high parity (i.e. a high number of births per woman), which can increase a woman's risk of haemorrhage, which is in turn a major cause of maternal death in the South.[33] The decline of haemorrhage-related maternal deaths in the North can be attributed to the introduction of oxytocic drugs for the control and prevention of haemorrhage; also, 99% of women have a trained birth attendant, good nutrition, availability of blood transfusions, and emergency transfer.[34] That all women worldwide do not have access to these state strategies for prevention and treatment of haemorrhage means that haemorrhage is still a leading cause of maternal death in the South.

Greater care needs to be taken to ensure that family planning strategies are not assumed to be the answer. Difficulties associated with implementing planned parenthood programs are also structural and socio-economic. Due to high rates of illiteracy and the low status of women globally, 'success' of these programs may rest on denying the women's right to make an informed decision. Specifically, imposing the Western trend of small families on Third World women is oppressive, as many women value their ability to bear children.[35] Another point is that there are major concerns about using the Third World as "an important laboratory for human testing."[36] Many are concerned that the IPPF (International Planned Parenthood Federation) may play a significant role in not only introducing wanted contraceptive services but, in a more negative light, promoting population control policies at the expense of dealing with wider forces undermining women's health.[37]

One force that directly affects women and newborns is Acquired Immune Deficiency Syndrome (AIDS). HIV infection and AIDS are now ubiquitous in many underdeveloped regions. There is great concern over the spread of the virus, full-blown AIDS, and opportunistic diseases associated with AIDS in much of the South. "In the first half of 1992, nearly half of the one million newly-infected people were women. Millions of infants escaping infection are destined to become AIDS orphans."[38] In Carol Hird's M.A. thesis research, nine midwives who worked in the South were asked about HIV/AIDS services. Three of the nine midwives reported that there were *no* services for people infected with HIV. Poverty, embarrassment to admit HIV exposure or infection, and a general lack of access to contraceptive devices and health education were highlighted.[39]

Ectopic pregnancies (pregnancy occurring outside of the uterus, usually the fallopian tube, rupturing and causing internal haemmorhage during early development of the pregnancy) are also a factor in maternal deaths, often related to increases in pelvic inflammatory disease (PID). The incidence of ectopic pregnancy has increased, especially in the United States and Europe. Two and three-fold increases in ectopic pregnancy make it the leading cause of maternal death in the United States and Europe. The major causes of maternal death in the United Kingdom (1985-87) were (in descending order): hypertensive diseases of pregnancy, pulmonary embolism, ectopic pregnancy, haemorrhage, amniotic fluid embolism, abortion, sepsis, anaesthesia-related deaths, and ruptured uterus. The total number of maternal deaths in the United Kingdom between 1985 and 1987 was 265, averaging 88 deaths annually for a maternal death rate of .42/100,000. Again, these deaths are very much the exception to the norm of maternal safety in labour and delivery in western societies.[40]

Many countries also report on issues, which are directly and indirectly influenced by women's status in her society and community. In the national and international literature, *predisposing factors* — which increase risk of maternal death — include poverty, adolescent pregnancy, pregnancy in older women, illiteracy, and race.[41]

EFFORTS TO REDUCE MATERNAL MORTALITY

Those favouring a primary healthcare model seek to establish the "basic needs of health education, immunization, primary prevention, a basic balanced diet, clean water, safe childbirth, family planning advice, and the ability of individuals and communities to take control of their health care needs."[42] This model of health care is endorsed by the World Health Organization as a strategy to assist communities to achieve "Health For All by the Year 2000." Sociologists, economists, epidemiologists, and demographers attribute health improvements — including decreased maternal mortality — to improved sanitation, clean water, greater educational attainment, and increased family income. These health improvements can be developed in the context of community-based midwifery. The midwife is a caregiver in many countries where social and economic inequities are dramatic, and the low status of women impedes positive health changes at the community level. In some African and South Asian countries (e.g., Ethiopia, Uta Pradesh province in India, Bangladesh, and so forth), the midwife has little status.

AN EXPLORATORY STUDY OF SAFE MOTHERHOOD INITIATIVES

In Carol Hird's M.A. thesis research for Thames Valley University, surveys were sent out to 35 midwives who were working, or had worked, in the South. Nine midwives completed and returned the questionnaire. This section provides some findings from this exploratory research.[43] Eight of the midwives were female, with one male respondent from Africa. This accords with the predominantly female nature of midwifery globally. The midwives were primarily working in Africa and Asia-Pacific regions. Their ages ranged from 31-60. The respondents were primarily senior midwives. All nine respondents were registered general nurses. The sample was evenly divided between those currently working predominantly as a nurse (4), and those working in another capacity (4) One respondent did not provide this information. Where numbers total less than nine, this means that not all midwives responded to specific questions. Nearly all of the midwives had been working as midwives for over a decade. Years of practice as a midwife ranged from 4 years (1 midwife), to 10-19 years (4), and 20-22 years (2 midwives). Six of the midwives had attended over 1,000 births.

Asked if "the status of women in your country has an impact on the rate of maternal mortality" all the midwives said that it had.

> In our country women have a low status because of the strong culture we have and though women are only beginning to speak their rights, it's difficult. Men seemed to be the predominant characters. (Papua New Guinea)

> Women are left to do a lot of work from dawn to sunset. Apart from their work in the office, the[y] labour all day trying to feed, cook, and look after their own families and the relatives which is common in this country, and [they] have little rest. (Papua New Guinea)

> Women in the country are treated like second-class citizens. They have no right to their reproduction, food. They work hard since childhood, even during pregnancy and old age. They eat little [compared to] boys in the family. They do not own land except to reproduce many babies — too soon, too early and too many. (Tanzania)

> High illiteracy rate leading to failure to comprehend health information effectively. Low socio-economic status leading to inaccessibility to health facility or time for prompt diagnosis of risks and Rx [treatment]. (Zambia)

Four midwives described their practice as both clinical and teaching. This is consistent with the mentor/apprenticeship model of teaching student midwives. Five out of nine midwives had additional education in safe motherhood. Of the remaining four: one midwife is a researcher in safe motherhood, another midwife facilitates and plans Safe Motherhood Programs, one midwife felt that the principles of safe motherhood were entrenched in the curriculum of midwifery education, and only one midwife cited lack of funding for the failure to receive additional education.

Safe Motherhood requires an end to barriers to safe care for expectant mothers. Some of these barriers have been identified in previous studies of Safe Motherhood Programs. In Carol's survey, several barriers were noted by midwives. These included:

Ignorance/Lack of information. For some women, it varied according to seasons because [the women] move from villages to fields during ploughing season. (Botswana)

Transport was a problem, distance from where the patients live; staff nurses, doctors and other health personnel's attitudes. (Papua New Guinea)

Lack of knowledge on the importance of attending antenatal clinic. (Tanzania)

The programme was just new, and mothers had to get proper information as many were still in doubt. (Papua New Guinea)

One respondent had not investigated this aspect of SMPs. She noted, however, that "it is not so much the frequency but appropriate timing and *content* of care at 4-5 specific points in pregnancy."

Eight midwives have taken part in advanced/life-saving skills programmes. The one midwife who responded negatively did perform four out of the five listed advanced skills. Use of advanced skills in the survey sample was inconsistent. The commonest advanced skills utilised were manual removal of placenta, rehydration with intravenous fluids, and suturing of cervical and perineal tears. Eight of nine respondents cited these interventions. The midwife from Sudan did not have preparation in advanced skills and this midwife is a coordinator for nursing and midwifery service development. This does not mean that life skills training is not available in Sudan; rather, this particular midwife may not have had need for such training as an administrator.

Other advanced skills included dilation and curretage for retained products of conception. One midwife had advanced training to perform Caesarian sections. Seven of nine used vacuum extraction (primarily for prolonged second-stage maternal exhaustion and fetal distress). Only one midwife cited administration of blood transfusions as a life-saving measure. One midwife identified administration of antibiotics and use of sedatives and hypotensive drugs in pre-eclampsia and eclampsia. All respondents used oxytocin, but only four used it routinely. One midwife indicated that oxytocin was used for multiparous women, and two midwives used oxytocin to control haemmorhage. Referrals to medical centres were established in seven sites surveyed. The two respondents who indicated referral was *not* in place were from Sudan and Indonesia. One-third of the sample indicated that there was no provision for transportation to the first referral level for complicated births. Six midwives mentioned that such transportation was established, but one respondent qualified this, noting that this depended on specific countries' policies.

All midwives reported that they were involved in health education in their communities. Antenatal care (ANC) was emphasized, and some mentioned working against traditions deemed harmful to women and girls (e.g. female genital mutilation).

> Educating community and individuals on risk factors and warning signs to make one seek medical advice, importance of antenatal care and delivered by trained personnel. (Tanzania)

> Health education is given on nutrition, family planning, breastfeeding, women's health issues. (Papua New Guinea)

> Health education on various obstetric and gynaecology topics to women's groups, church groups. Antenatal family planning and postnatal mothers. (Papua New Guinea)

> Nutrition for mothers and children, including breastfeeding initiatives. Motivation and educational talks on: family planning services, safe water and sanitation, environmental and personal hygiene, and value of ANC. (Zimbabwe)

> Midwives are educated on family planning in the hospital and clinics. Midwives go out to the community for antenatal care where they give health education and also in Maternal Child Health Services. (Zambia)

> Early registration for ANC, hospital delivery supervised by trained personnel. Reporting bleeding during pregnancy or other issues related to pregnancy. (Botswana)

> Some sisters and H.V.s [health visitors] are trainers for [eliminating] harmful traditional practices, especially female circumcision and I am one of these trainers. I did my session and my training to fight against these traditions. (Sudan)

Services for adolescents were not universally available. Four responded that such services were effective:

Teenagers will delay the next pregnancy and will explore avenues for integrating into normal education again. Adolescents delay their first pregnancy. (Botswana)

There are antenatal and prenatal complications in regard to this young age, e.g. toxemia, premature labour, inadequate pelvis. (Sudan)

Prevents unsafe abortion, successful in lowering maternal mortalities. (Indonesia)

No experience, but where I know of them — Tanzania Mexico, they are effective. (Midwife worked in several countries)

The majority of respondents checked "no," these services were ineffective. Two mentioned a lack of such services in Papua New Guinea. A Tanzanian midwife indicated that "the problem is still existing."

Remote areas from the urban areas, the services are inadequate and not integrated. (Zimbabwe)

They are not effective due to customs and cultural differences varying from country to country. (Zambia)

Six midwives reported that HIV/AIDS services were available under the SMP in their countries. Prevention of HIV infection is a major priority for many underdeveloped countries, especially those where AIDS is endemic. One respondent with wide experience in the underdeveloped world checked "yes" but she did not believe that "SMP programs generally include HIV/AIDS counselling, but that community care of AIDS patients is effective." Three midwives reported that SMPs in their communities did *not* provide services for people infected with HIV. Financial difficulties were highlighted.

There is lack of finance and lack of team system; also, there is a special program for eradication of HIV. (Sudan)

Inadequate funding by the Ministry of Health. (Zambia)

One problem with the questionnaire is that it rarely captured reasons that may underlie inadequate funding, such as financial crisis in the country, or ostracism of people with AIDS/HIV. (Questionnaires that are too detailed and demanding are unlikely to be filled in, or returned.)

The sample was divided on the issue of how effective HIV/AIDS programs were. Four indicated that such services were effective; four other midwives disagreed, noting that the services were not effective. Specific comments about the effectiveness or ineffectiveness of HIV/AIDS programmes were:

This is a collaborative effort between health workers and the community. There are midwife trainers who train others and do preservice education to trainees. (Botswana)

These counsellors are especially trained in counselling skill, in both basic counselling and HIV/AIDS counselling. (Papua New Guinea)

Depends what they set out to do! For example, community care of AIDS patients was effective. (Several countries)

The four midwives who indicated that these services were ineffective emphasized the role of greater education, and also overcoming inhibitions in discussing HIV/AIDS infection. "A lot still needs to be done to be advanced toward home-based care — education of caregivers and support services." "Victims are not educated enough to see the importance of services or [are] too embarrassed." Some respondents believed that such services were not reaching people, shown by rising rates of HIV infection.

Midwives were asked if the SMP provided "measures to improve women's status (in terms of social/educational/economic status)." Six respondents indicated that SMPs provided such measures. They cited access to education, fostering women's groups, financial benefits such as loans and gardens. A midwife from Papua New Guinea answered "yes," but cautioned that many women are excluded from SMP opportunities. "Educational opportunities are given to most women and especially those literate and those living in metropolitan areas. Majority of women live in rural areas and have little access to such services." (Indonesia)

A Tanzanian midwife applauded the creation of a government ministry for women, increased educational opportunities for women, allowing "soft loans" for women, and "empowering women to make decisions on their reproduction." An Indonesian midwife credited SMP with reducing rates of illiteracy among women by providing "basic education." She also mentioned how training skills such as sewing and handicrafts could increase the "economic status" of women. Other responses were:

Educational opportunities for all as they made sure everyone try to get the message. (Papua New Guinea)

Educational opportunities for women, equality [for women], [greater income for women], in this order. (Zimbabwe)

Health education — vegetable garden to eat and sell the surplus — Encourage women to participate in women's groups — literacy classes to curb the problem of illiteracy — sensitize about Government's income-generating policies. (Botswana)

Feminists have documented ways in which women are disadvantaged relative to men. Except where some women have unusual economic or social power, patterns of gender inequality are evident globally.[44] In their atlas of women's lives, Seager and Olson put this bluntly:

> Everywhere women are worse off than men: women have less power, less autonomy, more work, less money, and more responsibility. Women everywhere have a smaller share of the pie; if the pie is very small (as in poor countries), women's share is smaller still.[45]

The questionnaire also asked about the impact of the status of women in underdeveloped countries. The midwives were asked if women's status influenced maternal death in their countries. Eight midwives checked "yes." The one midwife who indicated "no" nevertheless implied that women's status affected mortality rates (this may reflect a misunderstanding of the questionnaire). Respondents often wrote about low income, long hours of work, (including responsibilities for families and in-laws), poor nutrition, exclusion of many women from formal education, and major barriers receiving proper health care. Some responses are outlined below.

> Educated women have less children, making antenatal care more often and delivered in safe hands. (Sudan)

> In urban rather than rural settings drought and HIV/AIDS are frustrating the effects of SMP. (Zimbabwe)

> Childbearing in this country begins early. One quarter of teenagers have borne a child by the time they reach 16 years. Most of the women are illiterate, thereby don't know the importance of antenatal care and are subject to unsafe and unclean deliveries in some parts of the country, especially rural areas. This results in maternal mortality because of their status. (Zambia)

One midwife said: "Generally maternal mortality is higher among women of low SES (socio-economic status]."

> A working woman can afford better food/meal for her and her family. An educated woman can care better [for] her health compared to an uneducated woman. This helps to reduce maternal mortalities. (Indonesia)

All midwives believed that better resources — education, money, higher social status — correlated with better outcomes for women. Midwives working at the grassroots level recognized the effects of underdevelopment, while this was not tapped directly in the questionnaire.

Midwives were asked to describe events surrounding the last maternal death in their practices. Some midwives were not directly involved in attending births. One midwife listed 1980 as the last year she witnessed a maternal death. Two midwives — from Zambia and Indonesia — had no experience of such deaths. For the remaining midwives, such deaths were a part of their practice. Six midwives had witnessed a maternal death. The following years were noted for the last maternal death seen by these respondents: 1993, 1994 (two respondents), and 1995 (three respondents). Maternal deaths, regarded as exceptional cases in western countries, are part-and-parcel of pregnancy and birth in many underdeveloped countries. Specific cases of maternal deaths noted in the questionnaires affirmed that these deaths are usually preventable, often stemming from malnourishment, lack of treatment services, and sometimes direct violence against women.

Haemorrhage. The woman started bleeding after delivery in the village. She did not get transport to bring her to the hospital early. She managed to reach the hospital after two days of bleeding. Although blood transfusion was given, the woman died after [a] few minutes in the hospital. (Tanzania)

[Very] severe anaemia HG 36% [3.6G]. (Malawi)

Wife bashing — husband bashed her when she was 7 months pregnant, killing both her and the fetus. (Papua New Guinea)

Postpartum haemorrhage and puerperal sepsis [infection following the birth of the baby, a condition readily treated in the developed world by antibiotics]. (Indonesia)

She was about 31 years old and she had 2 previous sons delivered by Caesarean section. The fetus was jaundiced and died. After 3 days the mother became febrile with distended abdomen. So she died after 7 days as a result of severe infection. (Sudan)

Ruptured uterus. Mother had transverse lie. Unqualified staff attempted internal podalic version and caused a uterine rupture. There was a delay in transferring the mother to hospital. (Zambia)

The final item on the questionnaire was open-ended. Respondents were asked to comment on their "practice as a midwife and experience with Safe Motherhood and/or maternal death." These comments help to capture their experiences and recommendations for change with SMPs:

SMP has to an extent reduced maternal deaths because the community in general has been educated and are aware of the importance of antenatal care and family planning. More traditional birth attendants have been trained and those who were trained a long time ago have received [a] refresher course. The major drawback is poor transport system to transfer the at-risk mother to the nearest referral. (Zambia)

Midwives find difficulties in providing quality care because of inadequate resources — financial, material, personnel — even when training has been adequate. (Zimbabwe)

Another respondent gave a detailed account of maternal injuries and an infant death:

...when she was 32 weeks she developed signs and symptoms of eclampsia at home, severe headache, epigastric pain, vomiting when she went to hospital. The young doctor in the casualty didn't know these signs of impending eclampsia so he gave her the injection of Cortigen B6 and sent her home. At home, she developed eclamptic fits then they returned her to hospital again and it was 8 hours from home. So the pregnancy was terminated by [Caesarean section] and the mother developed renal failure. Kidney dialysis was done 3 times. She was very ill for 2 months and then she recovered but she lost the precious baby and she goes into maternal morbidity. (Sudan)

An African midwife recommended that midwives should be able to give "integrated reproductive health" care, and that transportation systems for expectant women were inadequate. A midwife from Papua New Guinea praised the role of nurse-midwives in preventing maternal mortality. She highlighted the importance of midwifery conferences, peer support, and efforts to establish a midwifery association in her home country.

Once our midwifery association is formed, we will then clearly address the issues that are affecting our midwifery practice. We will also attend closely to maternal and perinatal problems and do our best to reduce maternal mortalities. Papua New Guinea... has the highest maternal deaths in the world.

Throughout the questionnaires the quality of the responses was striking and insightful. The candour of the midwives is very moving, and the over-whelming impression is one of sadness and regret that maternal deaths are part of their professional experience. It is encouraging to read that although midwives are part of women's larger experience of oppression by their own culture, they see a way through it in their own education and willingness to continue to care for women. Midwifery, an ancient resource throughout the world, could draw on traditional practices and international resources such as research, to reduce risks to many poor women. The point here is that midwifery is not a western invention which needs to be imported to under-developed countries; in fact, the potential for midwives to work effectively is often undermined by the thrall of obstetrical technology, and other aspects of medicalized health care. Differences between the North and South are striking: income, transportation, life-saving resources including medical sup-plies, access to education and contraception, are often lacking or inadequate in the post-colonial South.

There are many other examples of Safe Motherhood initiatives under-taken in difficult and oppressive conditions. In Magbil, Sierra Leone, Isha Daramy-Kabia, a midwife, established a community health centre in a village. This centre allowed the traditional birth attendants to receive training to improve their birthcare skills.[46] Another example is implementation of Safe Motherhood policies in Tanzania. Stella Mpanda, a midwife, was the catalyst for a national workshop to promote midwifery education and care, and thereby reduce maternal deaths. The point is that midwifery skills associated with developed countries need not displace all traditional practices in under-developed countries, and that merely applying technical skills will have a limited impact if overall political and economic conditions affecting women and families are not altered.

Many local initiatives in the South (e.g. Magbil, Sierra Leone) are funded by members of the International Confederation of Midwives (the Magbil initiative is funded by the Royal College of Midwives, London). Life-saving skills training in many African countries have been funded by the Foundation of the American College of Nurse-Midwives. Other member associations funding SMPs include: the Independent German Midwives Association (Bund Deutscher Hebammen) which has funded initiatives in Ghana and Sierra Leone; and the Netherlands Midwives (Nederlandse Organisatie van Verloskundigen) which has funded SMPs in Sudan. These are a few examples of numerous midwifery-led initiatives being made worldwide to ameliorate women's suffering in childbirth. Concerted efforts are being made at inter-national, national, regional, and local levels. To be effective, all planning must include policy dialogue, problem identification at community level, education, and improved communications leading to good referral and or-ganization strategies.[47]

POLICY IMPLICATIONS FOR MIDWIVES

The medical model does have its place in the diagnosis and treatment of diseases, but it should not have authority over social problems and should be considered in its place, along with other models of health care, instead of dominating and controlling all other participants.[48]

The low status of women in many countries in the world prohibits implementation of Safe Motherhood initiatives. In the South, higher rates of literacy, access to maternal health services, better nutrition, vaccinations, improved socio-economic status, and public health services have contributed to the overall improvement in women's health. A global improvement in women's status is recognized as the catalyst to attain the goal of Safe Motherhood for all by the year 2000.[49] Successful SMPs require teamwork and professional collaboration at all levels of implementation. Recommendations from the International Conference on Population and Development in September 1994 endorse the concept of Primary Health Care as a critical component of Safe Motherhood Programs. The causes of maternal death are known; the means of preventing these deaths are understood. We recognise that implementing preventive measures globally can achieve Safe Motherhood.[50] Publication of the WHO *Mother Baby Package*[51] offers a blueprint for Safe Motherhood Programs. Some strategies for SMPs are now used by many healthcare workers — including midwives — in the South. This collaboration cannot, however, take root without sufficient economic support from state regulatory bodies.

While there are continued efforts to fund SMPs by NGOs and other aid agencies, and thus assist implementation of SMPs at national and regional levels, it is the midwife and traditional birth attendant (TBA) who implement the program at the *community* level. Improvements in maternal and infant mortality have been reported in the Matlab area of Bangladesh, Sri Lanka, Thailand, and Indonesia.[52] SMP implementation in these countries took several forms:

- Development of community midwifery
- Strengthening of midwifery education
- Establishing organization of care
- Implementing a support system for the midwives
- Midwives accepting the inclusion of the TBA as a team member
- Developing a data collection system
- Provision of simple and sustainable birth supplies
- Establishing women's groups in the community to share education
- Empowering women to find solutions to community problems
- Provision of an emergency transport system

Politically, these strategies require sufficient resources to train midwives *and* to advance the status of women. SMP initiatives mean that midwives do not work in isolation, but as part of a multidisciplinary team. Nevertheless, the ideal of teamwork is often undermined in developed and underdeveloped countries where laws and state policies make for medicalized births, with a subordinated status for midwives within health services.

In North America, midwives have had a precarious legal status. There are concerns even where midwifery is legally recognized, or about to be recognized. In Canada, legalization of midwifery is established in Ontario, with Alberta and B.C. taking steps to secure legalized midwifery. Legalization has been accompanied by an examination of different models of practice. Since the formation of the Midwives Association of British Columbia (MABC) in 1980, their vision for midwifery practice has always been based on a *political and social* model of care. Concerns have been raised about the exclusion of independent midwives from the protected status of state-registered midwives, and limited access of aspiring midwives to accredited midwifery programs in Ontario. There are ongoing concerns over the bottleneck many aspiring midwives face through state-registration provisions in Canada, and serious concerns over class and race privilege, with an underrepresentation of women of colour in midwifery teaching and the midwifery student and practicing midwifery populations. In the United States, while recognizing midwifery as an important expansion of maternity and infant services, some caution that the politics of medical control often leads to a restriction on midwives' practices. Such restrictions in turn limit choices for expectant women.[53]

The principle that the midwife should be 'with woman' has guided their proposals for woman-centred care. Maternal and infant services should reflect this principle, as noted in the U.K. report, *Changing Childbirth*: "Maternity services must be readily and easily accessible to all women. They should be sensitive to the needs of the local population and based primarily in the community."[54] Support for this statement is found in international midwifery, feminist and sociological literature,[55] and reinforced in British Columbia by the *Seaton Report* on health care and costs.[56] This report endorsed policies of increased accessibility of health services through a return to community care, rather than institutionalized care. In the United Kingdom and some parts of Canada, government initiatives have resulted in changes in the delivery of healthcare services. The *Seaton Report* is subtitled "Closer to Home." The Expert Maternity group and the Seaton committee recommend health care in the community, where appropriate. The major shift in recommendations for future health policy is that in the U.K. care will be woman-centred. Care will follow the woman, rather than the woman having only the option of hospitalized birth.

There are numerous examples of SMPs initiated at the community level with Traditional Birth Attendants (TBAs), including education and upgrading of skills. Successful programs established the TBA as a team member. Often the midwife in the rural area visited the TBA in her practice on a regular basis, giving encouragement and supervision when appropriate. Where TBAs practiced in isolation, or where midwives were unwilling to include the TBA in the Safe Motherhood team, the results compared unfavourably with the programs where the TBA worked as an integral part of the team.[57] In 1992, WHO, UNFPA, and UNICEF agreed that the utilization and training of TBAs was not the ideal long-term solution for maintenance of SMPs. However, economic and political constraints have not allowed most countries in the underdeveloped world to establish midwives in a vital role in SMPs.

The concept of community-based care has worked effectively in Bangladesh and other areas where village midwives served women. Outcomes were compared with similar villages (but without midwives), and significant decreases in the number of maternal deaths were recorded, over a three year period, in the villages where midwives worked. The study suggests that posting midwives at the village level can improve maternal survival, if midwives are given proper training, resources, supervision as needed and emergency back up.[58] Similar programs at the community level in Akwa Iban State in Eastern Nigeria also decreased maternal mortality. However, in Indonesia and the Gambia, "trained birth attendants without skilled back-up and support did not decrease a woman's risk of dying."[59] Examples of safer outcomes attributable to midwifery care are also seen in the United States.

Improvements in the status of women are needed worldwide. These improvements include greater access to midwifery care, which can reduce maternal mortality rates. "There are literally thousands of small and large groups, collectives, coalitions, organisations... all taking action on the health issues that are important for women."[60] Women's status — "a composite indicator of cultural, economic, legal, educational, and political position"[61] — is best understood in the context of the woman's society or community.

This knowledge needs to stem not only from formal education of the midwife, but also an understanding of the social value of women in her community. Feminist writers have drawn our attention to disparities in formal education of girls, compared with boys, in many underdeveloped countries.[62] In the international midwifery community, some measures to improve maternal well-being have been made. Midwives are involved in education and support of women in their own communities. We believe that the future of women and midwives hinges on this movement to safeguard women during the childbearing years.

CONCLUSION

The redefinition of maternal deaths as a *political* problem helps to put women's status and mortality in a context that goes beyond physiology and medical intervention. Solutions to maternal mortality should not be restricted to enhanced medical resources and health resources generally. Worldwide, there is a movement to enhance women's status in their communities and wider societies. This takes many forms, all aimed at establishing new forms of work for women suffering from globalization and colonialist legacies.[63] Healthcare policies also need to take into account women's occupational statuses, and their roles as mothers, caregivers, and sisters. Educational opportunities and recognition of women as deserving human rights protection are two aspects that can be furthered through state auspices. Training of midwives through state-sponsored programs is another means of empowering women.

As Noga Gayle notes, the marginalization of black women (and women of colour generally), requires that black women move "from objects to subjects."[64] This means that the marginalization of women's experiences is acknowledged and reversed.

The invisibility of maternal deaths can be a serious omission in the emerging literature on Third World feminism. This seems to reflect a divorce between theorizing about women's status on the one hand, and the importance of establishing concrete resources for women at risk of maternal mortality. A synthesis of the two is in keeping with concerns of social class, race, and gender that are central to feminist theory and practice. The subject of maternal mortality, while not a taboo subject, has attracted little media or popular attention in the western world. Death during pregnancy, birth, and the postpartum period includes deaths under medical management, *and* also trauma and other aspects of women's experiences. Our argument here is that, if maternal mortality is presented as a problem of medical management and research, this obscures other, often very direct forms of violence directed against women.

Apart from social science articles and books on women, development, and maternal mortality, much of the available literature is written by physicians, with birth and death cast as medical events. Even the recent report on maternal deaths in the United Kingdom neglects such variables as women's socio-economic status, presenting instead a range of medical complications in explaining the phenomenon. While such explanations are important (not least of all in the North where women dying in labour has become a statistical rarity), it is important to allow for socio-demographic factors that may better explain patterns of maternal deaths. To understand the complexity of the issue of maternal mortality demands that midwives are well informed of the broader socio-economic cultural and political influences on women's lives.

It is critical that skilled midwives are available to women in the underdeveloped world. Kwast laments that

> Tanzania has experienced a decrease of 25% of midwives available for the increasing number of births brought about by a 2.6% population increase. I am convinced that this scenario is true for many countries. What was once envisioned as a pyramid of care has now become an hourglass with few midwives, skilled and available to provide essential maternity care.[65]

As we noted earlier in the essay, with few exceptions, feminist writing rarely touches on maternal mortality. This silence over women dying, may reflect the experience of Anglo-American feminist writers and activists, living in North American societies where maternal deaths are not nearly as frequent as in the South. Similarly, the general literature on maternal mortality rarely mentions feminism as a paradigm for understanding maternal deaths. Feminist thought and activism is often displaced by a seemingly more objective, medical model of problem solving. A possible bridge here is to use political economy, development, and gender as a combined paradigm for understanding women's status and life-chances. Theoretically, socialist feminism offers a critique of patriarchy and of capitalism, and is a framework for future work on this subject.

Feminist understanding of sexism, racism, and poverty has been profoundly deepened by Third World feminism, which articulates new outlooks from within underdeveloped countries. These outlooks include an appreciation of women in the context of religion, employment, legal rights, marriage, reproduction, and political life. It is also significant that these new theoretical outlooks have been complemented with active projects to improve women's well being in such areas. Feminist theory and action incorporates agenda setting by Third World feminists. This includes arguments against racism and imperialism, and for social justice for men and women.

> [I]t is not just a question of internal redistribution of resources, but of their generation and control; not just equal opportunity between men and women, but the creation of opportunity itself; not only the position of women in society, but the position of the societies in which Third World women find themselves.[66]

We recommend supporting midwives at a community level to promote women's health, and to provide information in culturally appropriate ways, rather than applying Western pedagogies of birth and safety.[67] Ways in which women's work is valued (or devalued) is also critical, including discrimination in paid employment. We must resist capitalist exploitation of human and other resources in the underdeveloped world. Maria Mies[68] outlines the damage caused by "overdevelopment" in the Third World, and proposes an "alternative economy" which counters labour exploitation, while bolstering self-sufficiency rather than economic dependency. Sari Tudiver, among others, criticizes the exploitation of resources in the South by wealthier nations, and outlines sharp pressures on women in underdeveloped countries to accept Western healthcare technologies, including new reproductive technologies.[69] Angela Davis shows how the poor and women have borne the brunt of state and private-sector policies designed to ensure "racial purity" and to stem the increasing population in underdeveloped nations.[70]

This politicized approach is a natural extension of the continuing work to enhance birth and reproductive choices for women throughout the world. Understanding violence against women — in the form of domestic violence, obstetrical routines, and embedded forms of discrimination against women — is an important starting point if women are to be empowered, not only 'rescued' from death. Sundari, reviewing studies of maternal death, links these deaths to structured inequality for many women, including lack of medical resources. Marginalized women must become a part of program planning.

> The prevention of maternal deaths requires far-reaching social and economic changes beyond the confines of the health care system. The factors that make

the natural processes of pregnancy and childbirth extremely risky and even fatal for poorer women are structural; so are the factors that influence the value women place on their personal well being, and those that influence their ability to seek health care for themselves. The last depends crucially on resources such as time, money, and information that women have at their disposal, and whether they have the authority for decision-making. However this does not absolve the health care system of its responsibility to make fundamental changes in both the structure and the delivery of health services.[71]

The World Health Organization[72] regards the midwife as the key person in the maternal healthcare pyramid. She can be a bridge between the community and health resources. In some parts of the world, the community midwife seeks relationships within the healthcare system which facilitate referral and promote more choices for expectant mothers. In underdeveloped countries, the maternity and infant care team includes midwives, physicians, nurses, social workers, educators, and researchers. The midwife may need to perform emergency obstetric procedures as a life-saving skill. Training of midwives to perform these skills can decrease mortality and morbidity. These skills include: antenatal risk assessment and treatment, monitoring labour progress, prevention and treatment of haemmorhage, rehydration with intravenous fluids, management of difficult deliveries, resuscitation, repair of episiotomies and lacerations, and management of infection.[73]

Midwives in the underdeveloped world have participated in policy and educational development at regional, national, and international levels. Their expertise and commitment to women's needs make them vital team members at the political level. If women's health needs are to be recognized, women must be represented on decision-making bodies where fundamental planning for health care occurs.[74] Inclusion of midwives in policy development for maternal-child health occurs as an artifact of state regulation. In countries where state regulation and full integration of midwifery services has been established, consultation with midwives and women has developed services which respect the choices of women and midwives. State regulation may of course undermine midwifery practice. For example, in the United Kingdom, following the Peel Report of 1970, women and midwives were persuaded that birth in hospital was safer than home birth, in spite of no research evidence with which to support this claim. The state, supported by the powerful medical profession, endorsed this report. The result of this universal hospitalization has been to decrease continuity of care and increase the speed with which medical intervention was accepted as "normal" practice.[75] Conversely, state regulation can support midwifery-led programs. In Sweden, state and midwifery support of the Baby-Friendly Hospital Initiative has resulted in the highest rates of breastfeeding mothers at six months postpartum in the developed world.

The low socio-economic status and lack of political power of many women and midwives in underdeveloped countries has slowed implementation of Safe Motherhood Programs. Empowering midwives and women must include state support of a *midwifery* model of care, one that is inclusive of traditional birth attendants, and articulated with resources that advance women's status as defined within their culture. Again, this is not a new initiative, for many of these arrangements have been established traditionally. The danger is that traditional practices will be outlawed, or otherwise sanctioned without reference to the communities concerned. Inclusion of midwives at *all* levels of health policy development is yet to be realised. Even if this is realized, there is serious concern that some aspiring midwives, including women of colour and/or first-generation immigrants from the South, will not meet admission criteria for formal midwifery training in Canada. There is an ever-present danger of reproducing marginalization of such women, leaving them outsiders in clinical, policy, and research aspects of midwifery, and losing their broader experience. Finally, prior to implementing midwifery-training programs in Canada or elsewhere, a failure to consider the legacy of colonialism in the South obscures structural forces of racism, poverty, and educational barriers that continue to place many women at risk. International recognition of the effect of these inequities should be the focus of Safe Motherhood Programs.

ENDNOTES

1. Ann Oakley, *Essays on Women, Medicine and Health* (Edinburgh: Edinburgh University Press, 1993).
2. World Health Organization, *Mother Baby Package: Implementing safe motherhood in countries* (Geneva: WHO/FHE/MSM, 1995); World Health Organization. *Maternal Mortality, Ratios and Rates: A Tabulation of Available Information* (3rd edition). (Geneva: WHO/MCH/MSM/Division of Maternal and Child Health and Family Planning, WHO Geneva, 1991); World Health Organization and International Confederation of Midwives, *Women's Health and the Midwife: A global perspective. Report of a collaborative pre-congress workshop* (The Hague: WHO/Maternal Child Health, 1987).
3. Starrs, cited in Barbara Kwast, "Safe Motherhood — The First Decade," *Keynote Addresses: International Confederation of Midwives, 23rd International Congress* (London: International Confederation of Midwives, 1993).
4. Carla Zahr Abou and Erica Royston, "Excessive hazards of pregnancy and childbirth in the Third World," *World Health Forum*, vol. 13, (1992).
5. World Health Organization, *Mother Baby Package: Implementing safe motherhood in countries* (Geneva: WHO/FHE/MSM/, 1995).
6. Human Rights Watch. *The Human Rights Watch Global Report on Women's Human Rights* (New York: Human Rights Watch, 1995).
7. Dara Culhane-Speck, *An Error in Judgement: The Politics of Medical Care in an Indian/White Community* (Vancouver: Talonbooks, 1987).

8. Carol Reid, "Sick to Death: The Health of Aboriginal People in Australia and Canada." In *Racial Minorities, Medicine, and Health*, B. Singh Bolaria and Rosemary Bolaria, eds. (Halifax: Fernwood Books, 1994).

9. Terry Wotherspoon and Vic Satzewich, *First Nations: Race, Class, and Gender Relations* (Toronto: Nelson Canada, 1993), 149.

10. Ronet Bachman, *Death and Violence on the Reservation: Homicide, Family Violence, and Suicide in American Indian Populations* (New York: Auburn House, 1992).

11. Joni Seager and Ann Olson, *Women in the World: An International Atlas* (London: Pluto Press, 1986), 106.

12. J.A. Fortney, "Implications of the ICD — IO Definitions related to Death in Pregnancy, Childbirth or the Puerperium," *World Health Statistics Quarterly*, vol. 43 (1990): 246-248.

13. Margaret Peters, "A Challenge for Midwives: the reduction of maternal mortality and morbidity rates throughout the world," *Midwifery*, vol. 4 (1988): 5.

14. Barbara Kwast, "Safe Motherhood — The First Decade," in *Keynote Addresses: International Confederation of Midwives, 23rd International Congress* (London: International Confederation of Midwives, 1993), 3.

15. Statistics Canada, *Health Reports Supplement No. 14: Births 1990* (Ottawa: Statistics Canada, 1992), 2.

16. Lelia Duley, "Maternal Mortality associated with hypertensive disorders or pregnancy in Africa, Asia, Latin America, and the Caribbean," *Journal of Obstetrics and Gynaecology*, vol. 99 (1992).

17. Deborah Maine, *Safe Motherhood Programs: Option and Issues* (New York: Center for Population and Family Health, 1991).

18. Barbara Kwast, "Safe Motherhood: A challenge to midwifery practice," *World Health Forum*, vol. 12 (1991).

19. U. Högberg, "Historical Aspects on The Role of Maternal Care in Reducing Maternal Mortality," *Maternal Health Care in an International Perspective* (WHO, 1992).

20. Mary Kensington, "Safer Motherhood — A midwifery challenge," in *Midwifery Practice: A Research-Based Approach*, Jo Alexander, Valerie Levy, and Sarah Roch, eds. (London: MacMillan, 1993).

21. Brian Burtch and Carol Hird, "A Case for Recognition," *World Health*, vol. 50, no. 2 (1997); Anne Scupholme et al, "Nurse-Midwifery Care to Vulnerable Populations: Phase I: Demographic Characteristics of the National CNM Sample," *Journal of Nurse-Midwifery*, vol. 37, no. 5 (1992).

22. Hani Atrash et al, "Maternal Mortality in the United States, 1979-1986," *Obstetrics and Gynaecology*, vol. 76, no. 6 (1990): 1058.

23. Jacquelyn Campbell et al, *AWHONN'S Clinical Issues*, vol. 4, no. 3 (1993); Judith McFarlane, "Battering During Pregnancy: Tip of an Iceberg Revealed." *Women & Health*, vol. 15, no. 3 (1989).

24. John Fildes et al, "Trauma: The Leading Cause of Maternal Death," *The Journal of Trauma*, vol. 32, no. 5 (1992): 644.

25. Hani Atrash et al, "Maternal Mortality in the United States, 1979-1986," *Obstetrics and Gynaecology*, vol. 76, no. 6 (1990): 974.

26. See Wendy Graham and Oona Campbell, "Maternal Health and The Measurement Trap," *Social Science and Medicine*, vol. 35, no. 8 (1992): 974; Elizabeth Comack, *Women in Trouble: Connecting Women's Law Violations to their Histories of Abuse* (Halifax: Fernwood Publishing, 1996).

27. Wendy Graham and Oona Campbell, "Maternal Health and the Measurement Trap," *Social Science and Medicine*, vol. 35, no. 8 (1992): 975.
28. Patricia Smyke, *Women and Health* (London: Zed Books, 1991).
29. John Paxman et al, "The Clandestine Epidemic: The Practice of Unsafe Abortion in Latin America," *Studies in Family Planning*. vol. 24, no. 4 (1993).
30. E. Royston and A. Lopez, "On the Assessment of Maternal Mortality," *World Health Statistics Quarterly*, vol. 40, no. 3 (1987).
31. Ann Oakley, *Essays on Women, Medicine and Health* (Edinburgh University Press, 1993); See also Dorothy Munyakho, "Poverty and ill-health go hand-in-hand," *World Health*, vol. 45, November-December 1992: 6-7, for a discussion of poverty in Nigeria, and efforts to improve literacy, health care, and sanitation.
32. Karen Harrison, "Maternal mortality in developing countries," *British Journal of Obstetrics and Gynaecology*, vol. 96, (1989).
33. Usha Stokoe, "Determinants of Maternal Mortality in the Developing World," *Australia and New Zealand Journal of Obstetrics and Gynaecology*, vol. 31, no. 1, (1991).
34. Irvine Louden, *Death in Childbirth: An International Study of Maternal Care and Maternal Mortality 1800-1950* (Oxford: Clarendon Press, 1991).
35. J. Caldwell and P. Caldwell, "High Fertility in Sub-Saharan Africa," *Scientific American*, (May 1990): 118-124.
36. Betsy Hartmann, *Reproductive Wrongs: The Global Politics of Population Control* (Boston: South End Press, 1995), 183.
37. Betsy Hartmann, *Reproductive Wrongs: The Global Politics of Population Control* (Boston: South End Press, 1995), 119.
38. Barbara Kwast, "Safe Motherhood — The First Decade," *Keynote Addresses: International Confederation of Midwives, 23rd International Congress* (London: International Confederation of Midwives, 1993), 15.
39. Carol Hird, *Midwives' Experiences of Safe Motherhood Programmes: A Literature Review and Survey* (London: Thames Valley University, 1996).
40. Richard Hebertson and Nelia Storey, "Ectopic Pregnancy," *Critical Care Clinics*, vol. 7, No. 4 (1991).
41. Ann Phoenix, "Black Women and Maternity Services," in *The Politics of Maternity Care: Services for Childbearing Women in Twentieth-Century Britain*, Jo Garcia, Robin Kilpatrick and Martin Richards, eds. (Oxford: Oxford University Press, 1990).
42. Rosemary Murphy, "Nurses as/and Mothers," in *Limited Edition: Voices of Women, Voices of Feminism*, Geraldine Finn, ed. (Halifax: Fernwood Publishing, 1993), 40.
43. Carol Hird, *Midwives' Experiences of Safe Motherhood Programmes: A Literature Review and Survey* (London: Thames Valley University, 1996).
44. Maria Mies, *Patriarchy and Accumulation on a World Scale: Women in the International Division of Labour* (London: Zed Books, 1991).
45. Joni Seager and Ann Olson, *Women in the World: An International Atlas* (London: Pluto Press, 1986), 7.
46. Isha Daramy-Kabia, "The Training of Traditional Birth Attendants for Safe Motherhood: Magbil, Sierra Leone," *Proceedings of the 23rd Congress of the International Confederation of Midwives: Volume I* (Vancouver: ICM, 1993); Mary Kensington, "Safer Motherhood — A midwifery challenge," in *Midwifery Practice: A Research-Based Approach*, Jo Alexander, et al, eds. (London: MacMillan, 1993), 126-127.

47. Barbara Kwast, "Safe Motherhood — The First Decade," *Keynote Addresses: International Confederation of Midwives, 23rd International Congress* (London: International Confederation of Midwives, 1993).
48. Rosemary Murphy, "Nurses as/and Mothers," in *Limited Edition: Voices of Women, Voices of Feminism,* Geraldine Finn, ed. (Halifax: Fernwood Publishing, 1993), 40.
49. Canadian International Development Agency, *Strategy for Health: Draft for Discussion* (Hull: CIDA, 1996).
50. E. Royston and S. Armstrong, "Preventing maternal deaths," *World Health Organization.* (Geneva: WHO, 1989).
51. World Health Organization, *Mother Baby Package: Implementing safe motherhood in countries* (Geneva: WHO/FHE/MSM/, 1995).
52. Duangvadee Sungkhobol, "Inspirational Talk: Precongress," *Keynote Addresses* (Vancouver: ICM, 1993).
53. Boston Women's Health Book Collective, *The New Our Bodies, Ourselves: A Book By and For Women* (Boston: Touchstone, 1992), 408.
54. Expert Maternity Group, *Changing Childbirth: Part I — Report of the Expert Maternity Group* (Department of Health: H.M.S.O., 1993).
55. Jenny Douglas, "Black Women's Health Matters: Putting black women on the research agenda," in *Women's Health Matters,* Helen Roberts, ed. (London: Routledge, 1992).
56. British Columbia, *Royal Commission on Health Care and Costs (The Seaton Report)* (Province of British Columbia, 1991).
57. Patricia Smyke, *Women and Health* (London: Zed Books, 1991).
58. Duangvadee Sungkhobol, "Inspirational Talk: Precongress," *Keynote Addresses* (Vancouver: ICM, 1993), 91.
59. Barbara Kwast, "Safe Motherhood — The First Decade," *Keynote Addresses: International Confederation of Midwives, 23rd International Congress* (London: International Confederation of Midwives, 1993), 13.
60. Patricia Smyke, *Women and Health* (London: Zed Books, 1991).
61. S. Thaddeus and Deborah Maine, "Too far to walk: Maternal Mortality in context," *Women's Global Network for Reproductive Rights Newsletter,* vol. 35, (1991): 24.
62. Jeanne Vickers, *Women and the World Economic Crisis* (London: Zed Books, 1993), 92
63. Sheila Rowbotham and Swasti Mitter, eds., *Dignity and Daily Bread: New forms of economic organising among poor women in the Third World and the First* (London: Routledge, 1994).
64. Noga Gayle, "Black Women's Reality and Feminism: An Exploration of Race and Gender," in *Anatomy of Gender: Women's Struggle for the Body,* Dawn Currie and Valerie Raoul, eds. (Ottawa: Carleton University Press, 1992), 237.
65. Barbara Kwast, "Safe Motherhood — The First Decade," *Keynote Addresses: International Confederation of Midwives, 23rd International Congress* (London: International Confederation of Midwives, 1993), 5.
66. Cheryl Johnson-Odim, "Common Themes, Different Contexts: Third World Women and Feminism," in *Third World Women and the Politics of Feminism,* Chandra Mohanty, Ann Russo, and Lourdes Torres, eds. (Bloomington: Indiana University Press, 1991), 320.
67. Brigitte Jordan, "Cosmopolitical Obstetrics: Some Insights from the Training of Traditional Midwives," *Social Science and Medicine,* vol. 28, no. 9, (1992).
68. Maria Mies, *Patriarchy and Accumulation on a World Scale: Women in the International Division of Labour* (London: Zed Books, 1991), 219-224.

69. Sari Tudiver, "Canada and the Global Context of the New Reproductive Technologies: A Cautionary Essay," in *Misconceptions, Volume 1: The Social Construction of Choice and the New Reproductive and Genetic Technologies*, Gwynne Basen, Margrit Eichler, and Abby Lippman, eds. (Hull: Voyageur Publishing, 1993).
70. Angela Davis, *Women Race & Class* (New York: Vintage Books, 1983), 220-221.
71. T.K. Sundari, "The Untold Story: How the Health Care Systems in Developing Countries Contribute to Maternal Mortality," *International Journal of Health Services*, vol. 22, no. 3, (1992): 524.
72. World Health Organization, *Mother Baby Package: Implementing safe motherhood in countries* (Geneva, 1995).
73. M. Marshall, "What Can We Do To Decrease Maternal Mortality? Life Savings Skills Training for Midwives," in *Proceedings: 23rd Triennial Congress, International Confederation of Midwives, Vol. III* (Vancouver: ICM, 1993).
74. Ministry of Health, B.C., *Policy Frameworks on Designated Populations* (Victoria, 1995).
75. Julia Allison, *Delivered at Home* (London: Chapman and Hall, 1996).

REFERENCES

Abou, Zahr Carla and Erica Royston. "Excessive hazards of pregnancy and childbirth in the Third World." *World Health Forum*, vol. 13, (1992): 343-345.

Adetoro, O.O. "A sixteen year survey of maternal mortality associated with eclampsia in Ilorin, Nigeria." *International Journal of Gynaecology and Obstetrics*, vol. 30, (1989): 117-121.

Allison, Julia. *Delivered at Home*. London: Chapman and Hall, 1996.

Atrash, Hani, Lisa Koonin, Lawson Herschel, Adele Franks and Jack Smith. "Maternal Mortality in the United States, 1979-1986." *Obstetrics and Gynaecology*, vol. 76, no. 6, (1990): 1055-1060.

Bachman, Ronet. *Death and Violence on the Reservation: Homicide, Family Violence, and Suicide in American Indian Populations*. New York: Auburn House, 1992.

Boston Women's Health Book Collective. *The New Our Bodies, Ourselves: A Book By and For Women* (updated, expanded edition). Boston: Touchstone, 1992.

British Columbia. *Royal Commission on Health Care and Costs (The Seaton Report)*. Province of British Columbia, 1991.

Burtch, Brian. *Trials of Labour: The Re-emergence of Midwifery*. Montréal: McGill-Queen's University Press, 1994.

Burtch, Brian, and Carol Hird. "A Case for Recognition." *World Health*, vol. 50, no. 2 (1997): 7-8.

Caldwell, J., and P. Caldwell, "High Fertility in Sub-Saharan Africa." *Scientific American*, (May 1990): 118-124.

Campbell, Jacquelyn, Catharine Oliver, and Linda Bullock. *AWHONN'S Clinical Issues*, vol. 4, no. 3 (1993): 343-349.

Canadian International Development Agency (CIDA). *Strategy for Health: Draft for Discussion*. Hull: CIDA, 1996.

Comack, Elizabeth. *Women in Trouble: Connecting Women's Law Violations to their Histories of Abuse*. Halifax: Fernwood Publishing, 1996.

Culhane-Speck, Dara. *An Error in Judgement: The Politics of Medical Care in an Indian/White Community.* Vancouver: Talonbooks, 1987.

Damary-Kabia, Isha. "The Training of Traditional Birth Attendants for Safe Motherhood: Magbil, Sierra Leone." In *Proceedings of the 23rd Congress of the International Confederation of Midwives: Volume I.* Vancouver: ICM, 1993.

Davis, Angela. *Women Race & Class.* New York: Vintage Books, 1983.

Department of Health. *Report on confidential enquiries into maternal deaths in the United Kingdom 1985-1987.* H.M.S.O., 1991.

Douglas, Jenny. "Black Women's Health Matters: Putting black women on the research agenda." In *Women's Health Matters.* Helen Roberts, ed. London: Routledge, 1992.

Duley, Lelia. "Maternal Mortality associated with hypertensive disorders or pregnancy in Africa, Asia, Latin America, and the Caribbean." *Journal of Obstetrics and Gynaecology,* vol. 99, (1992): 547-553.

Expert Maternity Group. *Changing Childbirth: Part I — Report of the Expert Maternity Group.* Department of Health: H.M.S.O., 1993.

Fildes, John, Laura Reed, Nancy Jones, Marcel Martin and John Barrett. "Trauma: The Leading Cause of Maternal Death." *The Journal of Trauma,* vol. 32, no. 5, (1992): 643-645.

Fortney, J.A. "Implications of the ICD — IO Definitions related to Death in Pregnancy, Childbirth or the Puerperium." *World Health Statistics Quarterly.* vol. 43, (1990): 246-248.

Gayle, Noga. "Black Women's Reality and Feminism: An Exploration of Race and Gender." In *Anatomy of Gender: Women's Struggle for the Body.* Dawn Currie and Valerie Raoul, eds. Ottawa: Carleton University Press, 1992.

Graham, Wendy and Oona Campbell. "Maternal Health and the Measurement Trap." *Social Science and Medicine,* vol. 35, no. 8, (1992): 967-977.

Harrison, K.A. "Maternal mortality in developing countries." *British Journal of Obstetrics and Gynaecology,* vol. 96, (1989): 1-3.

Hartmann, Betsy. *Reproductive Wrongs: The Global Politics of Population Control.* Boston: South End Press, 1995.

Hebertson, Richard and Nelia Storey. "Ectopic Pregnancy." *Critical Care Clinics,* vol. 7, No. 4 (1991): 899-915.

Hess, D.B. and Hess, W.L. "Management of Cardiovascular Disease in Pregnancy." *Obstetrics and Gynaecology Clinics of North America,* vol. 19, no. 4, (1992): 679-695.

Hird, Carol. *Midwives' Experiences of Safe Motherhood Programmes: A Literature Review and Survey.* Unpublished M.A. thesis, Degree in Midwifery Practice, Thames Valley University, London, England, 1996.

Högberg, U. "Historical Aspects on the Role of Maternal Care in Reducing Maternal Mortality" *Maternal Health Care in an International Perspective.* Proceedings, xxii Berzelius Symposium. Stockholm May 27-29, 1991. Uppsala University: WHO, 1992.

Human Rights Watch. *The Human Rights Watch Global Report on Women's Human Rights.* New York: Human Rights Watch, 1995.

Johnson-Odim, Cheryl. "Common Themes, Different Contexts: Third World Women and Feminism." In *Third World Women and the Politics of Feminism.* Chandra Mohanty, Ann Russo, and Lourdes Torres, eds. Bloomington: Indiana University Press, 1991.

Jordan, Brigitte. "Cosmopolitical Obstetrics: Some Insights from the Training of Traditional Midwives." *Social Science and Medicine,* vol. 28, no. 9, (1992): 925-944.

Kensington, Mary. "Safer Motherhood — A midwifery challenge." In *Midwifery Practice: A Research-Based Approach.* Jo Alexander, Valerie Levy, and Sarah Roch, eds. London: MacMillan, 1993.

Kitzinger, Sheila. "Why Women Need Midwives." In *The Midwife Challenge.* Sheila Kitzinger, ed. London: Pandora Press, 1988.

Kwast, Barbara. "Safe Motherhood: A challenge to midwifery practice." *World Health Forum,* vol. 12, (1991): 1-6.

--------. "Safe Motherhood — The First Decade." *Keynote Addresses: International Confederation of Midwives, 23rd International Congress.* London: International Confederation of Midwives, 1993.

Louden, Irvine. *Death in Childbirth: An International Study of Maternal Care and Maternal Mortality 1800-1950.* Oxford: Clarendon Press, 1991.

MacDonald, Martha. "Becoming Visible: Women and the Economy." In *Limited Edition: Voices of Women, Voices of Feminism.* Geraldine Finn, ed. Halifax: Fernwood Publishing, 1993.

McFarlane, Judith. "Battering During Pregnancy: Tip of an Iceberg Revealed." *Women & Health,* vol. 15, no. 3, (1989): 69-84.

Maine, Deborah. *Safe Motherhood Programs: Option and Issues.* New York: Center for Population and Family Health, Columbia University, 1991.

Marshall, M.A. "What Can We Do To Decrease Maternal Mortality? Life Saving Skills Training for Midwives." In *Proceedings: 23rd Triennial Congress, International Confederation of Midwives, Vol. III.* Vancouver: ICM, 1993: 1181-1195.

Maynard, Mary and June Purvis. *Researching Women's Lives from a Feminist Perspective.* London: Taylor & Francis, 1994.

Mies, Maria. *Patriarchy and Accumulation on a World Scale: Women in the International Division of Labour.* London: Zed Books, 1991.

Ministry of Health. *Policy Frameworks on Designated Populations.* Victoria, B.C. April 1995.

Munyakho, Dorothy. "Poverty and ill-health go hand-in-hand." *World Health,* vol. 45 (November-December 1992): 6-7.

Murphy, R. "Nurses as/and Mothers." In *Limited Edition: Voices of Women, Voices of Feminism.* Geraldine Finn, ed. Halifax: Fernwood Publishing, 1993.

Murphy-Black, T. *Identifying the Key Features in Continuity of Care in Midwifery.* Edinburgh: University of Edinburgh, 1993.

Oakley, Ann. *Essays on Women, Medicine and Health.* Edinburgh: Edinburgh University Press, 1993.

Paxman, John, A. Rizo, L. Brown, and J. Benson. "The Clandestine Epidemic: The Practice of Unsafe Abortion in Latin America." *Studies in Family Planning,* vol. 24, no. 4, (1993): 205-226.

Peters, Margaret. "A Challenge for Midwives: the reduction of maternal mortality and morbidity rates throughout the world." *Midwifery,* vol. 4, (1988): 3-8.

Phoenix, Ann. (1990) "Black Women and Maternity Services." In *The Politics of Maternity Care: Services for Childbearing Women in Twentieth-Century Britain.* Jo Garcia, Robin Kilpatrick, and Martin Richards, eds. Oxford: Oxford University Press, 1990.

Reid, Carol. "Sick to Death: The Health of Aboriginal People in Australia and Canada." In *Racial Minorities, Medicine, and Health.* B. Singh Bolaria and Rosemary Bolaria, eds. Halifax: Fernwood Books, 1994.

Roopnarinesingh, S., A. Ali and B. Bassan. "Is Adolescent Pregnancy Hazardous?" *West Indian Medical Journal*, vol. 42, (1993): 22-23.

Rowbotham, Sheila and Swasti Mitter, eds. *Dignity and Daily Bread: New forms of economic organising among poor women in the Third World and the First.* London: Routledge, 1994.

Royston, E and S. Armstrong. "Preventing maternal deaths." *World Health Organization.* Geneva: WHO, 1989.

Royston, E. and A. Lopez. "On the Assessment of Maternal Mortality." *World Health Statistics Quarterly*, vol. 40, no. 3, (1987): 223.

Scupholme, Anne, Jeanne DeJoseph, Donna Strobino, and Lisa Paine. (1992). "Nurse-Midwifery Care to Vulnerable Populations: Phase I: Demographic Characteristics of the National CNM [Certified Nurse-Midwife] Sample." *Journal of Nurse-Midwifery*, vol. 37, no. 5, (1992): 341-347.

Seager, Joni and Ann Olson. *Women in the World: An International Atlas.* London: Pluto Press, 1986.

Smyke, Patricia. *Women and Health.* London: Zed Books, 1991.

Stokoe, U. "Determinants of Maternal Mortality in the Developing World." *Australia and New Zealand Journal of Obstetrics and Gynaecology*, vol. 31, no. 1, (1991): 8-16.

Sundari, T.K. "The Untold Story: How the Health Care Systems in Developing Countries Contribute to Maternal Mortality." *International Journal of Health Services*, vol. 22, no. 3, (1992): 513-528.

Sungkhobol, Duangvadee. "Inspirational Talk: Precongress." (ICM/WHO/UNICEF) Safe Motherhood Workshop. International Confederation of Midwives 23rd International Congress. *Keynote Addresses.* Vancouver: International Confederation of Midwives, 1993.

Thaddeus, S., and Deborah Maine. "Too Far to Walk: Maternal Mortality in Context." *Women's Global Network for Reproductive Rights Newsletter*, vol. 35, (1991): 23-26.

Tudiver, Sari. "Canada and the Global Context of the New Reproductive Technologies: A Cautionary Essay." In *Misconceptions, Volume 1: The Social Construction of Choice and the New Reproductive and Genetic Technologies.* Gwynne Basen, Margrit Eichler, and Abby Lippman, eds. Hull: Voyageur Publishing, 1993.

Vickers, Jeanne. *Women and the World Economic Crisis.* London: Zed Books, 1993.

World Health Organization. *Maternal Mortality, Ratios and Rates: A Tabulation of Available Information* (3rd edition). Geneva: WHO/MCH/MSM/Division of Maternal and Child Health and Family Planning, 1991.

--------. *Mother Baby Package: Implementing safe motherhood in countries.* Geneva: WHO/FHE/MSM/94.11, 1995.

World Health Organization and International Confederation of Midwives. *Women's health and the midwife: A global perspective. Report of a collaborative pre-congress workshop.* The Hague: WHO/Maternal Child Health, 1987.

Wotherspoon, Terry and Vic Satzewich. *First Nations: Race, Class, and Gender Relations.* Toronto: Nelson Canada, 1993.

SECTION II

State Regulation of Midwifery Across Canada

Becoming Regulated:

The Re-emergence of Midwifery in British Columbia

J. Alison Rice

INTRODUCTION

In British Columbia, midwifery has become a self-regulated profession. The regulatory body, the College of Midwives of British Columbia (CMBC), has been established and initial regulations are in place. The first registered midwives will be practising in early 1998. As elsewhere in Canada, the struggle in British Columbia to establish midwifery as a regulated profession has been a lengthy process. The decision to seek status as a regulated profession was a deliberate one. This choice has already shaped and will continue to shape the profession as it re-emerges.

Two fundamental issues are interwoven into the story of the re-emergence of midwifery in British Columbia. These are: access to midwifery care and maintaining what can be described as the *spirit of midwifery*. Access to midwifery care means that childbearing women who want a midwife as their primary caregiver are able to have one. Access has a number of prerequisites including publicly funded midwifery services, culturally relevant and sensitive care, and an adequate number of midwives throughout the province. Midwifery education too, needs to be accessible to ensure a future supply of midwives.

The spirit of midwifery embodies what is unique about midwifery care, what distinguishes midwifery care from conventional medical care for childbearing women. The spirit of midwifery encompasses the values and beliefs of the profession. The model of midwifery care is based on these values and beliefs. In recounting the formal steps that have led to regulation in British Columbia, the challenges of creating a model that remains true to the spirit of midwifery and the provision of accessible midwifery care will be explored.

THE IMPETUS FOR THE RE-EMERGENCE OF MIDWIFERY

The history of midwifery in British Columbia parallels that of the rest of Canada. Both Aboriginal peoples and the immigrant settlers relied on designated community members to assist in childbirth. Apart from a few immigrant women, these midwives lacked any formal training in the regulatory sense.[1] With the rise of an organized and formally educated medical profession, attendance at childbirth was claimed by medicine as falling within its domain. Legislation regulating medical practice, and later entrenchment of the physician as the gatekeeper into the formal healthcare system under Medicare, effectively solidified a state-sponsored medical monopoly over childbirth.[2] Midwifery continued to be tolerated only where there were few or no doctors.

The re-emergence of midwifery in British Columbia has its roots in the social trends of the late 1960s and the 1970s: the resurgence of feminism, the women's health movement, the questioning of established social institutions expressed notably in the counterculture and consumerism. Women sought control over their bodies particularly in the area of reproduction. Grassroots organizations of lay women and a few health professionals began to question the medicalization of pregnancy and childbirth. The midwifery model began to take shape under these influences. A spirit of self-help added fuel to the midwifery movement.

Re-emergence of midwifery was most evident in segments of communities with a distinctive counterculture flavour, including the Gulf Islands and the West Kootenays. Although the number of midwives practising in these areas has varied over time, women in these communities have continued to seek the care of midwives. The greater Vancouver area, however, was and continues to be the centre for organized political activity. The counterculture roots of midwifery have a down side. Established healthcare providers have frequently dismissed midwives and their supporters as a 'hippie' fringe element. With such labelling it has been difficult for midwives to be taken seriously. Yet midwives have gained a political voice, lobbying with increasing sophistication, frequently surprising their opponents with a clearly articulated vision and research to support the vision. Midwives who have chosen the path of integration and regulation have learned to use the tools of the dominant medical culture particularly in arguing for home birth as a choice for women.

Midwifery Values

In some areas of British Columbia, counterculture ideals originating in the 1960s and 1970s have a persistent influence. These values included; rural life, self-sufficiency, and individual freedom. The distrust of technological approaches was evident not just in health care, but in many facets of life. Belief in the normal processes of pregnancy and childbirth combined with an avoidance of medical intervention was espoused. Many alternative approaches or complementary therapies that have come to be associated with midwifery and to be integrated into midwifery care originated in this earlier era. An example is the use of traditional herbal remedies rather than pharmacological agents. Other alternative and complementary therapies, for example aromatherapy, continue to be introduced and explored by midwives. But important to the spirit of midwifery is the nature of the relationship between the woman and the caregiver. Midwives were seen as the ideal practitioners to provide an alternative to conventional obstetrical care. Although women who seek midwifery care cannot easily be characterized, it is possible to describe a set of values and beliefs espoused by many of these women. These values and beliefs are generally shared by practising activist-midwives and their supporters. These include: the values of women's autonomy, and equality between the provider and the woman; beliefs about open communication, information sharing; respect for the natural processes of pregnancy and childbirth; and avoidance of unnecessary technology. Midwives describe themselves as the guardians of normal childbirth. In contrast to many countries where midwives have a role in the care of all childbearing women, high-risk as well as low-risk, Canadian midwives aspire to provide primary care to low-risk women. Involvement with women who seek midwifery care and later develop complications requiring medical management is limited to a supportive role, thus providing some continuity. This feature of the midwifery model of care — midwife as primary healthcare provider for low-risk women — excludes women who begin a pregnancy with conditions or with a health history that labels them as high-risk. Continuity of care is another midwifery value and frequently espoused as a distinguishing feature. To midwives this means a promise to the woman that the midwife attending her during labour and birth will be one with whom she has formed a trusting relationship. It is expected not only that the woman will know the midwife, but also that the midwife must know the woman well enough to understand her unique concerns. An essential facet of the relationship and a core midwifery value is woman-centred care. The whole experience revolves around the woman and her family as she defines it.

As we move into an era of regulation, midwives have been determined to remain true to these values and beliefs which constitute the *spirit of midwifery*. Although midwives do recognize that regulation will pose a challenge to some of these tenets of midwifery care, the paradox of seeking regulation as a means of gaining freedom to practise and choice for women has received little attention. Some express fear of what professionalization will do to midwifery and to midwifery care. Not all midwives in British Columbia support the goal of regulated midwifery. More will be said later about the opposition to regulation.

Legal and Practice Context

In British Columbia, unlike in Ontario and some other Canadian provinces, the law specifically prohibited midwives from practising their profession. Section 72, of the *Medical Practitioners Act*[3] gave the exclusive privilege of practising medicine, surgery and *midwifery* to members of the College of Physicians and Surgeons. Midwives practising in the community were practising illegally and risked being charged with practising medicine without a license. Burtch[4] details efforts by the state to control midwifery practice, most notably through coroner's inquests but in one case through criminal charges. Despite the constant threat of such actions by the state, midwives did practice and a small number of women chose midwifery care.

For most women, midwifery care in British Columbia has meant home birth and care outside the formal and regulated healthcare system. Women who lived in areas where midwives practised were able to contract for care and have access to midwifery care. Some were willing to travel long distances to have a midwife. Midwives generally charged a fee for an entire course of care, including the prenatal care, labour and birth care and postnatal care for the woman and her infant. Obviously, in the context of publicly funded, universally accessible health care, having to pay privately for midwifery care limits accessibility. Some families could not afford midwifery care despite accommodation by midwives with sliding fee scales and installment plans. When home birth was planned, the midwife acted as the primary care-provider throughout the childbearing cycle. However, if the woman chose to give birth in hospital, a physician acted as the primary caregiver for the birth. When a midwifery client had a hospital birth, whether planned or as the result of transfer of care, the midwife acted in a supportive role for the labour, usually referred to as a 'labour coach.' Direct involvement in care depended on a number of factors, such as the attitude of the nursing staff and the reputation of a particular midwife. Over time, some midwives established positive professional relationships, whereas others continue to be treated with suspicion and animosity by hospital staff.

Midwives and their clients relied on sympathetic physicians for back-up during pregnancy, during the birth and after, and for access to healthcare services that the midwife could not provide, such as laboratory tests. Usually this meant that the woman saw both her physician and her midwife or midwifery group during the course of pregnancy. In situations where a woman planned a home birth and a sympathetic physician was not available, she had two choices: keep her plans for birth at home secret or avoid medical care.

Few physicians actively participated in home birth. Both the College of Physicians and Surgeons of British Columbia and the British Columbia Medical Association opposed home birth. The current policy of the College of Physician and Surgeons of British Columbia[5] says, "there is at this time no place for planned home delivery in the province of B.C." Through their policies they were able to prevent physicians from participating in home birth. Risks of such participation for physicians included not being covered by professional liability insurance and the threat of professional disciplinary measures.

Hospital-based Midwifery

One midwifery service did provide hospital-based care. The Grace Hospital Midwifery Program, now the British Columbia Women's Hospital Midwifery Practice, has its origins in 1981 with two midwives and a supportive obstetrician at Vancouver General Hospital. Soon after, in 1982, four midwives with the back-up of four obstetricians began to practise at the then new Grace Hospital. Harvey, Kaufman and Rice[6] describe the development of this service and discuss the role that this and other hospital-based midwifery programs have played in the evolution of midwifery in Canada. Because of the legal situation in British Columbia, special permission was sought from the College of Physicians and Surgeons of B.C. to allow midwives to practise at the Grace Hospital. The College of Physicians and Surgeons allowed the midwives to practise in this one hospital but imposed conditions. They asked that all the midwives be Registered Nurses with recognized midwifery qualifications. The official voices for medicine continue to believe in a nurse-midwifery model. Medical control was further exerted by requiring direct supervision of the midwives by physicians. This was interpreted to mean presence of a physician at the birth as well as ongoing involvement by physicians in the care through chart reviews. Although the midwives have established collegial relationships with the back-up physicians, now Family Practitioners, this continuing requirement inhibits the true autonomy of the midwives. Within the midwifery community opinion is divided about the value of this hospital-based model. Although recognized as having elements of tokenism, the practice has a long record of providing care for women whose choice of birth place is the hospital. The Midwifery Practice at B.C. Women's Hospital continues to attract women and the demand continues to exceed the enrollment capacity. With regulation the organizational arrangements for the Midwifery Practice will change. What is not yet certain is whether the Practice will continue to have a presence in or an affiliation with B.C. Women's Hospital.

PERSPECTIVES ON REGULATION

Both community-based and hospital-based midwives in British Columbia have advocated the legalization of midwifery and have been active in working towards the integration of midwifery into the healthcare system. The principle of multiple routes of entry to the midwifery profession was staunchly promoted within the Midwives Association of British Columbia and has also been the stance of the Midwifery Task Force. Outside of these organizations there have been different visions of the future of midwifery, some of which prevail despite the establishment of the College of Midwives. The Registered Nurses Association of British Columbia (RNABC), although recently declaring support for an autonomous midwifery profession, long held the position that nurse-midwives should be allowed to practise midwifery and be regulated under the *Nurses (Registered)* Act 1979.[7] In January 1997, the RNABC shifted from this position and recognized that midwives will be regulated by the CMBC. Nurses are divided, still, on the establishment of midwifery as an autonomous profession. Those who have been active in the midwifery movement support the Midwives Association of British Columbia and College of Midwives of British Columbia model of midwifery practice. Others will continue to look to the RNABC to have their advanced practice skills recognized, but most show little interest in leaving secure nursing employment, particularly to make the shift from predictable work schedules.

Another perspective on the regulation of midwifery is put forward by a small group of women who practice in the Lower Mainland of British Columbia and call themselves the Community of B.C. Midwives. These women have called for decriminalization of midwifery rather than state regulation. This perspective recognizes that regulation will require midwives to adhere to practice standards and to practise within the scope of practice as defined by the College of Midwives of British Columbia. One of these women, Gloria Lemay, has been described in the press as a "controversial midwife."[8] The most outspoken opponent of regulated midwifery, Lemay has conducted her opposition largely through the media. In a letter to the editor she critiqued a spokesperson for Midwives Association of British Columbia (this author) for saying that registration of midwives is necessary to ensure public safety. She further attacked those working for regulation, challenging them to "quit going to meetings and start delivering babies."[9] In the same article Lemay says that her "dream is that B.C. will become the place in North America with the most choice in childbirth. Women will fly here from all over to avail themselves of these choices."[10] It is here, over the issue of midwifery care for home birth, that the compromises necessary for regulating midwifery become most obvious. To achieve greater access for all women, some women will not have access. Registered midwives will only be able to agree to care for women who are low-risk and who meet certain criteria. Additional criteria will apply to planned home birth. Midwives who fail to practise according to the standards of the CMBC risk professional disciplinary measures including losing the privilege of practising.

Accessibility to midwifery care then, is paradoxically limited under regulation. It appears that only a few women currently practising as midwives in the community hold the view that all women, regardless of risk factors, should have access to midwife-attended home birth. Members of both the CMBC and the MABC, bolstered by research describing the conditions which most favour a safe home birth, support the introduction of defined guidelines, standards and protocols. They see these as essential to gaining credibility and recognition as a legitimate profession. Nonetheless, debate continues on the extent to which women's wishes can be accommodated within a regulated system. The College now has a policy to guide registered midwives in caring for women requesting continuing care which would not be in accordance with the College Standards. This policy guides midwives in situations where the unacceptable alternative would be to abandon the woman.

The view that midwives must care for all women who seek their care and care for all women in the woman's choice of birth place has not prevailed. Those who espouse the decriminalization model rather than a regulated system have neither sought representation within the bodies dealing with the integration of midwifery into the healthcare system, nor articulated a credible alternative vision. The organized midwifery movement in British Columbia as represented by the Midwives Association of British Columbia has achieved cohesion on key issues. This cohesion has lead to agreement on the articulated midwifery model of care and has meant that energies of the movement have been harnessed towards the goal of legalization. Nonetheless contentious issues remain and other will undoubtedly arise. Among these is how to deal with unregistered practitioners.

EVENTS AND ACTIVITIES LEADING TO REGULATED MIDWIFERY

A pivotal event in the history of midwifery in British Columbia was the first "Midwifery is a Labour of Love" conference held in Vancouver in February 1980.[11] Various groups, including lay midwives and consumer organizations, called for the legalization of midwifery and the integration of midwifery services into the healthcare system. Energized by local and international speakers, midwives and consumers formed two organizations: the B.C. Association of Midwives (later renamed the Midwives Association of British Columbia, MABC) and the Interdisciplinary Midwifery Task Force (now called the Midwifery Task Force, MTF). The Association of Midwives set out to unite midwives and to promote the midwifery profession. The goal of the Association from the start was "to improve the quality of care available to the childbearing family, and to enhance the safety and flexibility of childbearing by promoting the legalization of midwifery."[12] The MABC, over time, promoted itself as the *de facto* professional organization. Policy documents intended to set standards for the practice and conduct of midwifery practice were developed. These included: a Philosophy of Midwifery Care, a Code of Ethics, Standards of Practice and Core Competencies, a Statement on Home Birth, Criteria for Medical Consultation and Transfer of Primary Responsibility.[13] A review process was instituted to inquire into complaints against member midwives.

Midwives from diverse backgrounds joined the Association. Some had both nursing and midwifery qualifications. Some had trained as direct-entry midwives and others came to midwifery through apprenticeship and self-study. Most have acquired more education and experience over time. The applicants for initial registration with the College of Midwives of British Columbia reflect this diversity of backgrounds. The implications of this diversity will be explored in relation to the activities of the College of Midwives of British Columbia.

The Midwives Association of British Columbia sought international recognition by applying to, and in August 1984 being accepted as a member organization of, the International Confederation of Midwives (ICM). It was undoubtedly an unorthodox step for the ICM to recognize a midwifery association that represented unregulated midwives and indeed an association in a jurisdiction where to practise midwifery was illegal. Nonetheless, promotion of midwifery internationally is one of the goals of the ICM. Membership in the ICM provided support and networking for the Midwives Association of British Columbia. This support has been drawn on in a number of ways, including to support the education for B.C. midwives.

The consumer voice in promoting midwifery and access to midwifery care has been represented by the Midwifery Task Force (MTF). Initially there was active involvement of healthcare professionals in the activities and the organization of the MTF. Over time, the work of the MTF came to be carried out almost exclusively by lay people, many of whom are consumers who have had midwifery care for a home birth. A number of the most actively involved women are both consumers of midwifery services and aspiring midwives. All along there has been a close liaison between the Midwives Association of British Columbia and the Midwifery Task Force. Both organizations actively promoted midwifery, both at the community level and by lobbying efforts directed at government. Both engaged in efforts to educate the public about the nature of midwifery care and its benefits.

Lack of political support for midwifery thwarted early efforts. Consumers continued to seek care and midwives continued to practise. Midwives who felt drawn to the profession but who lacked formal education took matters into their own hands by organizing a private midwifery school. With support from the Midwifery Task Force, the B.C. School of Midwifery took in two classes of midwives, in 1984 and in 1985. The school sought legitimacy for the program by getting accreditation in Washington State. Those who completed the program were able to write the Washington State licensing examination and apply for a license in that state. Those who successfully completed this process added the title 'Licensed Midwife' to their qualifications.

Formal Hearings
Prior to 1990, the provincial government did not respond to either consumer demands for midwifery care nor to the recommendations from Coroners' Courts that called for the regulation of midwifery. Without government support there had been no mechanism for achieving the necessary legislative reforms. In March 1990, the *Health Professions Act* was proclaimed. This Act established a Health Professions Council to hear applications from previously unregulated groups wishing to become regulated. The purpose of

regulation of health professions, under the Act, is to protect the public. The need for protection arises from a potential of harm to the public if the practice of the profession is not regulated. The need for reform in the healthcare system went beyond the area of professional regulation. Public dissatisfaction with other aspects of health care and concern about the cost and efficacy of care, prompted governments across Canada to study the healthcare system.

Royal Commission on Health Care and Costs

The British Columbia government appointed a Royal Commission on Health Care and Costs in 1990. The Commission held public hearings throughout the province. This was an opportunity for the Midwives Association of British Columbia to extol their vision for midwifery — to describe the spirit of midwifery. In their written submission, the Midwives Association of British Columbia called for "the legislative reform necessary to fully integrate midwives into the existing health care framework."[14] The MABC reminded the Commission of a recommendation from a 1988 Coroner's Court that midwifery be legalized as an autonomous profession to care for low-risk women. Other groups also made their views on midwifery known, including the RNABC and the Midwifery Program at the Grace Hospital. The Commission took notice of the developments in Ontario and the arguments for and against direct-entry versus post-nursing midwifery preparation. Noting the number of nurses with midwifery qualifications, the Commission recommended the introduction of nurse-midwifery as a logical first step. In all the Commission recommended that:

- pending the establishment of a College of Midwifery:
    a. nurse-midwives be granted an appropriate scope of practice under the *Nurses (Registered) Act*;
    b. the *Medical Practitioners Act* be amended to provide an exemption to midwives; and
    c. midwives be allowed to deliver babies in hospitals.
- upon application, the Health Professions Council approve the establishment of a college to regulate the practice of midwifery.
- nurses be permitted to be members of both the RNABC and the College of Midwifery.
- costs associated with midwifery care not exceed those associated with physician care.[15]

The Commission seems to have been impressed with the positions of the Registered Nurses Association of B.C., the B.C. Medical Association and the College of Physicians and Surgeons of B.C. Concerns about healthcare costs, too, are noticeable throughout the report. However, what the recommendations missed was the consumer perspective. The continuing alliance between the MABC and the MTF meant that involved consumers and politically active midwives had a vision of a fully autonomous midwifery profession and saw no need for the recommended nurse-midwifery alternative, even as an interim step. Many saw nurse-midwives as extensions of the medical model. Nurse-midwives, along with physicians, were characterized as authoritarian and interventionist. There had been an awareness, all along, that to call for nurse-midwifery might be more expeditious but the midwifery movement was clear on the longterm goal. Consequently there was no effective support for this interim step, to introduce nurse-midwives. The MABC did act on the recommendation to apply for status under the *Health Professions Act*. A change of government also meant that the political climate favoured the necessary public policy initiative. The New Democratic Party (NDP) had long espoused support for the legalization of midwifery. With the NDP now forming the government, the stage was finally set for some real progress. In a message from the Minister of Health, Elizabeth Cull, on International Midwives Day, May 5, 1992 the MABC was urged to begin the process of legitimizing midwifery by applying to the Health Professions Council.[16]

Health Professions Council
In the summer of 1992, the Midwives Association of British Columbia applied to the Health Professions Council for designation as a self-regulating health profession. As with every application, stakeholders were notified of the MABC's application and given an opportunity to critique the submission and to appear at the public hearing. The public hearing was held on January 25, 1993. Various professional groups and consumers made formal presentations and responded to questions from the Council members. The Midwives Association of British Columbia, as the applicant, spoke last, addressing the major concerns arising from the other presentations. There was no opposition, at this hearing, to some form of regulation. Home birth was the most hotly debated issue, with consumers groups advocating for choice, whereas the other professional groups called for midwife-attended births to take place in hospitals and birth centres.

The response to the MABC's application and the subsequent hearing came on May 10, 1993 in a dramatic venue. The MABC had organized and was hosting the International Confederation of Midwives 23rd International Congress in Vancouver. Midwives from all over the world attended. It was to this audience of 2,500 cheering midwives that Elizabeth Cull announced the recommendations of the Health Professions Council and the government's intention to adopt these recommendations and to integrate midwifery into the healthcare system. Midwifery was to become an autonomous profession with a regulatory College. The Health Professions Council[17] described a scope of practice — caring for healthy women through normal pregnancy and birth —

and called for necessary changes in the healthcare system to enable the integration of midwifery. On the issue of home birth the Council expressed concern about the "controversy surrounding the safety of planned home birth"[18] and recommended "a demonstration project on planned home birth."[19] In a politically clever compromise the Minister said that a Home Birth Demonstration Project would be conducted, "not to examine if home births should be allowed..., but how they should be administered."[20] The emphasis of the Home Birth Demonstration Project would be how best to integrate homebirth services into the healthcare system. In her speech, Cull's rhetoric was that of choice for women. She stated her belief that midwives "are an essential part of women's reproductive choices,"[21] and further said, the "government is committed to increasing choices for pregnant women while ensuring the health and safety of mums and babies."[22]

The mainstreaming of midwives also fits with other government health reform initiatives — called *New Directions for a Healthy British Columbia*. The New Directions plan follows many of the recommendations in the *Closer to Home* report. Several philosophical underpinnings of New Directions are consistent with the midwifery model of practice. Greater public participation in healthcare decision-making at all levels is an example as is the movement of care from institutions to the home or other community sites. One aspect of New Directions that will affect the integration of midwifery is devolution of healthcare planning and management from the central Ministry of Health to Regional Health Boards. Regionalization presents challenges to the integration of midwifery, particularly if Regional Health Boards have to fund midwifery services from their own budgets. Medical services will continue to be funded centrally. Thus, there will be a fiscal disincentive for Regional Health Boards to provide for midwifery services unless the province dedicates funding for these services.

The announcement that the government would act to establish midwifery as a self-regulated profession marked a concrete step for midwives in re-claiming what they believe to be their rightful place in the care of childbearing women. Yet despite this government commitment, the goal of a midwifery model that captures the spirit of midwifery was not yet achieved. Although describing midwifery as a choice for women, on the subject of funding for midwifery care Cull[23] said only that the government would review issues such as public funding and payment options. It was clear that the government wanted to legalize midwifery without adding any cost to the healthcare system. Midwives could hear the voices of other stakeholders in the comments on funding. The cost of health care is increasingly under scrutiny. Spending on health care constitutes the biggest portion of the provincial budget. Across Canada, provincial governments were making cuts to health-care spending in response to a decrease in federal-to-provincial transfer payments and government debt. The New Right's agenda of debt and deficit reduction seemed to be becoming a necessity for political survival. It was in the face of growing government and public concerns about healthcare costs that the funding issue had to be addressed.

The Midwifery Implementation Advisory Committee

Action by the government on the Health Professions Council recommendations included the formation of a Midwifery Implementation Advisory Committee (MIAC). MIAC's purpose was to advise the government on various aspects of implementation including the scope of practice and regulations. Composed of staff from several Ministry of Health departments, a representative from the Ministry of Skills, Training and Labour and representatives of relevant stakeholder groups, MIAC first met in September 1993. For the first time an interprofessional group, with wide representation, would be meeting regularly. It was now time to talk about how to integrate midwives. MIAC continued through 1996, and until the approval of the College of Midwives of British Columbia Bylaws were completed in the spring of 1997, to advise the Ministry on a wide range of matters related to midwifery regulation and integration. Initially MIAC had the task of responding to draft regulations which included the scope of practice and provisions for Aboriginal midwifery.

For the first time attention was directed to Aboriginal midwifery. The Aboriginal Health Policy Branch within the Ministry of Health began to address the needs and wishes of Aboriginal peoples, *vis à vis* midwifery, following the announcement in May 1993 of the government's intention to regulate midwifery. At this point it is useful to digress from the historical account of midwifery politics to elaborate on Aboriginal midwifery in British Columbia. It is also relevant to point out that Aboriginal women are not the only women whose needs had not yet been addressed in efforts towards legalization.

Aboriginal Midwifery

In pursuing the goals of legalizing midwifery and access to midwifery care, neither the Midwives Association of British Columbia nor the Midwifery Task Force addressed the wishes of Aboriginal peoples. There had been no attempts, within these organizations, to identify Aboriginal midwives. Neither the submission of the Midwives Association of British Columbia to the Health Professions Council nor the Health Professions Council's recommendations addressed the subject of Aboriginal midwifery.[24] Attention had been drawn to the healthcare concerns of Aboriginal peoples generally by the Royal Commission on Health Care and Costs.[25] Work on treaty negotiations and self-government, including management of health services, was underway.

The history of treaty rights and negotiations in British Columbia is a dismal one. Earlier governments effectively denied Aboriginal land claims. Only recently have serious attempts been made to deal with claims to land title and demand for self-government.[26] Self-government is seen to include assuming responsibility for health care.

Benoit and Carroll[27] describe the story of Aboriginal midwifery in British Columbia as a missing narrative. The history of Aboriginal midwifery is in danger of being lost. Benoit and Carroll[28] further recount the many negative consequences that contact has had on Aboriginal peoples. Traditional birthing care and practices were disrupted and discredited as a result of the imposition of a patriarchal medical model. More generally, public policy under the *Indian Act*, particularly the treatment of women and the removal of children from their communities to residential schools, caused widespread cultural alienation.[29]

British Columbia has over 30 linguistically distinct Aboriginal groups. Each has its own unique culture and traditions.[30] Consequently there is no one model of midwifery among First Nations groups. To address the question of Aboriginal midwifery, the Aboriginal Health Policy Branch sponsored two focus groups. At the first, participants were asked to talk about key aspects of Aboriginal women's childbirth experiences, cultural needs and the regulation and education of midwives.[31] Focus group participants talked about losses they had suffered in relation to birthing traditions. State repression of traditional practices had occurred. Women had become distanced from the traditional ways as a result of residential schools and evacuation from their communities to hospitals for birth. Not surprisingly with this history there was reticence on the part of participants to reveal traditional practices and for traditional midwives to identify themselves.[32] Although, as previously mentioned there is great diversity among B.C. Aboriginal peoples, themes arising out of the meetings were identified as:

- respect for life, teachings, and preparation for birth and health
- both men and women were midwives
- parents and elders were teachers of traditional birth practices
- pregnant women were highly protected by older women in their community and close family members
- diet, exercise, rest, cleanliness and safety were stressed
- caring for women had a spiritual as well as a purely practical dimension
- the afterbirth and the cord had strong cultural symbolism and meaning
- the present system of childbirth is not meeting the needs of Aboriginal women.[33]

Draft midwifery regulations were the main topic of the second focus group. The government, in the regulations, made provision for both traditional Aboriginal midwives and for a future that would include Aboriginal midwives regulated by the College of Midwives of British Columbia. The draft regulations were released for public review on November 10, 1994. Under the regulations, a Committee on Aboriginal Midwifery is to be established within the College of Midwives of British Columbia. Final approval of the regulations was announced March 16, 1995.[34]

Aboriginal Midwifery Regulations

The following definitions relating to Aboriginal midwifery are included in the regulations:

1. In this regulation 'aboriginal' means relating to the Indian, Inuit or Métis peoples of Canada;

'aboriginal midwifery' means

(a) traditional aboriginal midwifery practices such as the use and administration of traditional herbs and medicines and other cultural and spiritual practices,

(b) contemporary aboriginal midwifery practices which are based on, or originate in, traditional aboriginal midwifery practices, or

(c) a combination of traditional and contemporary aboriginal practices;

'home birth demonstration project' means a study and evaluation of planned home births in British Columbia administered by the Ministry of Health and the Ministry Responsible for Seniors;

'reserve' means a reserve as defined in the *Indian Act*.[35]

A subcommittee of the College of Midwives of British Columbia is to be formed to establish registration requirements and standards of practice. Traditional Aboriginal midwives will be permitted to manage home births on reserves.

According to the Aboriginal Health Policy Branch,[36] Aboriginal midwives want to be recognized and want both validation of current practices and a revival of traditional birthing practices. The regulations are designed to achieve both of these goals. Much is expected of both traditional practitioners and the formally educated Aboriginal midwives of the future. By reclaiming birth and encouraging women to give birth within their own communities, culturally appropriate care can be provided. The possibility of healing extends to the whole community and culture. Aboriginal peoples expect to be involved in shaping all aspects of their midwifery care. A working group is to be formed with the Nuu-chah-nulth Health Board, located in the Port Alberni region of Vancouver Island, taking a lead in future developments. The process is a slow one. Aboriginal communities have many issues to deal with, and midwifery does not appear to be a priority in the absence of financial support for education and for implementation. Midwives have recognized that women from marginalized groups, such as Aboriginal women, potentially will benefit the most from midwifery care. Yet, without additional resources and an ample supply of midwives, the neediest women will not have access.

COLLEGE OF MIDWIVES OF BRITISH COLUMBIA

As mentioned above, the government announced, on March 16, 1995, Cabinet approval of regulations governing midwifery and establishing the College of Midwives of British Columbia. A nine-member board was also appointed at this time. In making the announcement, the Minister of Health, Paul Ramsey, reiterated the commitment of the government to greater choice for women in their health care.[37]

The Board of the College of Midwives of British Columbia is made up of six midwives and three public members. Under the *Health Professions Act*[38] at least one-third of the members of all health regulatory boards must be public members. Of the midwives appointed to this first Board, one is an Aboriginal midwife. The remaining five members are all practising non-aboriginal midwives, most of whom have active community practices. All are members of the MABC. The decision of the Ministry of Health and the Ministry Responsible for Seniors to appoint these women who have been doing home births in defiance of the law, points to the strength of the commitment to homebirth services.

Midwives Regulations

The Midwives Regulations, in addition to the provisions for Aboriginal midwifery, establish midwifery as a self-regulated profession. The scope of practice, vigorously debated at MIAC, is:

Scope of Practice
4 (1) Subject to the bylaws, registrants may:
> (a) assess, monitor, and care for women during normal pregnancy, labour, delivery, and the post-partum period,
> (b) counsel, support and advise women during pregnancy, labour, delivery and the post-partum period,
> (c) manage spontaneous normal vaginal deliveries,
> (d) care for, assess and monitor the healthy newborn, and
> (e) provide advice and information regarding care for newborns and young infants and deliver contraceptive services during the 3 months following birth.[39]

Most hotly debated was the extension of contraceptive services to a full three months — beyond the traditional six-week postpartum period. Opposition to inclusion of a full range of contraceptive services and any well-woman gynaecology came primarily from family physicians.

The midwives regulations also set out *Reserved Acts*:

5 (1) Subject to section 14 of the Act, no person other than a registrant may, for the purposes of midwifery,
> (a) conduct internal examinations of women during pregnancy, labour, delivery and the post-partum period,
> (b) manage spontaneous normal vaginal deliveries, and
> (c) perform episiotomies and amniotomies during established labour and repair episiotomies and simple lacerations.

(2) Subsection (1) does not apply on a reserve to an aboriginal person who practised aboriginal midwifery prior to the coming into force of this regulation.[40]

Midwives are also required, by regulation, to advise women to have a medical examination in the first three months of pregnancy. The requirement for medical consultation in the event of deviations from normal is also set out. Additional regulations relate to home birth and the Home Birth Demonstration Project.

The Home Birth Demonstration Project

As previously mentioned the Health Professions Council in its 1993 recommendations called for a homebirth demonstration project. Despite the studies presented by the Midwives Association of British Columbia and the consumer voices calling for homebirth services, the Health Professional Council called for further study into the safety of home birth. Thus the government decided to mount a Home Birth Demonstration Project (HBDP), not to determine if home births should be allowed, but rather how homebirth services can be administered effectively.

Home Birth Demonstration Project Regulations

The regulations pertaining to home birth and the HBDP are:

6. (2) No registrant is permitted to manage a planned home birth except as part of the home birth demonstration project.
   (3) Subsection (2) does not apply on a reserve to an aboriginal person who practised aboriginal midwifery prior to the coming into force of this regulation.

Sunset Clause[41]

8. 6. Section 6(2) and (3) and the definition of "home birth demonstration project" in section 1 are repealed December 31, 1998.[42]

The regulations define the Home Birth Demonstration Project as "a study and evaluation of planned home births in British Columbia administered by the Ministry of Health and the Ministry Responsible for Seniors."[43] The purpose of the project is to determine the best administrative and organizational arrangements for midwife-attended home births, to assess protocols for emergency and non-emergency transfer and for transfer of care to a physician. Data will be collected on outcomes but the numbers will be too small to make any statistical inferences. Consumer satisfaction will also be studied. The project is being funded by the Ministry.

The Home Birth Demonstration Project will begin once there are registered midwives and they begin to practise. All registered midwives and their clients who are planning for a home birth will be part of the study. The restriction of home birth to within the context of the Home Birth Demonstration Project is, perhaps, the most obvious example of the effect of regulation on choice. Protocols for the HBDP will require that the midwife and the client engage in an extensive dialogue about home birth and the risks and benefits inherent in this choice. Planned home birth with a registered midwife is possible only for low-risk women. The conditions and complications which preclude home birth will be detailed in the consent process. Women must agree to comply with the protocols for the HBDP which include indications for transfer. The midwife must ensure that conditions which favour a safe home birth are met. These include certain equipment and back-up arrangements in the event that transfer, especially emergency transfer, is necessary. Most contentious is the distance from an obstetrical unit. Although the Ministry has not set a restriction on distance or travel time to a back-up hospital, some guidelines will inevitably influence midwives' advice and women's choices. The requirements of the project will exclude some women from the choice of planned homebirth care with a registered midwife as the primary caregiver. The inevitable consequence will almost certainly be continuing practise by a few nonregistrants, particularly those who already oppose such restrictions.

The mounting of the Home Birth Demonstration Project by the government represents a political compromise. Midwives argued eloquently for homebirth services as fundamental to the midwifery model of care and choice for women. The Health Professions Council called for a pilot study in selected communities in which "only specially qualified and experienced registrants"[44] would participate. Not satisfied with evidence from elsewhere of the relative safety of planned home births, they wanted B.C. outcome data as the basis for a definitive public policy decision on the issue of home birth. The government dealt with their recommendations by broadening the purpose of the Home Birth Demonstration Project and shifting the emphasis from safety to integration of midwife-attended planned home births into the formal healthcare system.

Funding of the HBDP by the Ministry will benefit the integration of midwifery generally. Development of informational materials for healthcare agencies and professions, work on emergency transfer issues and data collection tools are some concrete examples of useful components of the project. The Sunset Clause automatically ends the HBDP and restrictions on midwife-attended home births.[45]

FUNDING ISSUES

Of more urgent concern, following formation of the College of Midwives, however, was funding for midwifery services and for the work of the College. The *Health Professions Act*[46] requires health regulatory bodies to be self-funded by their registrants. Although, in the application to the Health Professions Council, the MABC suggested an interim regulatory body as a solution to allow for funding the early regulatory work, no such provision exists under the Act.[47] In the Council's *Recommendations on the Designation of Midwifery*,[48] reservations were expressed about the financial viability of a new College of Midwives given that the work would need to start before there were any registrants. Initially the government gave the College of Midwives a start-up grant of $75,000 and has continued to provide some funding. Prior to there being any registrants the MABC has been the only other source of funds. Members, at the 1995 Annual General Meeting, voted to donate a substantial amount which the MABC received after sharing the profits of the International Congress in 1993 with the International Confederation of Midwives. With the cost of running the Association and pending costs to support the integration of midwifery, the Association and the College were competing for these limited resources. While the College began work on required by-laws the MABC set about to secure public funding for midwifery services.

Funding for Midwifery Services

With the goal of establishing a College of Midwives accomplished in March 1995, the Midwives Association of British Columbia and the Midwifery Task Force turned their attention to the issue of funding. The government continued to repeat the rhetoric of choice for women. In the press release announcing the formation of the College, the Ministry of Health[49] said that, in regulating midwifery, government was providing choice and safe options for women. There was no mention of how midwifery was to be funded. "Support in principle" had been the catch phrase from government, but for midwives this vague promise was not enough. The MABC and the MTF throughout the rest of 1995 and into 1996, focused lobbying efforts on securing a commitment for publicly funded midwifery services. Using the government's own rhetoric of choice for women, both organizations emphasized that without public funding midwifery would not be a real choice for many women. The notion was also put forward that funding care provided by registered midwives would serve to discourage women from seeking care from nonregistrants. Both organizations sought meetings with government officials and politicians and encouraged letter-writing campaigns. Nonministry members of the Midwifery Implementation Advisory Committee also wrote key politicians and the Treasury Board. This latter support can be seen as a pivotal point in that key stakeholders, members of other regulated health professions, acted politically to support the integration of midwifery into the mainstream of the healthcare system. This support can in part be attributed to the group cohesion achieved after working on integration issues for over two years. Even more important, though, this type of support denoted that stakeholders had at last genuinely embraced the integration of midwifery and had a stake in its success. With a provincial election on the horizon, supporters of midwifery prepared to make midwifery funding an election issue. Just weeks before the election, the new Minister of Health, Andrew Petter, announced that the government would publicly fund midwifery care provided by registrants of the College beginning in 1996/97.[50]

A Remuneration and Benefits Working Group of the MABC had already started to meet with Ministry of Health officials to discuss how and how much midwives would be paid for providing midwifery services. For midwives, an important principle is that the funding must support the midwifery model of care. Despite government commitment to funding, little progress was made in the initial discussions because of a pending provincial election. There was great uncertainty over whether any commitment to funding would survive a change of government. This uncertainty ended when the New Democratic Party government was re-elected in May 1996. Work on funding midwifery care is continuing, with the goal of having the model clearly articulated and mechanisms in place for the first registrants.

The slim majority by which the NDP was re-elected was taken by many as a signal that economic restraint would be expected of the government. Healthcare costs, being such a large proportion of the provincial budget, will be carefully scrutinized. New programs are particularly vulnerable in this climate. One example is the disappearance of birth centres from the midwifery implementation agenda.

Birth Centres

The Royal Commission on Health Care and Costs[51] advocated the development of hospital-based birth centres. The Health Professions Council recommended that the "Ministry of Health encourage the organization of birthing centres in order to support the practice of midwifery, decrease costs, provide families with greater choice in health care services, and promote less interventionist health care."[52] Birth centres were being promoted, by these bodies and others, not so much as an additional choice but rather as an alternative to home birth. Formal agencies have considered the possibility of birth centres in British Columbia, including the Ministry of Health, Grace Hospital/B.C. Women's Hospital, and the Greater Vancouver Regional District. The latter body conducted a Birthing Centre Survey[53] which found a "high level of interest in birthing centres"[54] among childbearing women in the region. Despite this interest, birth centres have disappeared from the policy agenda most likely because of the capital costs involved. Although periodically groups of midwives had attempted to establish free-standing birth centres, midwives directed their efforts to ensuring that regulated midwifery care included home births. More important to midwives, at present, is the integration of midwifery into the current healthcare system and securing home birth as an option for women. As work of the College proceeds midwives also are preoccupied with their own professional futures.

COLLEGE OF MIDWIVES BY-LAWS

Early in May 1996 the Health Professions Council released, for public review, draft *Bylaws for the College of Midwives of British Columbia.*[55] These by-laws detail rules for conducting the business of the College, including: registration requirements, the inquiry and disciplinary process, Schedules of Drugs and Substances, and Screening and Diagnostic Tests. A minimum three-month period is required for public review of by-laws. The process took much longer. After responding to feedback from stakeholders and having been put through the Ministry of Health internal review processes, the by-laws received the required Cabinet approval on April 3, 1997.[56]

Midwives had been anxiously waiting to learn the process of and requirements for registration. These will have a major impact on the number of first registrants. Subsequent to the by-law approval, the CMBC invited potential applicants to begin the application process. There are to be two opportunities for midwives to apply under the initial registration provisions. The deadline for the first of these was June 20, 1997. The first applicants began, in the summer of 1997, to pass through a process of several steps to qualify for registration. These steps are: the assessment of the application file, a written examination, a skills examination, and an orientation program. Once successful in completing all of these steps, an applicant will become eligible to become registered as a midwife in British Columbia.

As was the case in Ontario, there will undoubtedly be some who cannot meet the requirements yet believe themselves to be competent to practise midwifery. Conflict and disappointment is inevitable. Much will depend on the availability of opportunities to fill in the gaps for those who fall short of the minimum qualifications. The hope is that some funding will be forthcoming for education and practice opportunities for these individuals. A step in this direction has been taken by the Ministry of Education, Skills and Training. A midwife was hired to assemble an inventory of resources that might be useful in helping midwives to upgrade or refresh their competencies.

One group, some of whose members feel wrongly excluded from eligibility to register, are nurses who have a midwifery qualification but who lack recent, full-scope experience. Many of these nurses are not well informed about the model of midwifery practice being introduced in British Columbia. Nevertheless, being a qualified midwife is part of their professional identity. It is hard for them to accept that in British Columbia they do not automatically qualify for registration nor will they be able to call themselves midwives. Most are trained overseas, particularly in the United Kingdom, but are not aware of the struggles of midwives and consumers there to reform childbirth services in ways that are consistent with the model being introduced in British Columbia.

As previously noted, the Registered Nurses Association of B.C. had long held that midwifery is a specialty of nursing and that they should regulate *nurse-midwives*. Although, as previously mentioned, RNABC recognizes that midwifery has been established as an autonomous profession in British Columbia with its own regulatory body, they now put forward the view that nurses with advanced skills in obstetrics should be able to "assist low-risk women to deliver babies in a controlled environment, such as a hospital."[57] This, the RNABC asserts, will provide an additional choice for childbearing women. In British Colombia there are many Registered Nurses who hold advanced obstetrical nursing or midwifery qualifications. Many of these nurses work in hospital maternity units where their previous training is an asset, yet they are restricted from practising to their full capability. It is too early to see whether the RNABC will have any success in promoting an expanded role for obstetrical nurses, or if women have an interest in planned, nurse-managed hospital births. Consumers, a driving force involved in the introduction of midwifery, support the model of midwifery as an autonomous profession.

Apart from their advocacy for a primary-care role for nurses with midwifery or advanced obstetrical nursing preparation, the RNABC has made positive contributions to the integration of midwifery. Their representatives have been active in MIAC and CMBC committees and have shown increasing comfort with the MABC and College of Midwives' vision and policies. An example of this cooperation has been on a MIAC subcommittee on nursing and midwifery relationships. This committee developed guidelines for communication between nurses and midwives both in the hospital and community settings during the prenatal, intrapartum and postpartum periods. This piece of work has been added to a B.C. Health Association manual for hospitals on the integration of midwifery. For nurses, the focus in the early period of midwifery integration will continue to be on nurse-midwife relationships — just one of a number of continuing issues.

CONTINUING ISSUES

Many challenges still lie ahead in integrating midwifery as a self-regulating profession in British Columbia. As a re-emerging profession, midwifery is entering a healthcare system that is under great pressure. Under New Directions many changes are already underway, such as regionalization. Governments are looking to reshape the way primary care is delivered and to ensure that care is both cost-effective and evidence-based. Some health workers are facing lay-offs as hospital beds are closed and budgets are cut. With the system in flux there are both opportunities and additional challenges for midwives. Undoubtedly funding is the biggest challenge, not just for direct midwifery services but also to support integration and education. Opportunities come from an increasing emphasis on consumer involvement in healthcare planning, and the movement of programs 'closer to home.' There are trends, too, to strengthen primary and preventive aspects of health care which fit well with the midwifery model of care. In integrating into this evolving healthcare system, midwives face the challenge of establishing themselves as competent professionals and members of the healthcare team.

Midwifery Supply

The number of initial registrants of the College of Midwives is likely to be small — fewer than 60 — including those who are granted conditional registration. Conditional registrants are those who do not meet all the registration requirements but who are close enough so that any deficits can be remedied with short courses or a period of supervised practice. An example might be midwives who have not attended a sufficient number of births in the last three years.[58]

Not all areas of the province will have registered midwives, limiting access for many women. Not only will there be an insufficient number to meet the expected demand, midwives will likely be clustered in a few regions, leaving large areas of the province with no exposure to regulated midwifery services. The initial number of midwives is a concern to midwives, to the government and to consumers. Midwives want to see their profession thrive and grow. With the focus of the College on the initial registration process, little attention has yet been paid to inter-provincial reciprocity or indeed to registration of midwives from other jurisdictions. In the absence of educational programs in British Columbia, new registrants will have to come from elsewhere once the in-province practising midwives have worked through the assessment process and achieved registration. Consumers are interested in having sufficient midwives to meet the demand. And demand is expected to grow once registered midwives are practising and publicly funded. The Ministry of Health is interested in numbers because of the obvious implications for funding midwifery services.

Integration

For midwives, integration means being able to provide care to women and their families in the community and attending women during labour and birth in the setting of the woman's choice, according to practice guidelines. It means having access to the same resources that would be available if the woman's primary caregiver were a physician. And it means being paid for their professional practice.

Both the CMBC and the MABC have been working to smooth the integration of midwives into the formal healthcare system. Integration committees are forming in some hospitals where midwives already have a presence. For midwives who have been working primarily in the community, encountering the bureaucracy and the institutional culture will be a challenge. Those accustomed to institutional settings will likely experience a new sense of freedom as well as the weight of responsibility for client care in the absence of institutional resources. But most midwives will be practising in groups and will provide support for other group members in both settings.

Some community midwives have already formed practice groups, while those new to community practice will have to form new groups or integrate into existing ones. Groups will have to accommodate members with conditional registration, balancing needs for supervision and continuity of care concerns. The rules of the College will have an impact on the organization of groups in that continuity of care is a standard that must be met. This means that practice group arrangements must ensure that each woman knows her primary midwife and the other members of the group who might provide care, especially those who may attend her in labour.

The funding model will affect practice arrangements, including support services for practices. Currently practising midwives are accustomed to frugality and doing without support staff to facilitate their work. They also are used to maintaining their own records but not to conforming with institutional record-keeping practices. The recording work of midwives is likely to expand dramatically to meet requirements such as peer review, interprofessional communication and quality assurance programs. Midwives will need new skills to take care of the paperwork demands. Many details still need to be worked out, such as data collection for the Home Birth Demonstration Project and tracking caseloads and transfers of care.

The greatest challenge, in the integration process, involves other health professionals. All the categories of reproductive healthcare providers must become familiar with the scope of practice of midwives in British Columbia and with the midwifery model of care. Now outdated notions about midwives and in particular about home birth will have to change. Other professionals will have to become convinced about the benefits of midwifery care and about the skills and competencies of midwives.

Education

The predominant view on midwifery education in British Columbia is that it be at the baccalaureate level. Many ideals have been expressed about the attributes of midwifery educational programs, including flexibility and ease of access. The roots of many community midwives are revealed in a loyalty to apprenticeship models and the desire to retain the positive elements of the apprenticeship system in formal midwifery education.

Some women who define themselves as aspiring midwives take their inspiration primarily from their own birth experiences at home with community midwives. They represent a diverse group impatient to begin their education. Their educational needs are diverse. Some already have university degrees, while others lack postsecondary education and favour nonacademic settings for their own midwifery preparation. In the absence of any government support for a provincial midwifery education program aspiring midwives have no access to formal education in British Columbia. Some are pursuing routes in other jurisdictions without any firm assurance that the preparation will be acceptable for registration in British Columbia. Achieving a program in British Columbia will certainly be a focus of political activity once the first registrants encounter the demand from women for midwifery care.

Remaining Challenges: Regulatory Perils

In British Columbia, little attention has been paid to the paradox inherent in a previously unregulated group seeking regulation as a way of gaining the freedom to practise. Some who actively support the establishment of a regulatory College of Midwives may be excluded from practising, and undoubtedly others who have not been involved will benefit from their work. The title midwife is, by regulation, a protected title in British Columbia. Thus, the mechanism seen as legitimizing midwifery will make it illegal for those who are not registered by the College to call themselves midwives or to practise as a midwife. Some who are now practising illegally according to the *Medical Practice Act* will also have the Midwifery Regulations, under the *Health Professions Act*, prohibiting them from continuing to practise.

A more problematic paradox is the belief, by midwives, that regulating midwifery is the best way to establish a women-centered midwifery profession, one that will truly be responsive to childbearing women and their families. In our regulated environment this appears to be the only way to gain admittance to the formal healthcare system, but the extent to which midwifery may change in entering the mainstream is not fully appreciated. There is a certain amount of naiveté evident in the midwifery community. This is most apparent in midwives who have not, in their practice, worked as accepted members of institutions. The persuasiveness of the biomedical model in healthcare institutions requires of midwives a constant struggle to adhere to their values. Furthermore, such institutions are still fundamentally patriarchal in character and largely unresponsive to agendas which do not fit with the dominant medical paradigm. Midwives, in gaining hospital admitting privileges to care for women who chose to give birth in hospital, will be subject to the rules of the institutions. Over time they will undoubtedly help to reshape the institutions, but compromises are inevitable. It is not just the institutions which midwives want to change. The very culture of childbirth, as experienced by most women, must change if midwifery values are to become mainstream. Davis-Floyd[59] and Mitford[60] both describe this culture in the American context, which is not very different from that in Canada. While midwives frown on active obstetrical management there are women who, according to Davis-Floyd,[61] want and assert their right to "technocratic birth." It may be difficult for some midwives to support women's choices when those choices include using technologies which are not necessary for safe outcomes, and further when the technologies themselves increase the likelihood of operative delivery and its accompanying risks.

A further problematic area, with which midwives will have to grapple, is the proclivity of professional regulatory bodies to act in self-interest and not purely in the public interest. Gross[62] asserts that for the most part regulation fails to protect the public. Drawing largely on examples from the medical profession he likens self-regulation to the fox guarding the chicken coop. The B.C. Royal Commission on Health Care and Costs[63] stated as one of the "necessary components of a health care system" that, "professional colleges must always put the public interest ahead of their own or their members' interests." The Government has responded by increasing the public representation on all health profession regulatory boards. All, as with the CMBC, are now required to have at least one-third public members. Increased public representation on such boards and adherence to basic midwifery values, such as sharing of knowledge, may increase the chance that the public interest will come first — but can we be confident, that an organized midwifery profession will, over time, exemplify public accountability over self-interest?

A final concern about midwifery regulation is the specifics of regulations. Two areas of difficulty stand out. First, is the rigidity of regulations and protocols. Reissman and Nathanson[64] criticize the widespread use of risk-scoring tools as a basis for managing childbirth. Although of some use in the study of large populations, their reliability in assessing individual women is questionable. Yet they are at present the only available tools upon which to base certain protocols, for example when it is necessary to transfer a woman to the care of an obstetrician, or from home to hospital for birth. The Home Birth Demonstration Project will make use of such protocols, excluding women from the choice of a midwife-attended home birth if they have risk factors on the exclusion list. Obviously such protocols can interfere with individualized care and with the midwife's judgment. Furthermore, defini-

tions of risk change over time. Regulations and protocols may not keep pace
with such changes.

Unregulated midwives, should they continue to practise, will undoubtedly step in to care for women who are denied access to regulated midwives
because of their risk factors. The consequence is almost certainly that some
women with recognized risk factors will seek the care of less qualified
practitioners.

A second, and related area of difficulty, concerns research-based practice.
Here a double standard exists in standard medical discourse. Midwives are
required, in order to gain legitimacy, to provide scientific evidence of the
efficacy of their practice. The parallel expectation of physicians is less
stringent, despite the efforts of governments to call for evidence-based care.
Obstetrics has been described as the least scientific of the medical specialties
and the least likely to abandon practices which have not been shown to be of
benefit. New technologies are introduced without adequate research to demonstrate benefit or to identify risks. Many instances of iatrogenic practices
and failed technologies form part of the history of women's health care in
Canada and elsewhere. Prominent examples include DES and thalidomide. A
less obvious example is the adoption of routine electronic fetal heart-rate
monitoring in labour. Although midwives have opposed this technology for
years, citing reliable studies of lack of benefit and increased Caesarean
section rates, many units continue to use this technology routinely and
unnecessarily. Medical hegemony overpowers reasoned, research-based discourse, making it difficult for midwives to effect change. When midwives do
attempt to change institutionalized birth practices, there is remarkable resistance and a demand for research demonstrating the benefits of the proposed
approaches. Often these are not new technologies but rather long-standing
midwifery approaches in use in other countries where midwives practice, for
example, birthing stools. In contrast, when objective data, which do not
support the medical paradigm of childbirth, are presented the findings may
be dismissed or yet more evidence demanded.

The debate surrounding home birth perhaps best exemplifies this particular paradox and dispels any remaining *naive notion* that the facts are what
are important in the hegemonic medical discourse. In British Columbia, the
Home Birth Demonstration Project is evidence of the strength of a particular
prevailing medical view — that home birth is unsafe. Even though the
government cleverly shifted the emphasis of the project away from the safety
of home birth and on to the administrative aspects of homebirth services, the
political need for the project is rooted in the power of medical opinion. The
Sunset Clause in the Midwives Regulation[65] gives reassurance that midwives
will have more control over homebirth services after 1998. No doubt by then
midwifery will have gained enough of a foothold in the formal healthcare
system so that self-regulation will be a more meaningful reality.

CONCLUSION

Midwives are on the brink of a new era in British Columbia. By 1998 only registrants of the College of Midwives of British Columbia will be sanctioned as legitimate midwives. Publicly funded midwives will be in place and women will have the choice of a regulated midwife as primary caregiver. But many of the challenges will continue.

Choice will be limited because of the supply of midwives. Although midwifery care will be accessible without direct cost to women, access is not just about the cost of services. Frequently, marginalized women lack access to care alternatives because of lack of access to information. This is especially true for women who lack English language skills. The midwifery community in British Columbia has little history of reaching out to disadvantaged and marginalized women. Midwives will have to face this issue if they are to claim to be accessible.

Meaningful access to midwifery care for all who desire it is one value that will take some time to achieve. We will also have to wait to see the extent to which midwives in British Columbia are able to establish practices which exemplify their other traditional values and beliefs. Will midwifery practices empower women to make informed choices? Will midwives, once they have professional status, continue to have egalitarian partnerships with the women they serve?

The extent to which midwives remain true to the *spirit of midwifery* will depend on them and on others in the system. Ultimately, as more women experience midwifery care and work in partnership with midwives, it will be the childbearing women who will reshape the culture of childbirth.

ENDNOTES

1. Midwives, whether they practised in Aboriginal communities or with settlers and their descendants, undoubtedly learned in apprenticeship or informal relationships with experienced practitioners. In some communities this may have been formally recognized within the cultural context. It is in the Western educational and regulatory sense that lack of formal training is meant here.
2. Brian Burtch, *Trials of Labour: The Re-emergence of Midwifery* (Montreal & Kingston: McGill-Queen's University Press, 1994).
3. *Medical Practitioners Act*, R.S.B.C. (1979) c.254.
4. Burtch, *Trials of Labour: The Re-emergence of Midwifery.*
5. College of Physicians and Surgeons of British Columbia, *Policy Manual* (Vancouver: 1995), M7-1.
6. Sheila Harvey, Karyn Kaufman and Alison Rice, "Hospital-based Midwifery Projects in Canada," in *Issues in Midwifery,* ed. Tricia Murphy-Black, (Edinburgh: Churchill Livingstone, 1995).
7. Health Professions Council, *Recommendations on the Designation of Midwifery* (Victoria: Government of British Columbia, 1993).
8. Rebecca Wigod, "Midwife, Claiming Coroner Seeks to Blame, Waits for Court's Say on Baby-death Petition," *The Vancouver Sun* (June 26, 1995), A3.

9. Gloria Lemay, "Midwifery Must Deliver on its Promise," *The Vancouver Sun* (June 16, 1996), A20.
10. Ibid.
11. Maternal Health Society, *Midwifery is a Labour of Love* (Vancouver: 1981).
12. Ibid., 96.
13. Midwives Association of British Columbia, *Information Packet* (Vancouver: 1993).
14. Midwives Association of British Columbia, "Submission to the Royal Commission on Health Care and Costs" (Unpublished paper, Vancouver, 1990), 4.
15. British Columbia Royal Commission on Health Care and Costs, *Closer to Home: The Report of the British Columbia Royal Commission on Health Care and Costs, Volume 2* (Victoria: Ministry of Health and the Ministry Responsible for Seniors, Province of British Columbia, 1991), D-22.
16. British Columbia Health Minister, "Fax Message to be Read on Behalf of the Honourable Elizabeth Cull, Minister of Health and Minister Responsible for Seniors" [on International Midwives Day], (Grace Hospital, Vancouver: May 5, 1992).
17. Health Professions Council, *Recommendations.*
18. Ibid., 30.
19. Ibid., 6.
20. Elizabeth Cull, "Speaking Notes for the Honourable Elizabeth Cull, Minister of Health and Minister Responsible for Seniors," (Unpublished Paper, International Confederation of Midwives 23rd Triennial Congress, Vancouver Trade and Convention Centre, Vancouver, B.C., May 10, 1993), 11.
21. Ibid., 3.
22. Ibid., 6.
23. Ibid.
24. Health Professions Council, *Recommendations.*
25. British Columbia Royal Commission on Health Care and Costs, *Closer to Home.*
26. Paul Tennant, *Aboriginal Peoples and Politics: The Indian Land Question in British Columbia, 1849-1989* (Vancouver: University of British Columbia Press, 1990).
27. Cecelia Benoit and Dena Carroll, "Aboriginal Midwifery in British Columbia: A Narrative Untold," in *Persistent Spirit: Towards Understanding Aboriginal Health in British Columbia.* Peter H. Stephenson, Susan J. Elliott, Leslie T. Foster, and Jill Harris, eds. Canadian Western Geography Series 31 (Victoria: University of Victoria, Department of Geography, 1995).
28. Ibid.
29. Ibid.
30. Tennant, *Aboriginal Peoples and Politics.*
31. Aboriginal Health Policy Branch, British Columbia Ministry of Health and the Ministry Responsible for Seniors, *Aboriginal Midwifery in British Columbia,* (Unpublished Speaking Notes Presented at the Canadian Confederation of Midwives Annual General Meeting, St. John's, Newfoundland, May 6 & 7, 1994).
32. Ibid., 2.
33. Ibid.
34. Ministry of Health and Ministry Responsible for Seniors, *B.C.'s First College of Midwives Established,* (News Release, March 16, 1995, Victoria:

Communications and Public Affairs, Ministry of Health and the Ministry Responsible for Seniors, 1995).

35. Ministry of Health and Ministry Responsible for Seniors, *Midwives Regulations* (Victoria: Communications and Public Affairs, Ministry of Health and Ministry Responsible for Seniors, 1995).

36. Aboriginal Health Policy Branch, *Aboriginal Midwifery in British Columbia.*

37. Ministry of Health and Ministry Responsible for Seniors, *First College of Midwives Established.*

38. *Health Professions Act*, S.B.C. (1990), c. 50.

39. *Midwives Regulation,* B.C. Reg. 103/95 (1995).

40. Ministry of Health and Ministry Responsible for Seniors, *Midwives Regulations.*

41. A Sunset Clause is one that has a limited time period after which it is automatically repealed. Specific restrictions on home birth in the Midwifery Regulations have such a clause and automatically end on December 31, 1998, unless further regulation is passed by Cabinet. The Sunset Clause in the regulations pertains to the Home Birth Demonstration Project and the requirement that all home births attended by registered midwives are carried out within the Home Birth Demonstration Project. Given the length of time it has taken from the approval of the Midwifery Regulations to registration of midwives and the concomitant start up of the Home Birth Demonstration Project, it would not be surprising if this date is extended to provide for a longer project.

42. Ministry of Health and Ministry Responsible for Seniors, *Midwives Regulations.*

43. Ibid.

44. Health Professions Council, *Recommendations,* 34.

45. *Midwives Regulation (*1995).

46. *Health Professions Act* (1990).

47. Health Professions Council, *Recommendations.*

48. Ibid.

49. Ministry of Health and Ministry Responsible for Seniors, *First College of Midwives Established.*

50. Ministry of Health and Ministry Responsible for Seniors, *Registered Midwives to be Funded this Fiscal Year,* (News Release, April 16, 1996, Victoria: Communications and Public Affairs, Ministry of Health and the Ministry Responsible for Seniors, 1996).

51. British Columbia Royal Commission on Health Care and Costs, *Closer to Home.*

52. Health Professions Council, *Recommendations,* 6.

53. Greater Vancouver Regional District, "Birthing Centre Survey: A Report on Public Interest in Birthing Centres in the GVRD," in *Report of the Birth Centre Working Group* (Burnaby, B.C.: December 1992) Appendix B.

54. Ibid., V.

55. College of Midwives of British Columbia, *Bylaws for College of Midwives of British Columbia,* Draft (Vancouver: 1996).

56. College of Midwives of British Columbia, *Bylaws for College of Midwives of British Columbia* (Vancouver: 1997).

57. Registered Nurses Association of British Columbia, *Position Statement: Advanced Obstetrical Nursing Practice and Midwifery,* Pub. No. 75. (Vancouver: 1997), 1.

58. College of Midwives of British Columbia, *Bylaws for College of Midwives* (1997).
59. Robbie E. Davis-Floyd, *Birth as an American Rite of Passage* (Berkeley: University of California Press, 1992).
60. Jessica Mitford, *The American Way of Birth* (New York: Plume, 1992).
61. Robbie E. Davis-Floyd, *Birth as an American Rite of Passage, 282.*
62. Stanley J. Gross, *Of Foxes and Hen Houses* (Westport: Quorum Books, 1984).
63. British Columbia Royal Commission on Health Care and Costs, *Closer to Home.*
64. Catherine Kohler Riessman and Constance A. Nathanson, "The Management of Reproduction: Social Construction of Risk and Responsibility," in *Applications of Social Science to Clinical Medicine and Health Policy,* eds. Linda H. Aiken and David Mechanic (New Brunswick: Rutgers University Press, 1986).
65. *Midwives Regulation (1995).*

REFERENCES

Aboriginal Health Policy Branch, British Columbia Ministry of Health and the Ministry Responsible for Seniors. *Aboriginal Midwifery in British Columbia.* Unpublished Speaking Notes Presented at the Canadian Confederation of Midwives Annual General Meeting, St. John's, Newfoundland, May 6 & 7, 1994.

Benoit, Cecelia, and Dena Carroll. "Aboriginal Midwifery in British Columbia: A Narrative Untold." In *Persistent Spirit: Towards Understanding Aboriginal Health in British Columbia.* Peter H. Stephenson, Susan J. Elliott, Leslie T. Foster, and Jill Harris eds. (Canadian Western Geography Series 31). Victoria: University of Victoria, Department of Geography, 1995.

B.C. Greater Vancouver Regional District. "Birthing Centre Survey: A Report on Public Interest in Birthing Centres in the GVRD." *Report of the Birth Centre Working Group* (Appendix B). Burnaby, December 1992.

British Columbia Health Minister. "Fax Message to be Read on Behalf of the Honourable Elizabeth Cull, Minister of Health and Minister Responsible for Seniors, International Midwives Day." Grace Hospital, Vancouver, B.C., May 5, 1992.

British Columbia Royal Commission on Health Care and Costs. *Closer to Home: The Report of the British Columbia Royal Commission on Health Care and Costs. Volume 2.* Victoria, B.C.: Ministry of Health and the Ministry Responsible for Seniors, Province of British Columbia, 1991.

Burtch, Brian. *Trials of Labour: The Re-emergence of Midwifery.* Montreal & Kingston: McGill-Queen's University Press, 1994.

College of Midwives of British Columbia. *Bylaws for College of Midwives of British Columbia.* (Draft) Vancouver, 1996.

College of Midwives of British Columbia. *Bylaws for College of Midwives of British Columbia.* Vancouver, April, 1997.

College of Physicians and Surgeons of British Columbia. *Policy Manual.* Vancouver, June 1995.

Cull, Elizabeth. "Speaking Notes for the Honourable Elizabeth Cull, Minister of Health and Minister Responsible for Seniors." International Confederation of Midwives 23rd Triennial Congress. Vancouver Trade and Convention Centre, May 10, 1993.

Davis-Floyd, Robbie E. *Birth as an American Rite of Passage.* Berkeley: University of California Press, 1992.

Gross, Stanley J. *Of Foxes and Hen Houses*. Westport: Quorum Books, 1984.

Harvey, Sheila, Karyn Kaufman, and Alison Rice. "Hospital-based Midwifery Projects in Canada." In *Issues in Midwifery*. Tricia Murphy-Black, ed. Edinburgh: Churchill Livingstone, 1995.

Health Professions Act, S.B.C. (1990), c.50.

Health Professions Council. *Recommendations on the Designation of Midwifery*. Victoria: Government of British Columbia, 1993.

Lemay, Gloria. "Midwifery Must Deliver on its Promise." *The Vancouver Sun*, A20, June 16, 1996.

Maternal Health Society. *Midwifery is a Labour of Love*. Vancouver, 1981.

Medical Practitioners Act, R.S.B.C. (1979), c.254.

Midwives Association of British Columbia . *Submission to the Royal Commission on Health Care and Costs*. Unpublished paper. Vancouver, 1990.

Midwives Association of British Columbia. *Information Packet*. Vancouver, 1993.

Midwives Regulation. B.C. Reg. 103/95, 1995.

Ministry of Health and Ministry Responsible for Seniors. "College of Midwives to be Established to License, Regulate Profession." News Release, November 10, 1994. Victoria: Communications and Public Affairs, B.C. Ministry of Health and the Ministry Responsible for Seniors, 1994.

Ministry of Health and Ministry Responsible for Seniors. "B.C.'s First College of Midwives Established." News Release, March 16, 1995. Victoria: Communications and Public Affairs, Ministry of Health and the Ministry Responsible for Seniors, 1995.

Ministry of Health and Ministry Responsible for Seniors. *Midwives Regulations*. Victoria: Communications and Public Affairs, Ministry of Health and Ministry Responsible for Seniors, 1995.

Ministry of Health and Ministry Responsible for Seniors. "Registered Midwives to be Funded this Fiscal Year." News Release, April 16, 1996. Victoria: Communications and Public Affairs, Ministry of Health and the Ministry Responsible for Seniors, 1996.

Mitford, Jessica. *The American Way of Birth*. New York: Plume, 1992.

Nurses (Registered) Act. R.S.B.C., c.302, 1979.

Registered Nurses Association of British Columbia . *Position Statement: Advanced Obstetrical Nursing Practice and Midwifery*. Pub. No. 75. Vancouver, 1997.

Riessman, Catherine Kohler, and Constance A. Nathanson. "The Management of Reproduction: Social Construction of Risk and Responsibility." In *Applications of Social Science to Clinical Medicine and Health Policy*. Linda H. Aiken and David Mechanic, eds. New Brunswick, NJ: Rutgers University Press, 1986.

Tennant, Paul. *Aboriginal Peoples and Politics: The Indian Land Question in British Columbia, 1849-1989*. Vancouver: The University of British Columbia Press, 1990.

Wigod, Rebecca. "Midwife, Claiming Coroner Seeks to Blame, Waits for Court's Say on Baby-death Petition." *The Vancouver Sun*, A3, June 26, 1995.

Regulation:
Changing The Face of Midwifery?

Susan James

As midwifery practice is becoming regulated across Canada, the question must be asked: Will anything be 'lost'? Will it be possible to maintain the model and philosophy of practice which emerged through a grassroots 'demand' for an alternative to the medical system of obstetrical care? Can midwives enter into the healthcare system and yet remain an alternative to the system? We should not expect midwifery to remain stagnant with or without regulation. Midwifery has grown and evolved as the world around midwifery changes. Like the effects of life events on the appearance of individuals, we ought to expect that regulation will be reflected in the face of midwifery. The question remains, will those changes 'fit' the self-image of midwifery — the new lines and characteristics that show our maturity, our experience, our character? Or, will those changes be ones that lead us to search in the mirror for some semblance of the midwives we thought we were — puzzling at the dramatic changes created by regulation? I am writing primarily about the Alberta experience. At the time of the completion of this chapter, midwifery regulation was passed by legislation and 'in effect.' However, the registration process has not yet occurred, so that no midwife is obliged to practice under the authority of the legislation.[1]

MIDWIFERY WITHOUT REGULATIONS
There are approximately 20 midwives currently in independent practice in Alberta. These midwives practice primarily in the larger cities in the province. In addition, there is a nurse-midwifery project at the Foothills Hospital in Calgary which allows a select group of midwives employed at the hospital some level of autonomy. However, officially, they work under the direct supervision of physicians. Midwives in independent practice provide continuity of care throughout pregnancy, birth and the first several weeks after the birth. The majority of women using midwifery services elect to have their births at home. While the unregulated status of midwives presents some barriers to practice (e.g. obtaining hospital admitting privileges, actually

'doing' the birth when a woman chooses to be in hospital, arranging for some lab work), midwives have worked out ways of accessing the healthcare system in order to ensure safe and appropriate care for their clients. Midwives are able to arrange lab work such as blood group and antibodies, hepatitis screening and newborn metabolic screening, because they have discovered that these tests are funded through provincial programmes and do not require a physician-billing number. Most midwives have established friendly and supportive arrangements with local physicians who may facilitate additional access to healthcare resources. In recent years, most midwives report an increased cooperation from paramedics, nursing and medical staff when hospital transfers are required for mother and/or baby.

Currently, women select midwives with care, making direct contracts with their midwives. For some women, the decision to engage a midwife for her childbirth experience is a difficult one, challenged by friends, family and their usual healthcare providers. One woman told me, "My mother refused to talk to me. She was absolutely against it. She said that I was taking my baby's life in my own hands and that I had no right to do this." Another woman recalled, "My family, well, they were never really negative toward it, but, they weren't supportive of it either. They just thought that I'd smarten up and change my mind and go into hospital, like where I belonged, by the end. They never believed that I would go through with it." Another couple wondered not only how their family would react, but whether their long-term family physician would refuse to treat them in the future.

The concerns voiced above reflect the general attitude toward midwifery in Alberta. We live in a conservative society where the cultural narrative of birth involves risk, technology, medicine and hospitalization. We have been taught to believe that the hospital is the only safe birthplace and that the physician is the only safe birth attendant. Further, the cultural myths about the dangers of midwifery are perpetuated by powerful stakeholders such as physicians, who perhaps have the most to lose if midwifery becomes accepted across the province. It is not surprising that, when women or couples challenge these cultural tenets by choosing midwifery (and home birth), they are met with criticism. Pregnancy and childbirth is a time of great vulnerability for a woman or couple. They want to be seen as good and responsible parents making good and safe choices for themselves and their children. For many couples, this is a big step into the responsibilities of the adult world, perhaps the first time that their decisions have such a direct bearing on someone else — their child. This is also a time when family support is very important. The decision to have a midwife in the face of these challenges requires maturity, confidence and strength.

The difficult nature of the decision may be further complicated by the exclusion of midwifery services from any form of third-party payment. In a culture where insured healthcare services are considered to be a right, the cost of midwifery care (ranging from $800 - $1500 per course of care at the time of writing) can influence a decision toward the alternative medical services which are covered by the Alberta Health Insurance Plan. For many young families, the cost of midwifery is a burden that is accepted, yet still difficult.

Both women and midwives experience a strong commitment to one another through this decision process. Women are paying for a service from a midwife who they have come to trust through their discussions with the midwife and from recommendations of other women. The midwife also develops a sense of trust in the woman — that she will provide the midwife with enough information to provide safe and competent care; that she won't sue her at the least deviation from the 'perfect birth.'

The relational aspects of midwifery become central to the entire caregiving experience. While knowledge and skills are important to safe and appropriate care, it is within the context of a deep commitment to the woman that the midwife performs these competencies. The moral impulse of the midwife is focused on the woman. The concerns of significant 'others' such as partners and family are part of the woman's 'story,' yet the woman remains central. Midwives claim that the relationship that is established between the midwife and the woman enhances the safeness of their practice. Women express a confidence in themselves that comes from knowing their midwife well and feeling that their midwife knows and respects them. One woman recently commented, while sitting naked in a swimming pool in active labour, "Birth is not a first date situation. I don't think I could relax and let my body do this with strangers around me."

An informed choice model of decision-making which is often identified as the hallmark of Canadian midwifery relies on the strength of the relational aspects of midwifery. A simple definition of informed choice is the active involvement of both the woman and the midwife in gathering information and in coming to decisions. However, informed choice is an extremely complex concept, difficult to capture in definitions. Robbie Davis-Floyd[2] refers to a holistic view to which midwives working within an informed choice model ascribe. Within this view, professional relationships are seen as reciprocal partnerships rather than authoritarian; the experience of the particular woman is the centre point for decision-making rather than a generalized norm; and many forms of knowledge beyond empirically derived theory are considered not only valid but essential to understanding a woman and her situation.

The role of the 'modern' midwife in Canada evolved through traditions of women helping women, and of a questioning of the mainstream healthcare system. Through these traditions, midwives and women share values and beliefs about pregnancy and birth.[3] Pregnancy and birth are considered to be normal experiences, combining physiological, social and spiritual dimensions. Mother and child are inextricably linked, physically, emotionally, and spiritually. There exists a general trust that when the woman makes decisions for herself, those decisions are also good for her child. The mother is the 'expert' source of knowing what is good for self and child. Midwives and women use a wide variety of types of knowledge in their work together. While objective, scientific knowledge has a place in midwifery, emotions, intuition, and narrative are examples of other forms of knowledge which are sought and valued.

SEEKING LEGISLATION

Midwives have sought legislation with ambivalence. On one hand, midwifery regulation is viewed as being important for protecting the public through ensuring high standards for preparation and practice. Legislation and its ensuing regulation bring credibility, status, and a rightful place and voice within the healthcare system. Midwives regard legislation as a way of further developing the knowledge and practice base of midwifery, of ensuring greater accessibility for women, and of improving their own working conditions.

Others, like Stanley Gross,[4] question the effectiveness of regulating and licensing healthcare professionals. While the general belief is that regulations protect the public, the structures that support regulations such as professional associations, colleges, and limited-access education programmes, may make it difficult for the public to challenge the power of the professional group.

> Professionalism in medicine is nothing more than the institutionalization of a male, upper class monopoly. We must never confuse professionalism with expertise. Expertise is something to work for and to share; professionalism is... elitist and exclusive, sexist, racist and classist.[5]

Even when there is a mandate to include consumers in processes such as peer review, a minority consumer voice may do little to reduce the power of the professional group. There have been examples where the consumer voice is hardly representative of the general public. Consumer representatives may be retired professionals, spouses of professionals or members of other health-care professional groups. Their alliance may rest with the professional group rather than with the public. At a recent meeting of midwives, consumers and government representatives at the Alberta Ministry of Health, midwives and consumers were told that the primary function of consumers is to be a 'watchdog' for unacceptable midwifery practice. While both groups felt comfortable with the concept of both consumers and midwives having re-sponsibility in ensuring an acceptable standard of practice, neither were comfortable with the adversarial nature of a 'watchdog' process. If the key players in an important process of ensuring public safety are uncomfortable with the process, we must wonder how effective that process can be.

Regardless of midwives' ambivalence about regulation, it appears that the regulation process is inevitable in Canada. Midwife and consumer groups explored regulatory options in various jurisdictions in Canada for several years, however, the major impetus for legislation and regulation may have been the recommendations of coroners in Ontario and British Columbia.[6] In the final report of the Health Workforce Rebalancing Committee in Alberta,[7] mandatory registration, controlled acts and defined scopes of practice will be required for all healthcare professionals.[8] The inclusion of midwifery in the list of healthcare professionals indicates that midwifery would have been regulated at some time in the future, even without consumer and midwifery encouragement.

CHALLENGE: MANDATORY CONSULTATION

With midwifery regulation, it is possible that choice could be restricted for women by the very fact that regulations direct that certain women are unsuited to midwifery care. For example, in the Alberta *Standards of Competency and Practice*,[9] the mandatory physician consultation lists may prohibit a woman expecting an eighth child from having a home birth or require that a woman with history of postpartum depression be seen by a physician.

Although the consultation lists are purposely written as very general guidelines, their very existence causes a challenge to much of what has been highly valued within midwifery tradition. Rather than providing an alternative or challenge to the canons of medical care, midwives will now be required to be accountable to medicine. The decisions made in the relations formed between midwife and the woman (and her family) will be subject to outside, so-called 'objective' influence. Visible or invisible, physicians enter into the relationship and have the potential to influence the decision-making process.

Some may argue that the consultation lists are just good common sense. What midwife who is committed to providing safe and competent care would question the advisability of seeking physician input when a woman's condition becomes complicated beyond her abilities? The principles of consultation and shared or transferred care are well accepted by midwives. Midwives welcome the legitimate route to consultation and transfer that accompanies regulation. However, there are many subtle messages in the presence and wording of the consultation lists.

Underlying the consultation lists is a message which reinforces the traditional hierarchy within the healthcare system. The exclusive reference to physicians for consultation implies that medicine is indeed at the top of the healthcare hierarchy. An additional message may imply that midwives are not adequately prepared to know when it is appropriate to consult physicians. The absence of similar lists for consultation with other care-providers may imply that consultation with a lactation consultant, public health nurse, or homeopath, for example, is not critical to the provision of good care, or that the kind of knowledge required to make such consultations is not at the same level of complexity as that required to make consultations with physicians. How may these subtle messages impact the confidence and trust in the midwife, both by the midwife herself, and by women? Will women themselves continue to be considered the central source of knowledge, or will midwives find themselves relying more and more on the voices of medicine for directions as to how to act appropriately? Will midwives continue to seek a wide variety of healing traditions to offer as choices to their clients? Or will the relative silence of these alternatives in the shadow of the loud voice of medicine in the regulations result in a disappearance of the traditions of difference?

A further challenge within the consultation process is the lack of a definition of 'normal' with respect to pregnancy, birth, and the newborn in regulations and standards. This absence of definition may give the midwife the potential for greater flexibility in her decision-making processes with each individual woman. However, the lack of a defined 'normal,' accompanied by physicians' exclusive privilege to diagnose[10] creates a legislation 'loop-hole.' The autonomy that midwives sought could be limited by the ability of physicians to determine which women are indeed 'normal' and therefore which women are suitable for midwifery care.[11] Further complicating the lack of a definition of 'normal' is the pervasive belief in medicine that pregnancy is not a 'normal' condition. Pregnant women can be classified as being low or high risk, but never healthy or normal.

In Alberta, the consultation lists were purposely written using very general terminology. This was done to create some flexibility in a midwife's practice dependent upon her relationship with consulting physicians and perhaps on her experience. There was also an attempt to facilitate expansion of the scope of midwifery practice in the future. For example, rather than using breech presentation as an indication for mandatory consultation, the term 'abnormal presentation' was used. If at some time in the future, breech presentation is considered to be appropriate for midwifery care, there will be no need to open and change legislated standards. However, the general nature of these lists may in fact create local variations in how midwifery may be practised dependent upon interpretation by the physicians consulted. Using again the example of 'abnormal presentation,' a midwife practising in a particular region of the province may be required to consult for all posterior presentations should the physician consider that to be 'abnormal.'

The consequences of choosing not to follow the advice of the consultant physician are not clearly outlined. While there is a sense that the woman, midwife and physician ought to collaborate in the decision-making process, all described options in the course of care following the consultation with the physician are dependent upon the findings of the physician. The option that the midwife can refuse to provide care to the woman who decides against medical advice is addressed.[12] The option that the woman may not wish any physician consultation is not clearly outlined. The client's 'informed consent' is required prior to any transfer of care, however, there appears to be no obligation to use 'informed choice' prior to consulting with a physician. In effect, the woman is completely left out of this process until it is underway. How might the consultation process impact the relationship between women and their midwives? Women may feel obliged to follow physician advice rather than endanger the registration status of her midwife. Women may perceive little difference in the overall approach of midwives and physicians. Midwives may feel squeezed between the expectations to comply with regulations and their obligations to their clients. Will the influence of the medical model lead midwives to accept the medical technocratic view of the woman as container for her fetus, a container who may make so-called 'bad' or 'selfish' decisions?

Challenge — Healthcare Reform

Coming into regulated practice in the midst of radical healthcare reform in the province of Alberta poses further threats to the face of midwifery. Expectations that midwives will somehow 'solve' all the difficulties encountered in delivering maternity services to rural, native or underserviced populations; that midwives will be willing to be used as an example of fiscal responsibility for other care providers; that midwifery education will not be an additional cost to the province are all expectations we are sure to fail.

The delivery of adequate maternity services in rural Alberta has been a challenge in recent years. Many communities find it difficult to attract and keep physicians for a variety of reasons, including lower earnings and lifestyle. Over the years, many small rural hospitals have closed their maternity departments. Consequently, many rural women are faced with long distance travel for prenatal care and for their births. Some rural areas view midwifery as a way of resolving their maternity services problems. While some midwives in the future may be very interested in living and practising in rural Alberta, this is not a short-term solution. The midwives most likely to be eligible for registration in the next year primarily have established practises in urban settings. The midwives who require additional experience prior to being eligible for full registration will have to get that experience with the registered midwives in urban settings. In the future, midwives who may be recruited by a rural community may find the same challenges of low earnings, long-distance travel and lifestyle as physicians have in the past, and have a tendency to remain in these communities for only short periods of time.

In many areas of the province, there is an expectation that midwives will provide services to women such as those in low-income, specific immigrant and Aboriginal groups who have not been well served by the healthcare system to date. For example, in Edmonton, one of the proposals to implement midwifery revolves around restricting midwifery practice to an area of the city where the proportion of low-income families is very high. Historically, women from that area have not attended prenatal care consistently, tend not to have postnatal follow-up and have low child-immunization rates.

One of the reasons why midwives sought regulation was to make midwifery accessible to women such as these. Midwives have long been aware that midwifery care has not been accessible to all women both because of the necessity of paying for midwifery services and because of the barrier of midwifery's alegal status in Alberta's healthcare system. While midwives attempt to provide culturally sensitive care, the reality is that now and in the near future, midwives are primarily white, middle-class women. Regardless of the intentions or the actual practice of midwives, the perception that they represent a privileged group in Alberta may make the choice of midwifery unappealing to women of races or classes who feel oppressed or marginalized within the context of the white, male business-model culture dominant in Alberta in the 90s.

For some women and families, regulation may make midwifery a more acceptable choice. Women who are struggling to fit within their newly adopted culture may have chosen physician care only because it is the dominant and only legally recognized practice within Alberta culture. Regulation may give women who would have preferred midwifery care a legitimate choice. In addition, if funded services are part of regulated practice, financial barriers to the choice of midwifery will be removed. However, regulation may reduce choices for some women. Women who currently seek all or some of their maternity care from traditional midwives of their own culture may be prohibited from this practice if their midwife does not seek registration or is not found eligible for registration.[13] Women who engaged midwives precisely because they were not part of the legitimate healthcare system, perhaps feeling more intimidated by a 'professional' than a midwife who by her nonlegal status has some 'sisterhood' in marginalization in Alberta society, may feel that their choices are reduced as midwives enter into the 'professional' world.

Coming back to the Edmonton plan, the concept of placing midwives into an underserviced population has a certain appeal. Midwives would like to make their services accessible to all classes and cultural groups. Indeed, many midwives would identify women in this particular area of Edmonton as among those most in need of midwifery care. However, it is questionable whether midwives can totally address the issues of what the medical model system would label as "poor compliance" with health care. Access or 'compliance' issues related to poverty, marginalization, and culture cannot be addressed by the implementation of midwifery services alone. While some of the reasons why women do not attend prenatal visits may be related to discomfort with the physician, it is likely that lack of funds for childcare and transportation, language barriers, and work and family responsibilities play a greater role in influencing a women's lack of attendance. While services which may meet these needs could be included into a midwifery implementation plan, this would not be consistent with the pattern of social services cuts made in the last three years in Alberta. Generally, women have been expected to carry the burden of healthcare and social services reform in this province.

The other difficulty with the Edmonton plan is the lack of fit with the philosophy and principles of midwifery. Choice of care provider has been an important aspect of midwifery in the past. Women seek the care of a particular midwife or midwifery practice because they want to, not because they are assigned to do so. If women are told that they must see a midwife, the type of relationship, the style of caregiving, and the safety aspects of midwifery may all be compromised.

In our current climate of fiscal restraint, all healthcare services are being asked to cut back, to justify all expenditures and to demonstrate cost effectiveness. When making presentations to stakeholder groups, midwives and their consumers have often used the argument that midwifery will save taxpayer dollars. While it is true that women who currently seek midwifery care and have home births spend far less for their midwifery care than the healthcare system spends on women who have physician-attended hospital births, we cannot be sure what the cost of midwifery care will be in the future. Midwives who have struggled with their low earnings in the past are not willing to settle for a funding agreement based on the fees they currently charge to women. In Ontario, the midwives found that they had higher rates of consultations to physicians in their first year of regulated practice. Consultations represent a cost to the system. If midwives are expected to demonstrate cost-savings in the first year of regulated practice, they may feel coerced to make decisions about things which will increase the cost of their care, such as the use of lab work, transfer to hospital, or consultation with a physician based on finances rather than on clinical judgement.

The emphasis on cost-cutting has also created a mandate to demonstrate the effectiveness of any service. Midwives welcome changes to the system that expect evidence-based practice. Midwives and childbearing women are well aware that many obstetrical practices are based more on traditions of power and hierarchy than on evidence of superior outcomes (e.g. episiotomy, routine continuous electronic fetal monitoring, and routine use of ultrasound). However, there is concern that the randomized clinical trial is the only accepted form of evidence. This research method does bring some level of assurance about the reliability of findings, however, does not always fit well with midwifery philosophy and practices. Midwives may find it difficult to randomly assign clients to particular protocol groups when choice is a central aspect of practice. Midwives may be prohibited from using techniques, treatments or approaches that have not met the test of the randomized clinical trial.

In Alberta, healthcare reform has resulted in the division of the province into 17 regional health authorities. Each region is responsible for assessing their healthcare needs and totally funding all services offered, with the exception of physician services, which continue to be funded by the provincial health insurance plan. This means that all negotiations for midwifery implementation are done at a regional level. As a result, it is possible that some regions may decide not to implement midwifery as one of their funded services and that there can be wide variations in the way that midwifery is practised from region to region. For the individual midwife, the burden of nonpractice professional work increases with regionalization. For example, rather than having a few of the province's midwives sitting on province-wide committees, nearly every midwife will have to sit on committees in order to fulfill their obligations to the regional health authorities. The position of the regional health authority as the paymaster to the individual midwife may create a potential for experiencing a conflict of obligations — 'ought my priority go to my client or to the region health authority when both want me at the same time?' Midwives may find that they have less available time for their clients.

Healthcare reform in Alberta has also brought about a strengthening of the traditional hierarchies in healthcare. Physicians are the only named professionals within any regional authority business plan. All other professionals have become invisible, hidden in the language of services rather than service providers.[14] Once midwifery is fully implemented in the regions, consumers who have not been involved in the midwifery movement to date may not realize there are midwives in their region; and if they do know that there are midwives, they may perceive that they must go through a physician gatekeeper to access midwifery services.

Challenge — Formal Midwifery Education

With the development of formalized midwifery education, will the art and spirit of midwifery be transmitted or will individual creativity be stifled through a commitment to the acquisition of skills and knowledge? The competency-based structure of regulations and standards could result in a education program that emphasizes technical skills rather than relational aspects of midwifery. In Alberta, the structure of the first assessment process for determining eligibility for registration may provide a glimpse at future midwifery education. An evaluation expert[15] advised a subcommittee of the Midwifery Regulation Advisory Committee that only those aspects of midwifery that can be objectively quantified are valid for assessment. As a result, the assessment will take the form of multiple choice questions and structured objective skills performance examinations. The expert advised that any attempt at assessing 'softer' aspects of midwifery, such as approach to women, informed choice and tolerance, will not stand up to objective standards. The obligation of the government in registering midwives is 'only' to protect the public from unsafe practice. In their eyes, anything that cannot be tested in an objective format does not compromise public safety. Will this bias toward 'objective' measurement influence the development of a midwifery curriculum and therefore the characteristics of midwives in the future? Will consumers be able to have concerns about 'softer' aspects of practice addressed by a regulatory body?[16] Perhaps the absence of these aspects in the assessment process will send a message to consumers that midwives do not highly value these characteristics in a midwife.

Even if midwifery faculty wish to create a midwifery program that captures the essence of midwifery as it is currently practised, they may not have the power to implement such a program. Women in academia are already well aware of the biases existing in that community. University regulations, economic constraints and the expectations for rigour, both for students and faculty, may lead to course expectations and forms of scholarly work which are not compatible with current midwifery knowledge and practice.

Current cost-cutting in education has resulted in heightened competition within the university environment. There is a sense of urgency to develop a large program quickly: students mean dollars. There is concern that a program may take in more students than can be accommodated by midwives for student practice experiences. This would result in students having significant portions of their education with other professionals such as physicians, or in other jurisdictions where medical model midwifery may be prevalent.

In Alberta, there has been a recent emphasis on distance education for all postsecondary programs. There has been an explosion of distance-education technologies available. Distance-education opportunities will be needed in midwifery education. Many of the prospective midwifery students are women with small children who may find it difficult to relocate for their midwifery education. It is likely that the best strategy for having midwives who are interested in working in rural or remote areas of the province, is to educate midwives who are already settled and committed to those areas. However, the match between distance technology and the philosophy and practice of midwifery needs to be carefully studied. At a recent meeting of a midwifery education committee at the University of Alberta, a plan was proposed to utilize a variety of 'telemedicine' technologies[17] to make it possible for a student to stay in a remote community and get practice expereince without a midwife present in that community. The purpose of this proposal was to devise a way to have more students than there are registered midwives to provide placement sites. There seems to be a level of discrepancy between an educational approach where there is no face-to-face contact between student and teacher and a high use of complex technology, and midwifery where touch, relationships and 'natural' approaches are emphasized. What impact will distance technology have on the philosophy and practice of midwifery?

In the past, women became midwifery apprentices, not based on previous academic achievements, but on personal attributes and compatibility with the midwife or practice. The length of apprenticeship, expectations and experiences were individually tailored. While it is recognized that the apprenticeship model is fraught with problems, it has also led to a sense of mutual respect among midwives. Midwives and their apprentices were closely connected during the learning experience. The learning was not restricted to specific academically defined activities, rather the lives of the midwives and the apprentices became enmeshed — watching one another's children, helping with moving, cooking and eating together. Midwifery is a lifestyle as well as a profession. An apprentice 'became' a midwife not by completing a particular number of years of study, or by catching a particular number of babies, but because they were recognized as midwives by other midwives and by clients. Even midwives who complete formal programs before entering practice, identify early mentoring or supervised relationship with an experienced midwife and the learning from women, as their 'real' midwifery education.[18] Will a formal program be able to capture the strengths of the apprenticeship model?

In the past, women tended to enter midwifery gradually, perhaps first as a client of a midwife, or as labour support for friends. The idea of becoming a midwife may take time to solidify. The arrangements required to become an apprentice can be complex and involve a number of difficult decisions for the apprentice and perhaps for her family. The arrangements are entirely the responsibility of the apprentice. Once the woman identified herself as a midwifery apprentice or student, there is a connection between the 'whatness' of midwifery and the 'I-ness' of her own role. In many formal professional education programs, it takes students a prolonged socialization period to identify themselves with the professional role. With regulations, midwifery education will be a direct-entry degree program. Students entering midwifery may have little or no prior contact with midwifery, its practices and philosophy. Although these students may gain all of the skills and factual knowledge of midwifery, the embodied sense of midwifery, the connection of self with the role may be difficult to accomplish within formal education programs. Is it possible to assess applicants for their potential to capture the 'spirit of midwifery?' Can this 'spirit' be taught or assessed?

Challenge — Gaining Access to Healthcare Resources

A strong motive for seeking legislation has been related to gaining access to healthcare resources. These resources include labs, pharmacies, hospitals, health units, and remuneration for services. Some believe that access will ensure that midwives are able to carry out their full scope of practice, and improve continuity, choices and 'working conditions' for midwives.

Most midwives currently live below the poverty level, often relying on a partner's income to pay bills. Midwives long for a regular income that matches the intensity of their work. However, will there be a price to pay for that income? Becoming an 'employee' of the government may legitimize expectations that midwives will work within the medical model. Weitz and Sullivan[19] found that once licensed, lay midwives tended to use intuition less and to be more likely to interpret events through the medical model. An emphasis on the medical model and its technologies may result in deskilling of midwives, with a loss of traditional midwifery skills and knowledge.[20]

Will salary or contract change the relationship between the woman and midwife? Even with the best will or intentions, it is possible that the nature of the partnership may change. Reid[21] found that, once lay midwives in the United States began to charge for their work, the relationship changed from that of a woman friend to a professional, with a focus on the pregnancy, rather than on the woman's life. An increase in the incidence of complications accompanied this change, perhaps because the midwife had less personal knowledge of the woman, and the woman abdicated much more responsibility to the midwife. The situation in Alberta (and the rest of Canada) is slightly different than that studied by Reid. Most unregulated midwives charge for their services. Regulation may ensure that third-party payment is available for midwifery care, making the direct cost to the woman free or minimal. Perhaps the critical point of Reid's research is the change from "woman friend" to "professional." We have many experiences outside of professional health care where we exchange funds with others for goods and services without that exchange interfering with our relationships. It is probably not the charging for services that makes the difference in the relationship. The tendency to give responsibility to the caregiver has been encouraged within medicine. The similarities in funding and regulated connections with medicine may result in similar patterns of abdication of responsibility to the midwife.

The incentive of income and the possibility of an on-off call schedule may attract midwives who do not regard the relationships between the midwife and woman to be central to caregiving. In a recent discussion with a group of nurses who have foreign midwifery credentials but have never practised as midwives in Canada, I was told that the close relationship is actually a negative influence in caregiving. In their view, it is important to maintain an objective distance from women, particularly in matters of decision-making. The midwife should not feel any need to attend the birth of any particular woman, and it should not matter to the woman who it is who attends her birth. While this perspective on midwifery care is common in some countries, it is closely aligned with medical-model care and very incompatible with current midwifery practice in Canada. Although principles of midwifery practice, such as continuity of care are outlined in the *Standards of Competency and Practice*,[22] the descriptions have been left open to interpretation. In the example of continuity of care, the description states that it is usually achieved through a one-to-one relationship; however, it can be accomplished by a small group of midwives. How are we to interpret the meaning of a 'small group' — is this 2 or 6 or 16? Who decides what is a suitable size — the health region, the midwives, the women? How do we resolve differences in what the midwives might be willing to do in terms of being on-call, providing continuity of care, and what the women expect? Will the driving force for the principles of midwifery care continue to be the women who seek that care, or will they become redefined by the professional group? Regulated practice, if funded, will make midwifery accessible to many more women in the province. In the Ontario experience, the demand for midwifery far outweighs the supply of midwives. Will this imbalance of supply and demand encourage midwives to push the limits of their relationships with women, knowing that the women who have managed to contract their care consider themselves lucky just to get any midwifery at all? Will women who have not had previous contact with midwives 'know' what they are missing if their midwife is only on-call every fourth night, or if she must meet six different midwives in the course of her pregnancy? One woman told me:

> It is very interesting to compare the first and second home births. With the first, even though I had midwives, I still wasn't in tune with what that meant. I really treated everyone who was there as though they were still part of the medical profession and I was really afraid, certainly not because of their personalities or anything that they'd done, but I was timid about speaking up about something that I wanted. I didn't want to be a bother. And with the second, it was completely different. I wasn't afraid to say "I want this" or "could you get this?" It was like a bunch of friends sitting around. And it was a lot happier.[23]

This woman had sought midwifery care for her first pregnancy, yet did not fully understand the difference between midwifery and medical care. It wasn't until after she had experienced the full extent of midwifery care that she developed an appreciation of what she could expect from her midwives. In Alberta, there is a tendency to rely on a marketplace model for dealing with care providers who do not meet the expectations of consumers. Theoretically, this could be a strong consumer-driven model, where practitioners who do not practice according to midwifery philosophy and principles would simply cease to exist because eventually no clients would engage their services. However, as this woman noted, clients who have not had exposure to midwifery services may not know what to expect and may feel somewhat intimidated to criticize the care that they do receive.

The payment model itself can create new stressers within a midwifery practice. A strict salary model could mean that a midwife will have to say 'no' to repeat clients who book late, if she is already 'full' for that month. A model which may have payment differences dependent upon place of birth may encourage subtle coercion regarding choice of birthplace. A model with no built-in ceiling for number of clients per year may discourage a fair and safe sharing of clients. In order to save money, a regional health authority may decide that the second attendant[24] at a hospital birth should be a case-room nurse or should be an on-call public health nurse at home births. This may mean that a woman makes her choice about birthplace based on her tolerance of taking a chance as to which stranger comes to her home or to her room at a time of high vulnerability.

Access to healthcare resources carries a price. One part of that price is the clear obligation to the healthcare system, paid perhaps by sitting on committees, doing teaching for various healthcare groups, participating in fundraising ventures or doing research. Another part of the price is less visible. For example, in order to gain hospital admitting privileges, midwives may need to make compromises in their usual practice, even if that practice conforms with midwifery regulations. A hospital may have a "local rule" as to how long is acceptable for the second stage of labour before an obstetrician must be consulted.[25] Hospitals are strongly hierarchical institutions where it may be difficult for a few midwives to challenge a long-established power structure.[26] Gaining admitting privileges opens new choices in a midwife's practice, yet may restrict choice overall. If maintaining privileges is contingent on not 'rocking the boat,' the midwife may find herself following the hospital's party line regarding issues such as who if anyone is suitable for homebirth, the use of routine diagnostic tests such as glucose screening in pregnancy, and 'allowing' choice in matters of newborn care such as vitamin K, ophthalmic prophylactic treatment and immunization.

MEETING THE CHALLENGES — RECOGNIZING THE FACE IN THE MIRROR

As regulated practice becomes a reality across this country, it is vital that midwives continue to carefully examine how regulation will impact the face of midwifery, ensuring that we retain the aspects of midwifery that are highly valued by midwives and consumers. If we hope to preserve the face of midwifery, even in a more 'mature' form, we cannot become complacent, believing that the inclusion of a philosophy statement or the words "informed choice" in the regulations or standards of competency and practice will be an adequate safeguard. Our task is to discover ways that we can protect the definition of childbirth that evolved through unregulated midwifery practice from the threats posed by the very legislation that enables the full scope of midwifery practice.

While change cannot be regarded as negative, the difficulty of moving from a primarily domestic sphere of work to a public, professional sphere presents challenges and dilemmas to midwives and ultimately to the women with whom they work. Through this process of change, we must continue to remind ourselves of our heritage and our vision of midwifery. We cannot lose the radical nature of midwifery, nor the centrality of the relation between the midwife and the woman. There are so many ways that we could find ourselves in an adversarial relationship with our clients. We need to remember that midwives and consumers have worked together to bring midwifery to this point. We do not need to buy into marketplace and business models for our future relationships under regulation. We must learn ways of communicating our relationship models so that we can build on these, rather than abandon them because no one understands what we mean by the relational aspects of midwifery practice.

As we priorize our tasks for meeting the challenges of regulation, we need to choose our battles wisely. Across Canada, there are just not enough midwives to expend energy on every small issue. There may be some issues that are appropriate to 'give' to others. Consumers are more important than ever in facilitating the implementation of midwifery. Theoretically, at least, it is the consumer voice that is heard the loudest in the healthcare reform movement. We also must learn not to be intimidated by the 'big boys' of government and medicine. We must cautiously evaluate their offers to help us out, do it for us, take care of us. These early steps into regulated practice will set the tone for our future relationships with these powerful stakeholder groups.

The identification of excellent role models in practice settings is critical if the 'spirit' of midwifery is to be kindled in the future. Students, prior learning assessment candidates, and new practitioners will all benefit from experience with midwives who are able to fully incorporate the philosophy and principles of midwifery in their practice. Within midwifery education programs, risk taking and creativity will be essential to maintain a high value on practice experiences and traditional midwifery knowledge, while maximizing opportunities for students and the profession itself to build a strong knowledge base.

The regulation of midwifery practice must stay in the hands of midwives with a place for a strong consumer voice. Collaborative care with other professionals is essential to good, safe practice, but must maintain the spirit of collaboration and not become a form of control by another profession. We must acknowledge the influence of 'others' such as policy-makers and other professionals in the relations that develop between women and their mid-wives. The potential for radical influences by these 'others' on midwifery practice is great — we cannot ignore them, or permit them to become invisible. In jurisdictions where midwifery is a legitimate part of the health-care system, there is evidence of this influence.[27] Above all else, midwives must continue to do what Barbara Katz Rothman[28] calls "breaking the circle" of what is considered to be legitimate knowledge about pregnancy and birth. And we must find the courage to use that knowledge in our practice — both with the women who seek our care and in our interactions with other care-providers.

ENDNOTES

1. The MRAC's *Midwifery Regulation, Standards of Competency and Practice,* and *Recommendations for Midwifery Assessment and Education* were passed by a standing policy committee of the Alberta Legislature in November 1994, and went into effect August 1, 1995. The process to assess the registration eligibility of current practitioners and other individuals who have midwifery education and/or experience began in the spring of 1995 and is expected to be completed in the fall of 1997. It is anticipated that the earliest possible time of registration will be in early 1998.

2. Davis-Floyd, Robbie, *Birth as an American Rite of Passage* (Berkeley: University of California Press, 1992).

3. Margaret Reid, "Sisterhood and Professionalization: A Case Study of the American Lay Midwife," in *Women as Healers. Cross-Cultural Perspectives,* C.S. McClain ed. (New Brunswick: Rutgers University Press, 1989).

4. Stanley J. Gross, *Of Foxes and Hen Houses* (Westport: Quorum Books, 1984).

5. Barbara Ehrenreich and Deidre English, *Witches, Midwives and Nurses* (New York: Feminist Press, 1983).

6. Brian Burtch, *Trials of Labour* (Montreal: McGill-Queen's University Press).

7. Health Workforce Rebalancing Committee, *Principles and Recommendations for the Regulation of Health Professionals in Alberta* (Government of Alberta, 1995).

8. Under the MRAC *Midwifery Regulation* (1994), midwives only have protection of the title "midwife." This means that someone could offer all or some midwifery services and not be liable for prosecution as long as she did not call herself a midwife. Under the Health Workforce Rebalancing Committee (1995), the scope of practice of midwifery will also be protected. While supporters of regulated practice would argue that this is a positive addition to midwifery regulation, it does remove choices from consumers who may have wished to receive services from a particular individual who for a variety of reasons may not have been regulated.

9. *Standards of Competency and Practice* (Government of Alberta, 1994).

10. Throughout the *Midwifery Regulation* (1994) and *Standards of Competency and Practice* (1994), midwives are given the ability to assess and communicate the results of their assessment. Under current legislation in Alberta (and in other provinces), physicians are the only professionals who are able to "diagnose." While there may be a fine linguistic line between assessment and diagnosis, legislatively, diagnosis is considered to be a more authoritative act. Unless other professionals such as midwives are given

authority to diagnose, there will always be the risk that a practitioner could be charged with practising medicine without a license if their decision-making was seen to be based on diagnosis.

11. Elizabeth Massey, "By Her Own Authority," *Alberta Law Review*, vol. 31, no. 2 (1993): 349-390.

12. In MRAC's *Standards of Competency and Practice* (1994), a midwife is not obliged to continue providing care to a woman who decides against the advice of a physician. There is a "non-abandonment" clause to protect the midwife who decides to continue to provide care during labour and birth to the woman who decides against midwifery or physician advice. However, there is no such clause for the pre-and postnatal periods.

13. It is difficult to estimate the extent of traditional midwifery in the province. The fear of prosecution acts as a barrier to open communication about the roles assumed by traditional midwives of any culture. Unlike the Ontario midwifery legislation, Alberta's regulation does not have a clause to protect the practice of Aboriginal midwives. This was done at the request of the Indian Health Care Commission who wanted to ensure that it was clear that Aboriginal communities in Alberta are not accountable to provincial laws related to health care. While this was an important political act, the provincial government interpreted it to mean that the Aboriginal communities are not interested in midwifery, and therefore no plans for addressing integration and collaboration regarding midwifery for Aboriginal women have been included in the midwifery implementation plan for the province. The consequences for registered midwives, who elect to practise in some sort of partnership with traditional midwives in Aboriginal communities, remain unaddressed.

14. The Alberta Ministry of Health has mandated that each Regional Health Authority provide particular services. Maternity services are among the required services. With the exception of physicians, it is up to the region to decide who can best deliver the service. There is no mandate that any other particular provider be included. Accompanying the focus on services is an emphasis on competencies. There is a lack of recognition that there is more to the services provided by a particular professional group than a collection of competencies. For example, although midwives and physicians have many competencies in common, the way in which they enact these competencies may differ enormously. This is further complicated by a move toward a "multi-skilled worker" who can provide a service but is not necessarily regulated. Many healthcare professionals are concerned that this emphasis on services and competencies rather than providers will result in a disappearance of groups such as nurses and physiotherapists.

15. The Professions and Occupations Bureau of the Alberta Ministry of Labour directed that a subcommittee of the Midwifery Regulation Advisory Committee (MRAC) be struck to design the registration eligibility assessment process. The rationale for this was that there was a belief that the practising midwives on MRAC would be given an unfair advantage in the assessment process if they were involved in its design. A "testing consultant" on contract to the government was asked to advise the subcommittee on matters of test validity and reliability. This individual has a background in psychometrics and is a member of the Faculty of Medicine at the University of Alberta.

16. Initially, the regulatory body for midwifery will be a "Midwifery Committee" under the Health Disciplines Board. Five midwives will be a part of the Committee. Under the MRAC's *Health Workforce Rebalancing* (1995), it is

likely that a College of Midwives will eventually be responsible for regulation. However, it is unclear how and when a College will be formed.

17. 'Telemedicine' technologies include teleconference, videoconference and Internet linkages. A practitioner in a remote site can perform a number of assessments and treatments under the 'supervision' of another practitioner many kilometres away by hooking into the technologies. There are even gloves (something like virtual reality) that the practitioner in the remote site wears to perform an assessment. The supervisor can put on a pair of these gloves and 'feel' what the practitioner is feeling. This has been a very positive move in healthcare, where it may be months before a particular consultant is able to travel to a remote community or where the cost of moving a 'patient' to a tertiary centre to wait for an assessment or treatment is high. It is unclear how effective these technologies are when being used to teach students. The physical and emotional effect of the use of such technologies on the clients (and in the case of midwifery care, on the fetus) has not yet been studied.

18. Alice Ouwerkerke, "Uniting Vocation and Avocation," Masters thesis, University of Alberta, 1995.

19. Rose Weitz and Deborah Sullivan, "Licensed Lay Midwifery and the Medical Model of Childbirth." *Sociology of Health and Illness*, vol. 7 (1985): 36-54.

20. Margarite Sandelowski, "A Case of Conflicting Paradigms," *Advances in Nursing Science*, vol. 10, no. 3, (1988): 35-45; P. Thompson, *The Nature of Work* (London: MacMillan Education Ltd., 1989).

21. Margaret Reid, "Sisterhood and Professionalization," op. cit.

22. *Standards...*, op. cit.

23. From interview conducted by Susan James for "With Woman: The Nature of the Midwifery Relation," Ph.D. diss., Universtiy of Alberta, 1997.

24. In the MRAC's *Standards of Competency and Practice* (1994), the second attendant at a birth is ideally another midwife. However, in order to ensure that midwives can practice in rural or remote areas where it may not be feasible for two midwives to practice, there is an exception saying that when another midwife is not available, another person can be the second attendant at a birth as long as they have adequate knowledge and skills to fulfill that role.

25. In the MRAC's *Standards of Competency and Practice* (1994) prolonged second stage is an indication for mandatory consultation with a physician. Prolonged second stage is not defined in the document. Because this is a controversial area of knowledge and practice, it is open to wide interpretation. While one hour of second stage has often been considered the limit in obstetrical active management of labour, midwives tend to use far more flexible guidelines for second stage, taking the condition of the individual mother and baby into consideration. The implications for women of this arbitrary definition of second stage is that the outcome of consultation is usually the use of interventions such as episiotomy, vacuum, and forceps delivery.

26. Mavis Kirkham, "A Feminist Perspective in Midwifery," in *Feminist Practice in Women's Health Care*, C. Webb, ed. (New York: John Wiley and Sons, 1986).

27. An article written by an Australian midwife, Maggie Lecky-Thompson, "Homebirth Midwives," *The Lamp*, vol. 45, no. 2 (1988): 10-14, about her homebirth practice is preceded by a strong warning by the General Secretary of the New South Wales Nursing Association that this article does not reflect

the views of the association and that any midwife who steps outside the association regulations will be disciplined.

28. Barbara Katz Rothman, *Recreating Motherhood* (New York: W.W. Norton, 1989), 178.

REFERENCES

Burtch, Brian. *Trials of Labour: The Re-emergence of Midwifery.* Montreal: McGill-Queen's University Press, 1994.

Davis-Floyd, Robbie. *Birth as an American Rite of Passage.* Berkeley, CA: University of California Press, 1992.

Ehrenreich, Barbara, and Deirdre English. *Witches, Midwives and Nurses: A History of Women Healers.* New York: Feminist Press, 1983.

Gross, Stanley, J. *Of Foxes and Hen Houses: Licensing and the Health Professions.* Westport, CT: Quorum Books, 1984.

Health Workforce Rebalancing Committee. *Principles and Recommendations for the Regulation of Health Professionals in Alberta: Final Report of the Health Workforce Rebalancing Committee.* Government of Alberta, November 3, 1995.

Kirkham, Mavis. "A Feminist Perspective in Midwifery." In *Feminist Practice in Women's Health Care.* C. Webb, ed. New York: John Wiley and Sons, 1986.

Lecky-Thompson, Maggie. "Homebirth Midwives: Powerful Pioneers or Ratbag Radicals?" *The Lamp,* vol. 45, no. 2 (1988): 10-14.

Massey, Elizabeth. "By Her Own Authority: The Scope of Midwifery Practice Under the Ontario Midwifery Act, 1991," *Alberta Law Review,* vol. 31, no. 2 (1993): 349-390.

Midwifery Regulation Advisory Committee (MRAC). *Midwifery Regulation.* Professions and Occupations Bureau, Government of Alberta, 1994.

Ouwerkerke, Alice. "Uniting Vocation and Avocation: Becoming a Midwife in Alberta Prior to Regulation." Master's thesis, University of Alberta, 1995.

Recommendations for Midwifery Education and Assessment. Professions and Occupations Bureau, Government of Alberta, 1994.

Reid, Margaret. "Sisterhood and Professionalization: A Case Study of the American Lay Midwife." In *Women as Healer: Cross-Cultural Perspectives,* C.S. McClain, ed. New Brunswick: Rutgers University Press, 1989.

Rothman, Barbara Katz. *Recreating Motherhood: Ideology and Technology in Patriarchal Society.* New York: W.W. Norton, 1989.

Sandelowski, Margarite. "A Case of Conflicting Paradigms: Nursing and Reproductive Technology," *Advances in Nursing Science,* vol. 10, no. 3 (1988): 35-45.

Standards of Competency and Practice. Professions and Occupations Bureau, Government of Alberta, 1994.

Thompson, P. *The Nature of Work.* London: MacMillan Education Ltd, 1989.

Weitz, Rose, and Deborah Sullivan. "Licensed Lay Midwifery and the Medical Model of Childbirth." *Sociology of Health and Illness,* vol. 7 (1985): 36-54.

Ontario Midwifery in Transition:

An Exploration of Midwives' Perceptions of the Impact of Midwifery Legislation in its First Year

Mary Sharpe

HISTORICAL PREFACE

This preface focuses principally on events in the greater Toronto area of Ontario. Recent Ontario midwifery legislation embodies a discourse and an image of midwifery that has become prominent in the last twenty years. While it illuminates a particular form of maternity care, now enshrined in government documents, it can shadow, by exclusion, other manifestations of midwifery, both historical and current. When I[1] speak of midwives in this chapter, I will be referring to a small, predominantly white middle class community of women, who, in concert with a strong consumer body, crafted a model of midwifery which became accepted by the Ontario government and implemented in the Midwifery Act in 1994.

The episode of legislation under discussion exists within a long history of many generations of women helping women with their birthings on this land that is presently called Ontario. In many First Nations, Aboriginal midwifery developed from a holistic cultural world view that wove together concepts of mind, body and spirit. Many Aboriginal midwives played a central role in their community with their birthing wisdom and particular spiritual connection to the family.[2] Neighbour women[3] or foreign-trained midwives working within their ethnic communities were usually specially chosen and respected as the primary helpers at births. As well, numerous women in Ontario, over the years, out of choice or necessity, birthed alone.

The agency of midwives in Ontario was disturbed by the gradual medical takeover of birth and by the transportation of women to centres where hospital delivery was available. Framing women's work around birthing and reproduction as illegal was a powerful means of suppressing these midwives. It lead to persecutions, investigations and inquests, particularly when the interests of the medical profession and these women practitioners were at odds. In the late 19th century, doctors attended births in larger numbers; by 1935, half of the births in Ontario occurred in hospital and by 1960, practically all. After this time, home births were occasionally attended by Aboriginal or foreign-trained midwives, especially in the north where physician services were scarce. Within two generations, midwife-attended births had almost completely disappeared in Ontario.

Consumers began to critique the medicalization of childbirth in the 1950s, and by the 1970s the women's movement was actively attempting to demystify knowledge around reproduction and birthing. Women helped others individually or through self-help groups. They worked alegally and illegally, usually voluntarily outside the system, to accomplish what women wanted and needed. They struggled to obtain safe abortions and to permit choice over place of birth, particularly home births.[4] Among the sites of political action were childbirth classes,[5] breastfeeding support groups and women's health groups. Women, insisting that they were not experts, learned skills to help women with abortions, to give birth and to breastfeed. Ontario lay midwives in the late 1970s and 1980s were involved in these activities.

Much feminist work centred on preventing sexual violence against women and supporting women when it had occurred. Obvious links were noted between sexual violence and the male-dominated obstetrical practices of intimidation, procedures done without information or permission, episiotomies and unnecessary instrumental deliveries. Early lay midwives attempted to interrupt these practices by empowering women to validate and protect their bodies and their experiences.

Several Ontario lay midwives helped mount a pilot gynecological teaching project by working as professional patients instructing medical students.[6] These women were trained and well paid to teach vaginal examinations to the students and to evaluate the students' abilities. This was an opportunity to teach medical students interpersonal skills and raise awareness about the importance of discussion, sharing information, participatory care, and obtaining permission before any procedure.

Many foreign-trained midwives, who may have preferred to continue to work in their previous role as midwives, were working as labour and delivery nurses in Ontario hospitals. The subsequent professional development of midwifery in Ontario occurred with the active participation of only two or three of these women,[7] and only one of these midwives was in the first group of licensed midwives in Ontario. In 1973, some of these midwives formed the Ontario Nurse-Midwives Association (ONMA). This group wanted improvements in maternity services for women but few attended home births or supported them publicly.

In the early 1970s, a small number of family physicians were still attending home births, usually assisted by nurses from the Victoria Order of Nurses (VON). In 1976, government funding for this service was discontinued as an unnecessary expense. A group of consumers and professionals created the Home Birth Task Force to protest this action. Home birth had became popular as a reaction to restrictive hospital policies where babies were often delivered instrumentally in cold rooms and routinely separated from their mothers. A growing understanding[8] of the importance to the baby of gentle birthing practices, and of the infant's need for continuous nurturing contact with his/her mother, inspired this group.

Without the VON, the new need for assistants to physicians at home births was met by women aspiring to become midwives. For the most part, these assistants were childbirth educators, women who had given birth at home or those wishing to realize a personal philosophy around maternity care. In addition, they were usually privileged enough to be able to sustain the risks of working alegally.

The task force actively supported home birth by organizing educational events, most notably a workshop with a lay-midwife educator who encouraged the women in attendance to consider and name themselves "midwives" and if possible attend her training centre in Texas.[9] Evolving from the activities of the Home Birth Task Force, the Toronto Birth Centre Committee began work to lobby for another venue for birth in free-standing birth centres. By 1979, lay attendants had begun to network and established study groups and informal midwifery clinics in their homes.

Typically, at these clinics pregnant women, who had learned of the clinic by word of mouth, would gather one morning a week in one of the lay midwife's living rooms, bringing snacks to share. Herbal tea was usually warm on the kitchen stove. On a shelf, there was a donation jar for a small fee to help pay for the midwives' expenses, and a collection of books women could borrow. The morning was like a drop-in where children played with each other and women talked together while they waited to see the lay midwife of their choice in one of several bedrooms upstairs. At noon, the lay midwives would gather in the kitchen over a pot-luck lunch and discuss what they had learned from the morning contact with the women and make plans for educational activities. In 1981, these lay midwives and others created the Ontario Association of Midwives (OAM).

Many of these lay midwives developed allies among certain medical professionals who were willing to step outside their usual roles. These professionals contributed such skills as suturing, obtained antihaemorrhagic drugs essential for midwifery practice, signed birth certificates, and were available for consultation. By 1980, most physicians[10] at home births expected lay attendants to 'catch' the baby and be active in other medical procedures. Although legally responsible and usually present at births, most home-birth physicians supported the attendants' participation; they had often developed trusting relationships with them and appreciated their labour attending skills and their ability to spend time before and after births. Women taking charge of their health care increasingly requested these lay attendants at home and in hospital. For some lay midwives, this work became a full-time vocation.

In 1982, the College of Physicians and Surgeons of Ontario declared home birth unsafe and discouraged support for lay midwives, warning that it was professional misconduct for a member to permit, counsel or assist any person not licensed as a physician to engage in the practice of medicine. Hospitals threatened to withdraw privileges from physicians who attended home births and by 1983, few doctors offered this service. Although concerned consumers at that time wanted the choice of home birth to remain open, some felt that this could be accomplished only through the support of home-birth physicians; others, inspired by midwives from British Columbia, considered that birthing options for women could best be realized through legislated midwifery. It was in this latter context that the Midwifery Task Force was created. In response to the lack of physician attendants, lay attendants became primary caregivers at home births. They began to call themselves midwives, formed cooperative arrangements and took on apprentices. Until the midwifery legislation of January 1994, the role of these 'midwives' at planned hospital births was limited to labour support, with the doctor responsible.

Two Ontario inquests into baby deaths following midwife-attended home births in 1982, and the stories of the persecution of midwives in the United States and British Columbia, were powerful organizing forces for Ontario midwives. The Ontario Minister of Health formed the Health Professions Legislative Review and the ONMA and the OAM, jointly "The Midwifery Coalition," submitted a brief requesting midwifery regulation. In 1983, the Midwifery Task Force of Ontario, comprised primarily of midwifery clients, began to lobby for legalization of a model of midwifery care with informed choice, choice of birth place and continuity of care as core principles.[11]

In the mid 1980s, the Ontario government funded a hospital-based nurse-midwifery project at McMaster Medical Centre. At its inception, this service did not offer continuity of care nor home births but prenatal care and nurse-midwife-attended births. The director of this project and the chief of obstetrics who supported it subsequently became key consultants and leaders in the process towards legislated midwifery.

In 1984, at the Midwives' Alliance of North America Conference held in Toronto, the ONMA amalgamated with the OAM to form the Association of Ontario Midwives (AOM). Following another inquest in 1985, the jury recommended the regulation of midwifery to protect the safety of the public, recognizing that home birth would continue underground in any case. The Ontario government appointed the Task Force for the Implementation of Midwifery Care in Ontario to investigate midwifery internationally and accept proposals and submissions from many interest groups. Its 1987 report recommended direct-entry[12] autonomous midwifery for Ontario.

A group of Ontario consumers and midwives who understood the necessary ingredients of professionalism[13] and its processes developed standards and regulations so that the AOM would be recognized as a self-regulating body. Many of their documents were used as a basis for decisions of the Interim Regulatory Council of Midwifery and its successors, the Transitional Council and ultimately the College of Midwives. In May 1991, the Midwifery Integration Planning Project, mandated by the Ministry of Health in 1990, completed the outline of a midwifery education program, a four-year baccalaureate degree.[14] In October 1992, 72 Ontario midwives began a one-year pre-registration program and assessment period run by the Michener Institute in Toronto. And in January 1994, when the Health Professions Legislative Act which included the Midwifery Act was enacted, 58 Ontario midwives began practising as publicly funded, regulated health professionals.

Responding to efforts of Aboriginal women and midwives lobbying for acknowledgment of the cultural significance of traditional Aboriginal birthing practices, and supported by the Equity Committee[15] of the Interim Regulatory Council on Midwifery, the Ontario government exempted Aboriginal midwives from the registration process in Section 35 of the Midwifery Act. These midwives[16] are recognized by the Ontario government as practitioners within their communities.

We see in the energetic struggle to recreate midwifery, a meaningful feminist endeavour and triumph. Ontario midwifery provided a model that is different from and challenges current obstetrical practice, and thus represents a significant paradigm shift from male-dominated maternity care to woman-centred care provided principally by female caregivers.

TRANSITION TO LEGALIZED MIDWIFERY

Midwifery now moved into the mainstream of Ontario health care. The Midwifery Act in January 1994 required the establishment of new work structures, processes and relationships. Midwives asked themselves: What will legislative regulation mean for our lives, our practices and our relationships with the women for whom we provide care? How will the midwifery model we have crafted be altered? Might legislation be the only way to prevent other professional groups from taking control of midwifery?[17] Could our model be preserved and possibly expanded to provide women with better and more accessible midwifery care? It was this widespread mixture of doubt, ambivalence and excitement about new possibilities in myself as a midwife and in others, that led me to study this transition.

I engaged in a case study,[18] based on interviews with Ontario midwives, to examine the impact of legislation on their practices. Have midwives' worst fears or brightest hopes come true? Sixteen of the 24 licensed Ontario midwives who had been practising in Ontario for at least five years prior to and during the first year following legislation, were interviewed. This group of midwives was homogeneous with respect to race and class: all were Euro-Canadian middle-class women; a more diverse seed group of midwives would have more appropriately represented a province whose largest city is the most multicultural in the world. Eligible participants were selected from eleven practices and six geographical areas, both rural and urban: one midwife was in solo practice; the others were in shared practices of from two to five midwives. This chapter is an attempt to give voice to a wide range of these midwives' feelings and perceptions. Most midwives were interviewed only seven months after they had moved into offices and ten months after legislation. It was acknowledged that as midwives attempted to make sense of this new situation, the struggles and difficulties might dominate their discussions. It was recognized as well that in this sensitive period of adjustment, midwives might have perceptions and observations that would later be lost as they became accustomed to these changes.

AN OVERVIEW OF MIDWIVES' PERCEPTIONS

Midwives felt variously delighted, freed, satisfied, acknowledged, frustrated, overworked, anxious and cautious about the changes that legislation had brought. Among their responses, common themes and areas arose, but the ways in which midwives regarded these differed. Most often mentioned were:
1. changes in the relationship with the client,
2. the new role of the midwife as primary caregiver:
    a) with an expanded role in prenatal, intrapartum and postpartum care,
    b) with increased paperwork and responsibilities in hospitals,
    c) with new interprofessional relationships,
3. an alteration in work arrangements with colleague midwives,
4. changes in clinic settings and administration,
5. government remuneration for midwifery services.

The least change was noted in the caregiving for women choosing home birth, the home being seen by midwives as the crucial site where the essence of midwifery care could most be preserved. The majority felt that regulation protected the existing model of care and that their expanded role as primary caregivers in hospital and in prenatal care somewhat increased their ability to provide care closer to the midwifery ideal. However, most midwives expressed uneasiness and the need for vigilance in the years to come since changes had necessitated a new interaction with professional procedures, behaviours and language that might shift midwifery work more towards current manifestations of the medical model.

ONTARIO MIDWIFERY MODEL

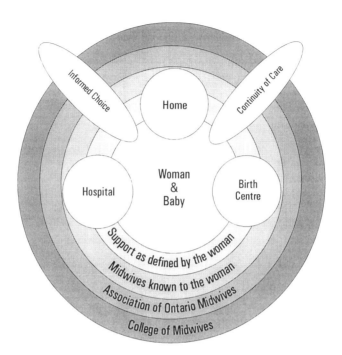

Here is a model representing the situation in which Ontario midwives currently work. The model consists of concentric circles representing a variety of relationships. Central is the woman and her baby, surrounded by her personal supporters *as defined by her*. Midwives *known to the woman* (usually two but no more than four) surround them and provide *care that is continuous* and *nonauthoritarian* for the woman and her baby, during pregnancy, the birth and for six weeks postpartum. Visits of between half an hour and an hour are arranged between the woman and midwife so that a *relationship develops over time*, and information is shared so the woman can make *informed decisions* around her care. These concepts of *continuity of care* and *informed choice*, which are highly significant to all involved in the woman's care, are represented by ellipses. Three circles overlapping the 'family' and midwife group are the settings in which *women choose to give birth* and where midwives work: the home, the hospital, and where available, the free-standing birthing centre. Around the group practice is the professional association, the Association of Ontario Midwives, and finally the regulatory body, the College of Midwives. Not included in this model are the webs of interaction that occur between the medical profession, the midwife and the family especially when there is a need for consultation or referral of a midwife's care to a physician.

INCREASED DEMANDS

The following lists attempt to illustrate the proliferation of tasks, duties and responsibilities of the Ontario midwife after legislation.

PRE-LEGISLATION

Most midwives' tasks were:

- acting as primary caregiver at home births
- documenting care for home births
- serving as back-up midwife at home births
- acting as labour supporter and advocate at hospital births
- providing prenatal and postpartum care but not as the primary caregiver
- educating oneself through reading and attending courses

In addition, some midwives were:

- attendees at weekly organizational meetings with their practice group
- active committee members of the Association of Ontario Midwives
- members on government planning committees
- educators for the public
- graduate students seeking credentials

The following tasks that midwives had performed have not continued after legislation:

- providing initial contact with the woman and scheduling appointments
- choosing to work with an apprentice midwife

POST-LEGISLATION

In addition to most of the above, midwives' tasks usually include:

- acting as primary caregiver at hospital births
- documenting care at hospital births
- providing prenatal and postnatal care as the primary caregiver
- ordering of prenatal testing and prescriptions of certain drugs
- preparing necessary paperwork for the funding organization
- attending regular meetings on hospital committees to ensure admitting privileges
- attending educational presentations at hospital
- participating in workshops to satisfy requirements of the College of Midwives

- preceptoring responsibilities for assigned baccalaureate program students
- interacting with office administrators

As well, some midwives presently may be:
- faculty members in the midwifery baccalaureate programs
- committee members and registrars of the College of Midwives
- colleagues with nonmidwife second attendants in small practices

IMPACT ON MIDWIVES

With legislation, the midwife has been catapulted into a new status, role and context. Many noted that stress, increased work load and an increased sense of responsibility affected their midwifery care. Most said they were undergoing some form of adjustment which appeared, for some, to be related to the details of their working situation before legislation. For example, for those few midwives who had always worked in an office rather than in their homes, who had office equipment and an established working relationship with their partners, the adjustment was not as dramatic. Midwives in Ontario who had helped design the changes wrought by legislation seemed more prepared for these changes and less anxious than those who were more distant philosophically or geographically from the locus of this process.

Government funding increased requests for midwifery care in most parts of Ontario. Some midwives, especially in rural areas, found that their previous modest caseloads approached maximum numbers. However, regardless of whether their caseloads increased or decreased, all midwives reported more time spent on bureaucratic responsibilities.

Many changes had to be made rapidly: moving clinics from homes into offices with support staff; creating and spending start-up budgets for offices and equipment. Midwives now became primary caregivers for clients and their babies until six weeks postpartum and were responsible for prenatal testing. Now, as primary caregivers in hospitals, they immediately had to master hospital procedures, including extensive documentation.

The ongoing public education and political work necessary to maintain the gains of legislation, and the continuing demands of mounting and developing the new baccalaureate program added considerably to the stress for many midwives. Here are some quotes from midwives illustrating the intense demand of the first year of legislated midwifery practice:

The year has been so fraught with adjustments at every level.

In a sense, I think that one of the hardest things for us in this first year has been that we have not had the luxury of being able to do one thing at a time.

I am on a big learning curve. I'm much busier.

It's been about a year now and with the incredible speed of the additional demands... I'm sort of surfacing.

I feel that I'm in a pressure cooker all the time. I feel that I never catch up to the work and that there is no way to catch up to the work and so all of that impacts on how I practice as a midwife.

I am stretched and stressed a whole lot and I know that affects my client care.

I am so stressed out I can hardly remember who I have had as clients this year.

That just makes us a little bit more stretched. Many days I think, if only I had another couple of hours when I was alert and full of energy. We just need more time.

I'm working harder. Maybe it's accumulated tiredness. There is more clinical work and lots of systems work. There are many little things but not major changes.

More impact on me and my life... The thing that shocks me the most is I didn't anticipate it; it surprised me.

People are dealing with a grumpy midwife and they're dealing with a grumpy mum... I find that I don't have the same level of patience.

CLINIC SETTING

Prior to legislation, midwives usually saw their clients in their homes. Many aspects of the midwives' new role required that they now work out of offices: for example, laboratories pick up requisitions and specimens, instruments need to be autoclaved, faxes sent and received. Midwives reported that the new provision of offices, equipment and administrators were significant supports for their work. Some appreciated the division of home and work that this new arrangement brought. For some, this new setting felt more "professional."

It's good to have the kind of facility and equipment and supplies and support to work in a much more professional way... I have a place I can go to. Support at the place where I see people. Office staff, someone there who can be helpful to people when they come in, answer the telephone, help us with the load of documents we have to deal with on a daily basis. It feels really special.

In contrast to a home clinic setting, the atmosphere seemed more like a doctor's office with a receptionist, a waiting room, telephones ringing and more busyness. One midwife felt that there was more possibility for interruptions during visits with clients in the office, and that there she was less considerate of her clients.

Now, I find that I do know I'm not so considerate of them in terms of their time. There is this thing of being a professional. Now I find that I know I'm in the office, so especially if there's a doctor who needs to phone me or someone I'm having difficulty getting in touch with, I know I'm here so I allow myself to have my visits with my clients interrupted, or postponed, because I need to get these people during working hours. This happens much more often. The other thing is other people in the office..., knocks at the door, meetings to attend, another midwife. There are a lot more interruptions. One of the nice things about being in the office is having another midwife to consult with immediately, but it also does change the nature of your visit if you have somebody else come in or knock at the door. The clients now, they must find it different.

Another midwife was making a special effort to protect her client from disturbances of the office.

I may be thoroughly rushed and overworked in all of the work I am doing, I still have to be very careful to protect that time with the woman. That means when she comes and the door closes, I have to compartmentalize that I am with her now and we're all concentrating on her. My goal has been to insulate the individual client from any of the new stuff I have to do.

Another respondent felt ambivalent about this change; however, she appreciated not having her space intruded upon.

The other thing is seeing people in an office setting. Again this is so interesting but there are these subtle changes... When someone comes into my office, they're not in my home. They're not in my space. [On the other hand,] it's a relief not to have to clean my house for clients and to think some of them may overstep the minimum boundaries: for example, with their children getting into my children's things.

Yet another midwife noted that clients had expressed sadness and missed the visits in her home and even in some cases had turned down midwifery care after legislation because of this change in setting. Another felt there was less intimacy since she was no longer able to welcome clients into her home.

It's not as intimate and you have to work harder to create that intimacy. Having people waiting in the waiting room. At home I spaced my appointments and never really had that much conflict in time. I'd give myself a couple of hours, spend time with the kids again, then see somebody again. It was a much more free flowing thing. I feel almost more medicalized with this: Okay, next woman coming in!

Somehow hugging somebody in your own home is very different than standing in the office hugging someone. Not that I feel different, but there is already a distance created by the space.

In moving to an office, one midwife felt she lost her autonomy.

> My sense of loss of autonomy coincides, of course, with losing the clinic space in my house and becoming part of a practice and working out of an office.

Many midwives and the women whom they served were predominantly middle class. It was noted that the office setting provided an equalizing effect for midwives who had differing life styles, and worked to the advantage of those who did not formerly feel comfortable having clients in their homes.

> In a way, working in an office is an equalizer for the midwives. It is an interesting thought because there are midwives who are very well off who can afford to have housekeepers and not worry about what things look like because it's taken care of. And there are midwives who are not so well off who always had to worry about — was the home reasonable to have people coming in? It is beginning to feel that we are more equal and I don't ever get the sense at this point that a client chooses her midwife because she lives better or worse. And there was some of that feeling at times. Certain women would be more comfortable with a particular midwife because of her lifestyle.

NEW ACCESSIBILITY TO MIDWIFERY CARE:
POSSIBILITIES AND CHALLENGES

All the midwives observed that after legislation, requests for midwives' services had increased dramatically: in some cases, three or four times the number of requests were received than practices could accommodate. A large percentage of women requesting midwifery care were repeat clients who were delighted that they now didn't have to pay. Some midwives noted that many women seeking midwifery care for the first time were younger and much more culturally and socially varied than before. Midwives felt very positive about the greater accessibility and felt that public funding and the current legitimacy of midwifery made this possible.

> Our clientele has definitely changed to access more of a multicultural community. Some women have told me that they couldn't have chosen to have a midwife in the past because it didn't feel secure enough. It felt too radical... It feels good to be more accessible.

> The women who mostly sought us out in our practice were in their mid-30s, educated, and generally financially fairly well off; people who were more vocal and demanding in terms of what they wanted out of their childbirth experience and critical of hospitals... Now our clientele is basically often young women, women without the benefits of a lot of education or financial backing or a settled home and many with very difficult social situations.

Midwives expressed concern that after legislation, some women seeking care were not clearly committed to the midwifery model in which birth is considered normal, were in general less concerned about their health, weighed their decision to have a midwife less carefully, wanted the midwife to make decisions for them, and in general seemed more closely aligned to the medical model.[19] Some women seeking midwifery care were reluctant to relinquish an ongoing connection with a physician or were unclear that midwifery care now meant that the midwife would remain the primary caregiver unless circumstances indicated a referral to a physician. In the past, midwives were considered part of the counterculture and outside the system, and many clients had identified with this stance. Now the midwife, as a part of the healthcare system, was considered more mainstream and it was felt that the new client population perhaps reflected this. Some midwives felt co-opted by changes in hospitals.

> People who don't have the same commitment to their own health and being responsible for their own well-being are coming to midwifery care now for a variety of reasons.

> I miss having clients who really want the natural, who know they can birth, are willing, and aren't afraid.

> When I started I had women who would do anything to keep from going to the hospital. You don't have that same kind of pioneering spirit among people anymore. Consumers aren't fighting anymore because hospitals have changed.

For some midwives the change in the nature of the client provided some challenge and some extra effort. Some said it was important to select or actively discourage potential clients, or to clearly declare their own preferences around birth options. Others felt it necessary to educate potential clients about the midwifery model so that women could be clear about their choice of midwifery care. Still other midwives felt that it was important to educate themselves about their clients' needs and to work with clients in more creative ways to respond to those needs: for example, developing strategies to work with linguistic barriers, offering certain clients more clinic time than others, and preparing materials to make information more accessible.

> We are taking more care to explain things so that they really know what they are going to be working with.

> Flexibility is needed to make meetings with the midwife longer than an hour if someone wants to talk about something more.

> There is a need to restructure much. In the past we relied on a lot of written things. Even talking about reading things can be kind of threatening because it reminds them of school work. We need to rework our handouts to be briefer so the people can explore as they want to, but so they don't feel overwhelmed or threatened by them.

Some midwives, overwhelmed with requests for midwifery care, wanted to be available to those who were more aligned with the midwifery model, and therefore preferred clients choosing home birth. A midwife's mandate is to respect a woman's choices. However, if from the outset of her care a woman declares that she will be making choices which place her squarely in the 'camp' of the medical model, does it make sense for the midwife, who supports birth as a normal physiological event, to take this woman on as a client?

Client selection was seen as an ethical dilemma needing further study. Most midwives spoke of how their practices struggled with a selection process. Midwives seemed aware that in the past they had accessed primarily a white middle-class population and wished to develop affirmative action policies to make midwifery care an option for diverse groups of women. Some midwives noted that they had to learn how to limit clientele and that this was a new experience for them. Strict selection on a first come, first served basis was not seen to be necessarily fair. Other considerations such as the woman's need, her cultural or social situation, her choice of birth place and commitment to natural birth and the midwifery model, influenced client selection.

> Ethically how can you say to someone, 'You haven't thought this through enough.' We are a publicly funded service. Can we really select clients? It's tricky.

> Now we prioritize for home births. We need to make an effort for home births. We save one spot a month until 28 weeks for teens, Native women. Those are things that have come fairly recently.

Midwives were concerned that the very consumer values that had helped shape Ontario's midwifery model might change and shift the midwifery model closer to the medical model.

> The client base that came to us led to the development of the model. Our consumers have really led the model... It's changing. That's what will change the base of midwifery and moreover, we have to continue to have that really strong relationship with consumers who care about the same model: the women who want the same thing. Their voice really made a difference for us in getting to where we are and it's their voice that will make the difference in keeping us who we are.

FUNDING

Funding midwifery care was seen as consonant with 40 years of healthcare history in Ontario. Midwives were delighted that women didn't have to pay for their services and saw funded midwifery as a strong public response towards respecting women's choices.

Access to free health care is so deeply embedded in people's minds that the idea of charging automatically disqualified people from investigating it. Since it is now free, people who wouldn't have considered midwifery are going for it .

Many midwives began their work as part-time volunteers, supported by their partners' incomes or through other occupations such as teaching, nursing, childbirth education or community work. As they gained experience, they offered more care and began to charge. Immediately before legislation, most midwives' maximum fee had risen to $1000-$1500, a fee which covered an average of over 40 hours with each client and helped defray expenses. Most midwives also used sliding fee scales, created arrangements for skills' exchanges and often provided free care.

Midwives unanimously rejoiced in the personal advantages of being publicly funded. One reported that being a paid professional affected her self-esteem; another found that being paid well gave her new energy so that she liked her work again.

It was an extremely exhausting lifestyle. It certainly does help [to be salaried] because there's only so many years that you can go on providing that care with almost no holidays and virtually no income and nothing for retirement.

One midwife who had formerly felt that she needed to do work as a "saint" out of the "goodness of her heart" and felt guilty if she was unwilling, welcomed being able to acknowledge rough spots in her work now she felt she was paid appropriately. For one, there was less worry about getting and keeping clientele, more freedom to just "be who I am" and "stand my own ground." She felt that she hadn't always been honest or straightforward with clients about her limits, for fear of losing their business. One interviewee felt that clients who paid privately for her care felt they had ownership over her and that she was at their "beck and call." Another, by contrast, felt that a woman who paid for her services treated her as "valuable," and in response she "would go all out" for her client.

A midwife felt that pre-legislation, the payment she received from her client directly related to her reputation and to the service she provided; now she felt more identified with her profession than with her client. Another said that the relationship with her client felt less intimate.

I am no longer being paid for the service that I give. That I excel at what I do was important. My work used to be based on my reputation. I feel I have moved into anonymity.

It's a more intimate contractual relationship between that person and you. They're paying you money to get your care. Not to say that money is necessary to create that intimate relationship....

Some saw altruism as a valuable quality in a midwife and worried that future midwives might choose the profession primarily for the salary. Before legislation, accessibility to midwives was limited not only by linguistic and racial barriers but also by the payment factor. This was also a mechanism, which had screened the client base for commitment.

In the context of the economics of reproduction, structural power and the global under valuation of women's work,[20] the legalization of midwifery in Ontario made an important statement: women count. Public funding of midwifery overturned the situation of unpaid or poorly paid support of women by women in this particular area. The salary range for the Ontario midwife now falls between that of a nurse and a general practitioner. Midwifery is no longer just another poorly paid female profession.

Some Ontario midwives had overworked because they couldn't afford to turn away women who asked for their services.[21] The additional income accrued by taking on extra clients helped compensate for being underpaid and helped to rationalize the time that some midwives spent away from their families. Now midwives are paid adequate salaries for a reasonable caseload and are not paid more if they work over their quotas. Legislation allowed that midwives be paid for clinic appointments of between a half hour and an hour's duration. The funding system was intended to ensure that midwives take time with their clients because there would be no financial incentive for them to take on more clients.

RELATIONSHIP WITH COLLEAGUE MIDWIVES

Before legislation, most midwives worked as independent practitioners with their own clientele. They would request that another midwife meet with their client at least once for back-up purposes. If the client was planning a home birth, the back-up midwife would assist at the time of the birth. Hospital births required only one midwife because the physician was the primary caregiver at the birth, and the midwife was the labour supporter and advocate. Arrangements among colleague midwives ranged from tightly organized collectives to casual cooperatives.

After legislation more involvement and contact with partner midwives was needed. Midwives now became primary caregivers at hospital births and were assisted in this setting by another midwife from the practice. Since the practice group now wrote checks from government funding for midwives' salaries and equipment, a new level of organization and group decision-making was required within the practices.

In addition, legislation made each midwife in a practice legally responsible for the actions of every other midwife in the practice. This created a norm that a midwife avoid making decisions that could negatively affect the others. Colleagues needed to spend more time with each other working out the details of their practice relationship. Some midwives felt there were advantages for midwife and client in this closer working relationship[22]: protection and support for one another, greater group strength and efficiency. Others considered this increased communication with partners to be time consuming and personally limiting.

> I think working together is something that improves everybody's communication skills. I think that it improves care. I value our practice so much; what you have are people's strengths and weaknesses. The strengths of all affect all the women. I enjoy that environment.

> There are mutual responsibilities under our liability insurance and under the midwifery act. I'm responsible for what my partners do. It's so codifying and limiting. To actually practise and know that with every move you're making, you are responsible to the other members of your practice. You can no longer make an individual decision; you are making it as part of a collective. I can feel a lot of feeling lying up in my chest about this. There's a part of me that's feeling duped.

The principle of 'continuity of care' encourages the development over time of a relationship between the client and midwife. For some midwives, the increasing time commitment to partners has somewhat shifted their focus away from client-midwife relationships to intercollegial relationships.

Most midwives moved into a 'shared care' model: after 28-weeks gestation, a woman's visits would be shared between two midwives. This created the possibility of some time off-call for individual midwives, yet required more effective communication among partners about the care for women in their practice. Some midwives experienced acceptance of, and increased comfort with, sharing care following a significant event in their own lives for which they had to leave their client: for example, when a close family member was ill or died. They were reassured that even under these circumstances their client would be well cared for. Others, however, felt 'shared care' interfered with the development of a one-to-one relationship with their clients. Under this new arrangement, would the midwife be less caring, or more ready to serve and care for her client? A midwife in one practice where the care was not shared yearned for the advantages that such an arrangement would bring.

> The sense I have in our group is that there's reluctance to let go of those last vestiges of the independent midwife — not wanting to succumb to the group or the shared care, on the one hand, yet on the other hand, we need more time off.

The assessment process for the regulation of currently practising midwives encouraged some, who had been working intermittently and often alone, to see midwifery as a full-time future profession for themselves. They became more active and began to connect with other midwives to build their birth numbers in preparation for assessment. However, regulation disqualified other midwives who did not have the required numbers of births within the stipulated assessment period, effectively stopping their practices, temporarily or permanently. For one midwife the rearrangement of midwives to new practices resulted in isolating her from midwives with whom she had previously associated.

EXPANDED ROLE AS PRIMARY CAREGIVER IN PRE- AND POSTPARTUM CARE

Legislation decreed that midwives be the primary caregivers for women and their babies throughout the pregnancy and up to six weeks following the birth, necessitating that midwives perform physical assessments, order prenatal tests, connect with laboratories and make proper referrals to specialists when necessary. Most felt that this expanded role enhanced the client relationship towards more continuous and holistic care.

> The care is less fragmented. The continuity is really a continuity because we have access to that piece the doctors were doing before. That's the big change for us.

> Some old clients who come to us now don't know they don't have to go to a doctor. 'You mean you can do everything!' They are thrilled.

> If anything, I think I can provide my clients with something a little bit more. They don't have to run around to two caregivers. I think it's changed in a positive way. I am way more accessible.

> There is a warm fuzzy feeling when you are a recognized caregiver. When the lab people know that, yes, it's appropriate for you to have the results and order the lab tests and it's so nice that the pharmacists know that we can prescribe certain things.

For some midwives this role gave them a new status as autonomous caregivers. Being the primary caregiver clarified the scope of their practice. It was no longer shared with a physician, but it was accompanied by a new weight of responsibility. Some now better appreciated the role that physicians assume.

> There is a stronger sense of responsibility because you are the one she relates to during the pregnancy.

> I feel the weight of the responsibility terribly now. I had a way of pedalling around the surface and kind of half knowing what was going around a lot of things without ever fishing in and saying, 'What is this really all about?'

> It is like your whole range of vision has to be enormously wide, and you need a certain kind of emotional clarity for that.

Several midwives noted with dismay that their clients lacked trust that the midwife alone without a doctor could fulfill her new expanded role as primary caregiver for all aspects of normal prenatal and postpartum care for the mother and baby. However, it was appreciated that, just as the midwife was adjusting to an expanded role, so the client was adjusting to the midwife's new scope of practice. The perception by some that clients were now more interested in a medical model of care than before may be due to the midwives' new role which exposed them directly to requests for testing and medical technology.

The midwifery principle of providing information to support informed decision-making by the client took on a different form. No longer were midwives primarily emphasizing the alternate view that had not always previously been offered by the physician, but now they needed themselves to incorporate views that reflected the community medical standard as well. This led to a dilemma for some who felt that their describing tests to clients might be construed as condoning these tests. Some were anxious that they might forget to talk about possible genetic testing in time. Midwives felt that the requirement to offer testing shifted their care towards a focus of *verifying* rather than *assuming* pregnancy to be normal and that midwives themselves might be moving away from a 'wellness' model towards a pathology-oriented model which relied on ultrasounds and an increased use of the 'system' with less time spent on woman-generated material relating to the woman's feelings, questions and circumstances. The use of technology varied amongst midwives. How were midwives utilizing the principle of informed decision-making with their clients? To what extent was the particular bias of a midwife now relevant to client choices?

> I always say that my presenting this does not make it legitimate. I only feel obligated because, if a month down the road you hear about it and you say, 'Why didn't my midwife talk to me about this?' I feel I need to make sure that clients know what is out there.

> I feel myself sliding more into the use of technology in the accepted medical standard. I see the changes in the trends and I am unsettled by them.

> The list of tests grows and will continue to grow because science provides us with more ability to detect things. It's a cumulative thing and the normality of pregnancy is being lost even on the majority of women I think, in terms of being able to believe that it's normal. This is us changing since legislation.

> How insidious the whole thing has been in just working its way into my definition of my midwifery care antenatally. It comes with ordering all of our lab tests and ultra sounds. I would love to see a study of how many ultrasounds midwives in this province are ordering now, and lab tests and lab results, and how much we're using the system now.

Although they had systems of record-keeping before, some midwives were bothered by the amount of paperwork and documentation required for each client after legislation. Some midwives found that their attention was given more to their notes than to the mother and baby. Standardized prenatal and postpartum forms were thought to be constraining in that they dictated aspects of care: that is, if a place on the form is not filled out, the record is incomplete. Furthermore, it was felt, records cannot capture much of the affective care that is provided.

As partners became legally responsible for each other in sharing care for clients, many more clinical details needed to be remembered and attended to during visits. The focus of the meeting could not be primarily getting to know the woman. One midwife felt that, although the content of the clinic visits had changed, women still felt cared for by their midwives. Some midwives said that they needed to pay attention to how they provided clinical care in order to adequately address emotional and social needs and the participation of the woman's family. Some midwives reported that they were consciously working on balancing what they saw as good midwifery with the changes, and looked forward to increased adaptation to their new expanded role.

> What's really changed is taking on the full primary responsibility for the woman. We're the main one who has to detect if things aren't so straightforward and confer and consult. But at the same time, we need to make sure the care she receives is a woman-centred care and involves informed choice — the philosophy that's always been at the basis of midwifery here. I want to keep a lot of the old approach because that's why we got midwifery legalized in the first place — from what women wanted.

> We had to think this through as in the past and come up with a style that we felt really respected the woman, treated her with dignity, allowed her to feel an equal relationship with us — and how to do these other new things in that context.

> The way you do hands-on care is important and how you involve the family. Health reform initiatives encourage more active involvement in their care by the users of the healthcare system. It would be a tragedy if any kind of legislation undermined our ability to spend enough time to do that kind of participatory care.

MIDWIFE AS PRIMARY CAREGIVER AT HOSPITAL BIRTHS

Moving into the hospital system was recognized by midwives as an extraordinary and unprecedented event in health care in Ontario, which broke the medical monopoly over admitting privileges in hospitals. Most midwives seemed delighted with their new role and status in this setting.

Legislation stated that midwives should provide choice of birth place for their clients in the home, hospital or birthing centre, and that they be 'confident' and 'competent' in all these settings. In order to keep their registration with the College of Midwives, they must annually attend a minimum number of births in both home and hospital. Midwives at present are funded by the Ministry of Health and, although not hired by hospitals, are able to apply for hospital privileges in the same manner as physicians. Two midwives attend the woman at each hospital birth, except in solo practices or exceptional circumstances; doctors and nurses are not in attendance unless a transfer of care occurs.

Some midwives felt that receiving admitting privileges and working within the hospital had required considerable courage and skillful communication by midwives with hospital staff. Many hospitals had included midwives on committees preparing for integration and had policies and procedures in place designed to facilitate this; some hospitals had actively courted midwives to apply for admitting privileges. In other settings, however, the initiation of and responsibility for the negotiations with the hospital fell primarily on the shoulders of the midwives. For the latter, the transition was very difficult; these midwives had to do much ground work to educate hospital staff about midwifery before hospital privileges were extended. In these hospitals, midwifery care was considered highly controversial. The nature of maternity care in hospitals varied greatly; some hospitals had facilities supportive of labouring women — for example, bathtubs, showers, birthing rooms — and others did not. In some hospitals, there were discrepancies between what the administration and the nursing and obstetrical staff wanted with respect to midwifery integration into the hospital. In most hospitals, midwives were required to be active on hospital committees and attend educational rounds in the obstetrical department.

Most midwives appreciated the increasing respect and cooperation both from physicians and from other health professionals and noted that healthcare workers were all better informed about midwives. Some midwives spoke about a new relationship with obstetricians — a relationship with no animosity, which allowed for honest exchanges about management possibilities with clients. Others, however, experienced the medical staff as unwelcoming and not always accommodating. Some midwives felt they were accepted whether obstetricians liked them or not. In the past, transports of a home birth to hospital often met with disapproval from hospital staff; now this was not such an issue because there were communication lines in place and the midwife could usually continue providing supportive care.

One midwife complained that when hospital births were not straight-forward and needed some intervention, she had to interact with technology in a more direct way. She did not enjoy being on staff in a hospital. In addition, midwives now had to arrange the setting and the necessary personnel to be there if there were complications; these were responsibilities formerly attended to by the physician or nurse in hospital.

I am struggling with: would it be more ideal if we had separate midwives, some who do births in the hospital and others who just do home births? I don't want to be caregiver of the machine.

Some midwives felt closely monitored and scrutinized in hospitals, and that the hospital staff was testing them, waiting to assess their level of competence. There was great pressure to be very careful about what they did; it was important to 'act professional' in order to be accepted by the medical staff and to maintain their hospital privileges. Proper documentation and the appropriate manner of making referrals were some 'professional' skills. In exchange for hospital privileges, some midwives felt compromised, being now required to comply with certain hospital rules with which they didn't agree — because they would be regarded as negligent if they didn't. Some midwives implied that they had to 'behave like good girls' and 'move into line' in order to get what they wanted for their clients in the hospital setting and to maintain their credibility.

Of their new relationship with nurses after legislation, midwives mentioned: more open communication which relieved stress, feeling safe to walk out to the nurses and ask for help, nurses who were willing to help and were supportive. Some experienced 'give and take,' others that the nurses were helpful if needed but not forthcoming. One midwife sensed that nurses were worried that involvement with midwives might be risky. Another felt that her occupation was misunderstood as being luxurious. Although there were orientation sessions for nurses and staff regarding integration, because of the size of hospitals, there might still be staff on shift who were not familiar with the midwifery model.

Some nurses who had considerable obstetrical experience or were trained as midwives in other countries wanted to become Ontario registered midwives. They expressed their disappointment to some current registrants that the College of Midwives' prior learning and experience assessment process required additional work, time and money. One midwife felt it important to reserve positive feelings about acceptance in the hospital, since this was perhaps the "honeymoon stage." Midwives felt a special responsibility to their new profession noting that how they behaved during this integration period might affect midwives' acceptance in hospitals in the future.

Midwives felt that their new situation of working in the hospital was very stressful and that they were on a steep learning curve with respect to: the orientation to hospital procedures, protocols, equipment and paperwork, as well as the new responsibilities of admitting a client to and discharging the client from the hospital. Excepting those who had previous nursing experience, most had found this overwhelming at first but with time were somewhat able to adapt.

Three roles around a woman's birth were recognized: primary caregiver, documentor and labour supporter. Most midwives wished to assume all three but felt that this was difficult to accomplish in the hospital where they were distracted from their clients and felt disjointed and disconnected from them:

> The hospital is the most disturbing situation to me because I'm finding it difficult to feel like I'm both fulfilling my expected role as a healthcare professional in the hierarchy of the system in the hospital as well as just being with someone — which is what I feel my primary role is.

> When I get into the hospital, I'm in admission mode, and it takes a good hour. It's hard to find my place again in the labour in a hands-on supportive way because I have those ongoing charting things.

> I'm just not able to be as focused on them individually or totally. There are many other things running in my mind at the same time.

> Now you have a legal document that has to be completed. You're going to have to separate yourself from that woman and give something else your attention.

> You can't leave the room and sit some place a little distant and give them some privacy and still be part of it. You have to leave the door open or be in the room.

> In the hospital, it felt like I was walking through a prescribed scenario and there wasn't a whole lot of me in it; that they [the family] had chosen a route and I accompanied them through their route. I'm still trying to deal with what that means to me.

For planned hospital births, midwives labour with the woman at home, come into the hospital for the birth and then often return home with the mother several hours after the birth. The journey to the hospital for the birth seemed for one midwife a hiatus in care: "It's not until we get home and get settled that I pick up on the old midwifery care."

Midwives needed to prepare women choosing hospital births for the challenge of administrative duties which might take them in and out of the room. Others bring their clients and/or a second midwife into the hospital early to allow for enough people to provide the necessary support and accomplish the admitting tasks. One midwife noted the tension that these new duties created, but found that she was still really clear that the needs of her client for her support took precedence over other tasks.

The definition of being a good midwife in the hospital had changed for one midwife: before legislation it had to do with her labour supporting skills; now, it had to do with her clinical care and charting. Another noted that experiences in the hospital were influencing how she worked at home births in that she didn't have as much "hands on."

It's more up to them. I think I'm giving more over to the dad to be doing the supportive one-on-one, or a close family friend or another family member.

A midwife felt that she was influenced by the hospital setting as in the past.

You feel yourself being sucked back into the medical model as you apply for privileges. It's an ongoing struggle to separate yourself... I've been in medicine and I've been in that role and it's real easy for me to get back into the lingo and the patter. Moving back into that setting, some of us are mimicking the behaviour of that setting, which seems to be accepted in that setting.

In spite of the clear preference of most midwives to attend women at home, they were glad that they could offer the hospital option. Having hospital privileges allowed midwives to respond more fully to their clients' preferences, expectations and needs in this setting. Formerly, the physician's 'delivery' style and the activities around labouring and birthing did not always correspond to what midwives thought were in the woman's best interests. Now as primary caregivers at hospital births, midwives spoke with relief of their new role of being able to continue care for the woman after they entered the hospital in a manner they felt was appropriate. A midwife noted that some clientele were attracted to midwifery care because midwives now had hospital privileges and were seen as more legitimate; some of these women later opted for home birth.

Midwives noted the possibility of influencing hospital protocols by working in the hospital and sharing the "art of midwifery" with hospital staff and medical students. The midwife's presence in the hospital setting could model the provision of woman-centred care.

LABOUR COACHES, BIRTH ATTENDANTS OR DOULAS

Midwives mentioned the use of especially designated labour supporters and advocates other than themselves as an issue that had arisen since legislation. Some midwives noted that they encouraged women to have other labour support especially at hospital births because they felt that they were unable to give the support they had previously offered themselves because of other bureaucratic responsibilities. Another midwife didn't welcome clients' use of "labour coaches" because she felt this was a role she had always fulfilled herself and wished to continue. Some midwives felt that there might be a danger in midwives' relinquishing the labour support role, in that they might move into a role that has been typical of physician care.

It could be that midwives are going to get so busy that we're going to be just like obstetricians and rush in catch the baby and rush out again and the labour coach will do all the work.

STUDENTS IN PRACTICES AND THE BACCALAUREATE PROGRAMME
One midwife noted:

> We've got a College of Midwives; we've got our own teachers. The school is a good thing. And the teachers doing births; I think that's good.

The new Ontario Midwifery Education Programme appears to be a highly successful accomplishment according to a recent report by external reviewers[23] who note that:

> The Midwifery Education Programme now in its third year and funded by the government of Ontario, is the pioneering university midwifery programme in Canada. For the first time in this country, midwifery graduates will be trained to practice as self-regulating, autonomous primary healthcare practitioners under the midwifery philosophy.... the programme combines apprenticeship with academics for midwifery... It demonstrates careful, intensive planning to meet the special geographical, multicultural and public health needs of the Ontario population... the programme exhibits consciousness of, and sensitivity to, Native issues... the programme is... current, relevant, and progressive. It has these components: small class size and self-directed learning..., broad based learning that relates to society at large..., diversity of student backgrounds.

Midwives mentioned that the educational program and the presence of students had created a change in their practices. All of the midwives interviewed are acting as paid 'preceptors' or clinical teachers of student midwives who spend fifty percent of the baccalaureate program training in midwifery practices. At the time of the interviews, students were doing course work and were not present in practices; perhaps as a consequence, students were rarely mentioned in the interviews with midwives. Some midwives noted that their relationship with clients had changed because care was being shared not only with other midwives but also with students. Another midwife said that it was a challenge to figure out how to provide care that is based on continuity and a relationship with the woman and at the same time encourage the woman to bond with a student as her care-provider. In addition, midwives needed to learn how to develop appropriate relationships with the students.

> There is a big responsibility for us to be there for women but at the same time step far enough back to allow the student who's following this woman all the way through to bond with her as her primary caregiver.

Involvement with students increased midwives' overall work load, requiring yet another task to be accomplished. Many said they enjoyed the presence of students who brought new ideas and learnings to the practice. Some saw students as important supporters for the practice, especially during labours in the hospital.

When we have students with us that definitely helped to fill the gap with labour coaching role — for the woman's sake, having three sets of hands helped.

One midwife predicted that issues around students would be "enormous" for midwives in the future. Contrary to the pre-legislation apprenticeship system in which the midwife would have chosen her apprentice, students currently are assigned to preceptors; one midwife felt this situation was like an arranged marriage.

I have a student now who I had never met before and she is going to be with me for a year. This is an arranged marriage. She is ultimately going to be doing all my care. I have taken a student out of professional responsibility, not because I want one. I want to provide that care myself. I want to do hands-on midwifery. The changes are just beginning.

MIDWIFE-CLIENT RELATIONSHIP: FRIENDS AND PROFESSIONALS?

It is important to note that midwives repeatedly said that they had not noticed major changes in their relationships with clients especially once the client had been accepted for care. However, the midwives spent more time discussing this theme than any other and all midwives could identify areas, some obvious and some more subtle, where the relationship had altered.

I mean, I am often sitting there with one of those early visits, and again you used to spend most of your time chatting, and now you are filling in forms and writing things and ordering things, doing tests and so on. And I often comment to them and say, 'You know, we used to spend this time chatting,' and you plow your way through a visit that takes an hour because there is so much to do and you really haven't remembered to say, 'How are you feeling?' But, I don't know that that translates into such a huge difference for the clients either though, because whatever you talk about is the surface level of the communication anyway. If you are talking about your kids or your plans or your hopes around the birth, for them the emphasis is on the fact that you are taking care of them. That underlying communication is still the same; they are interested that you are taking care of them. So, I don't think that it is actually all that different.

Formerly, most midwives were personally chosen and, barring exceptional circumstances, committed themselves to care for their clients themselves. Initial and ongoing appointments were arranged through direct communication between the midwife and the woman. Now midwifery offices have administrators who take on these roles; as women become clients of the practice, distance may be created between the woman and the midwife at the outset.

That expectation that we were there 100% for these women I truly believe was an unrealistic expectation on both sides because you could never be there 100%

for anyone and I think it was a bit arrogant of us to think that we could. Because, in doing so, we didn't anticipate the needs that these clients would have if that eventuality came to pass and we couldn't be there.

Appointments in the midwife's home pre-legislation had provided an opportunity for clients to observe a part of the midwife's personal life; this kind of sharing was no longer possible. Nonetheless, midwives still observe and participate in the personal life of clients. Now there may be more of an imbalance around who in the client-midwife relationship is being observed and monitored, which may create a different kind of exchange.[24]

Although most midwives welcomed shared care, some noted a loss of personal closeness with the woman as a disadvantage. Becoming friends with their clients often had been about having something in common; for instance, having children at the same time. Some midwives found this past situation satisfying. Others felt that a close emotional relationship had been a drain on time and energy, especially if clients contacted midwives socially outside of clinic time. One midwife felt that the relationship she had experienced with clients previously was "co-dependent." For some, former relationships didn't allow space for, or even intruded on, other activities in the midwife's life.

> Maybe we've had too much of that kind of feeling. I don't know. Too much attachment to their midwife. Sometimes I think we may be too much attached to the women.

> I don't think that the midwife should be so close to her clients that she doesn't see what is going on. We were too unselfconsciously friend and supporter of the mother. I think that there is a necessary distance, your own life has to be separate from your work. Your own relationships, spirituality are hampered by having too many relationships. I feel I carry around with me a kind of sadness about all of those relationships I had in the past with clients that I couldn't really develop. I am saying that now the distance is good.

The nature of the care provided to clients is a powerful issue with which many midwives struggle. At times, women seek the support of midwives because their own mother is distant and they wish the midwife to take on a mothering role. However, the midwife's position as a professional interfacing with patriarchal structures and procedures may bring a different aspect of the midwife more into play. One midwife noted that with the increased responsibility, her clients are now more in her thoughts than her feelings and that this for her was a significant shift. Perhaps the post-legislation role of the midwife is evolving towards a creative balance of both feeling, nurturing mother figure and professional caregiver with attributes such as authority and rationality.[25]

My clients are more in my thoughts now than they used to be, even though I am not as emotionally connected to them. Less in my feelings, more in my thoughts. I will go home and think, I must remember to do such and such for so and so.

They are much clearer about what my role is. They don't confuse me with their friend and their mother. They relate me only to the pregnancy, so they don't call me when they're bored or lonely, which I used to find was very time consuming and draining.

Now, because clients had come to her through the public domain, one midwife felt she hid behind that professional role, thus affecting the amount of hands-on care she was willing to give. Some felt that the nature of their contact with the mother was different because of where the midwife was when she initially connected with her client; some midwives saw themselves now positioned on the inside or at the centre of the medical care system rather than on the outside or at the margin. In the past, women often requested things that were outside the scope of medical practice and came to midwives for that care. One midwife now felt this service in some respects was impossible to offer. The woman and her family are considered to be central decision makers. What if their decisions run counter to the midwife's view and her sense of appropriate care? Within what kind of limits can the midwife simply chart that the woman has 'refused' a certain kind of care?

I find now I can hide behind the mask, the face of the professional. I'm now a professional midwife. It presents itself on a very basic level with the amount of hands-on care I give.

Another midwife who had previously appreciated the spiritual aspect of her work, noted that new duties of professionalism deflected her from this.

I feel that we are now cast upon a dry land; that there are now jobs to be done; rather than before being in that water that flows within some primordial sea, with eyes closed, tapping into instinctual wisdom with the heart chakra open, nothing more important than the sacredness of this 'being with woman.'

As midwives move into a more 'professional' role, they seem currently to be searching for a balance in their relationship with clients that make the working relationships optimal not only for the client but also for the midwife. One midwife reported:

Midwives want to have families, they want time to live life and enjoy life and although the blessing of the work that we do can be wonderful when you're there, it's a short period of time that's with those people and you leave it, you move on. I think, if you're wanting to live life and you're making choices in your life to have a partner or have kids and spend time with them and watch them grow up as you get older, I think right now we're balancing that quite well with giving the kind of care women want.

MAJOR CHANGES BEFORE LEGISLATIVE REGULATION

Midwives were asked to discuss any major changes that had occurred in their midwifery practices before legislative regulation. It seemed that for some, legislation represented one of many significant points in the overall evolution of Ontario midwifery and it accelerated some processes and trends.

Midwives mentioned their increasing confidence over the years. They described feeling "more comfortable in my shoes" and "matured." Naming oneself a midwife and "coming out of the closet" increased comfort. For one midwife it was important not to be worrying about what others thought of her and her work. The fear of being considered unsafe had loomed large for one midwife. Accepting the possibility of legal action, as well as finding out that midwifery practice was alegal, not illegal, were significant milestones. Working without doctors, coupled with the pressures of inquests, had caused shifts towards taking on responsibility with an increased sense of intentionality and seriousness.

> The experience of seeing midwives going through inquests really made me feel strongly that the system had to be changed.

One midwife noted that due to the increased codification and defining of her practice and conformity to those codes, she found herself falling into the fears of the medical model.

> I have noticed an increased codifying and defining, determining what's right, what's not right, what's inside standards and what's outside of standards and gradually conforming to those codes. I've moved farther and farther away from all of that which we are also capable of knowing. I've fallen into all of the fears of the western medical model.

Standards and protocols based on research were being developed in the attempt to ensure midwives were safe practitioners. In addition, working in small practice groups and sorting out differences in approach amongst the member practitioners was a major change for some midwives.

> There was a slow evolution of practice from prenatal instructor and labour coach — key in our development and transition in becoming primary caregivers. An ever-increasing responsibility through the development of standards and protocols, and a willingness to work on those and make sure we were providing the best care and being safe practitioners.

A few midwives had their first children in their early years of practice, and that brought a new perspective and understanding to their work. For one midwife, moving from a concern of "what if" to assuming "all will be normal" and filling herself with positive experiences was a change. For another, working with continuity of care made her more confident.

It was amazing to realize by going through the continuity of a woman's pregnancy into her labour and postpartum you knew a lot more about that woman and the baby too, and that gave such an underlying confidence in your practice. I wasn't as nervous. I was much more confident because of the continuity of the care.

TOWARDS IDEAL MIDWIFERY CARE?

In spite of individual differences and emphases, there was considerable solidarity and congruity concerning midwives' definitions of ideal midwifery. The midwives interviewed all have very high ideals about the nature of the care they wish to provide, which corresponded strongly to the College of Midwives' document, The Philosophy of Midwifery Care in Ontario. Using the midwives' own words, these definitions have been distilled and consolidated; ideal midwifery care is:

The midwife on her own, or with a small group of other midwives whom the woman knows, being available and being able to spend time to provide a full spectrum of care to the woman who requires her services throughout the pregnancy, labour, birth and postpartum. Care which is a balance of many differing aspects. Care that is accepting and nonjudgmental, informative, supportive and sensitive. Care which involves a strong responsive emotional relationship in which the woman and her family can say what they want to say and that the [midwife] will be listening; where there is openness and there is trust. It is care that is not overwhelming or over-encompassing or imposing. Care which encourages the woman to be independent and to do her own problem solving and make decisions about her baby and about herself. Care that informs, offers a woman choices, and respects and supports the choices she makes. Care which is woman-centred, holistic, very personalized and respectful of the woman as an individual. Care where there is a balance of power in the relationship between the woman and the midwife. Care which looks after the woman and her family, with the midwife quietly in the background being very responsible with attention to safety. Care which involves using science and the best available knowledge. Care where birth and pregnancy are considered normal.

Professional distance and experience were noted as important. Ideal care depended on the midwife working in conditions where she could care for herself with improved working conditions: administrative help, an adequate salary and time off for herself. The uniqueness of the midwifery model as separate from the medical model was emphasized.

Some midwives mentioned as their ideal, aspects that are not enhanced by legislation. Legislation has given registered midwives the exclusive right to practice, and thus women's choices of primary caregiver for maternity care are now limited to physicians and regulated professional midwives. The neighbour woman, "the traditional midwife with a sixth sense," friend or unlicensed midwife now risks fines and imprisonment if caught intentionally assisting a woman during her birth. Some midwives wished for: drop-in clinics where mothers can choose if they wanted care or not rather than recommended regular visits;[26] two kinds of midwives: one attending home births and another attending hospital births; and a system where radicalization and change were always possible.

Some midwives were unclear as to whether ideal care was more possible after legislation and implied that, because of the shortage of midwives right now, it might be difficult for women to find their "ideal" caregiver. Some felt they had been providing ideal care before legislation.

> I think the way I've been doing midwifery care over the years is ideal. Over the years we've gotten into a system of the way it's best to do things.

Most other midwives felt that legislation contributed to more ideal care with: "universal" access to midwifery care; a midwifery educational system which uses practising midwives as teachers and provides students with an equal balance of clinical and academic experience; a funding system that supports long visits between the midwife and her client; assurance of the continuity of caregiver and more options.

Home birth was seen as the site where ideal midwifery care could most be manifested and could be used as a model for care at hospital births. Legislation created an exceptionally positive atmosphere for home births. Legislation preserved home birth, provided government sanctioned home birth, made home an accepted choice of birth place, and advocated home birth by requiring all midwives to maintain confidence and competence in the home setting. And finally, it was implied that home is the setting wherein creative midwifery care is made possible.

One midwife discussed how the political context for establishing legislated midwifery had been favourable and noted the complexity of the changes that had occurred.

> You can't say that legislation means 'x' and the consequence means 'x' because legislation is a complex social issue and it happens in a certain moment in history and in a certain political context, and I think that we have been incredibly lucky — angels were looking down on Ontario. Because we had this moment in history when the women's movement was having an effect, health reform was really apparent, the government was willing to take on medicine. Sociologists have pointed out problems like the loss of autonomy, I feel that we have more..., an expanded practice... I think it is an amazing coincidence of the personalities that have been involved that have helped us along.

That midwives must do home births by legislation has led to an amazingly favourable environment for people choosing home births. The fact that it was in regulation without question, it almost took the pressure off the midwife to say: 'I'm a home birth advocate.' She can now say, 'I don't have a choice, I have to attend home births.'

The Ontario model itself was seen as a framework for ideal care.

I don't think of anything as ideal because we are always reaching for something. The Ontario model gives us a framework. There is the flexibility for us to be individual practitioners, the time to really play out options and choices and it allows us to do a dance around so many issues. The ideal for me is to take the Ontario model and to strive to give it life and reality and I think that in some ways it is much more achievable now.

I think the basic ground stones that have been laid down for the foundation of midwifery in 1994 in Ontario are really excellent. Internationally, the world is looking at Ontario which I think is the leading province of ideal midwifery care in the world.

FOR FUTURE CONSIDERATION

The current manifestation of Ontario midwifery in its legalized form has drawn on the traditions of midwifery in other western countries[27] and is notable for the practices of continuity of care and choice of birth place. These practices are being replicated in some other countries and are admired by many midwives around the world. Thus Ontario midwifery reform has been not merely a local activity but one that has some global connections with other midwives and women supporting a similar philosophy and practice. However, the Eurocentric content in the rendering of Ontario midwifery, both pre- and post-legislation, may present some limitations.

It seems important to note that the values expressed by midwives in the study reported in this chapter, specifically those such as autonomy and choice in what is considered "ideal midwifery care," are an expression of western liberal individualism[28] and may not be practicable for midwives in nonwestern countries. Furthermore, there is likely an ethnocentric ignorance among Ontario midwives. They may at times romanticize midwifery and birthing practices in nondominant cultures, and in jurisdictions without legislation, without an understanding of how patriarchical oppression, poverty and difficult working conditions affect the health and choices of childbearing women and their midwives in some sites. In comparing studies of midwifery around the world, DeVries[29] notes great diversity in the status of the midwife: while their work is similar, their status is not. How much are Ontario midwives thinking and working within the Euro-Anglo-American cultural framework?

How well is Ontario midwifery doing at connecting with and supporting midwives in and from nondominant cultures?

When we come to the question of access to midwifery care and education, one wonders to what extent midwifery legislation in Ontario has simply provided luxury items for the privileged: good salaries for predominantly middle-class midwives, midwifery care and education for predominantly middle-class clients and students. Attention needs to be given continuously as to how resources can be appropriately distributed.

Although midwifery care is now potentially more accessible to a wider range of women, it seems clear from the midwives' responses that the demand for midwifery care far exceeds its availability. Furthermore, it seems that in some settings women were not able to access care because information about midwifery and the routes of access were not adequately or appropriately available to them. What are the ethics of client selection? What might be some means of taking affirmative action to continue to include a wider racial, social, class and cultural diversity of women and encourage their access to midwifery care in the future?

There is also concern about the lack of diversity amongst currently practising midwives. Future studies may reveal more diversity within the midwifery community, as midwives with varied backgrounds graduate from the Midwifery Education and the Prior Learning and Experience Assessment Programmes. However, at the time of publication, there are still few registered midwives in Ontario of non-European descent.

Accessibility to the Midwifery Education Programme is also a highly significant issue and one that receives considerable attention from faculty members. One wonders, however, how the categories to be examined in the application process might be racially biased towards the dominant culture. Students in the midwifery education program have taken up the challenge of raising interviewers' sensitivity to equity issues. They have met and developed an equity guide which interviewers are encouraged to read immediately before they engage in the interviewing process.

Does the recent re-emergence of midwifery and its legalization in Ontario reflect the feminist principles of sisterly connections based on mutual respect, effective kinship, and equality in relationships between women? As in most feminist projects, there remain troublesome contradictions and dilemmas.

Legalization was effected by a small group of midwives who equipped themselves with the necessary political skills. This group worked hard and achieved this amazing transformative work for women. They worked through committees in the Association of Ontario Midwives which invited participation from the membership and which operated according to a consensual model. According to Bourgeault,[30] who has explored the development of other professions, the clarity of vision of this small elite group of midwives and their maintenance of power was essential to the goal of achieving legislation.

The process of bringing about legislation demanded that midwives to be seen as a unified group with a common purpose. However, some midwives who were uncertain about this goal felt excluded, silenced, and even felt labelled as dangerous. Midwives working hard at legislative issues felt that politically uninvolved midwives excluded themselves from the process. This division created tensions within the midwifery movement, commonly reported in women's movements, which were felt by some to be the antithesis of feminist ideology.

It seems essential to acknowledge the efforts of many midwives and consumers working towards the social recognition of midwifery at the local level, particularly in rural areas far from the hub of the political activity in Toronto; and also the midwives who 'kept the home fires burning,' providing a stable and continued presence in midwifery practices so that others could do the political work.

The legislation of midwifery rendered illegal the activities of those midwives who, although unregistered, still engaged in the same work that Ontario midwives formerly did. Some midwives felt they had betrayed those presently unregistered caregivers who had been marginalized in this way. Others argued that standards for entry to practise had to be set and some would eventually be excluded.

Legalized midwifery has necessitated new bureaucratic and educational positions for midwives in the College of Midwives and baccalaureate programs. Will their assumption of new roles create a power differential in relationships among midwives? If so, how will the profession be affected? In an attempt to address these questions, the profession has made it a priority to ensure that both teachers and administrators remained practising midwives.

The current Ontario Midwifery Education Programme, the placement of students, and comparisons with the old apprenticeship model of midwifery education are areas which deserve attention. The development of a baccalaureate program for the education of midwives gave midwifery an academic status and made possible future access to graduate work in midwifery. In many caring professions, for example nursing, there has been an escalation in academic requirements and the necessity for updating one's credentials. This escalation may be a way for feminized occupations to achieve professional status, while at the same time increasing the marginalization of those with nonacademic credentials.[31] Will the baccalaureate program in fact prove superior to the old apprenticeship method of training midwives? Will graduate midwives from the Michener Pre-registration, the Midwifery Education and the Prior Learning and Experience Assessment Programmes be considered similarly qualified by the professional and lay community?

The nature of the new connections between faculty and student in midwifery academia and between the midwife preceptor and student in clinical placements are highly significant as midwifery training occurs. Difficulties arise when the establishment of standards and requirements necessitates the evaluation of student by teacher, one woman by another, especially if the evaluation is not positive. How can one establish an academic atmosphere where there is safety if not comfort? Self and group evaluation through peer review has been a part of the Ontario midwifery tradition. In addition, students are presently encouraged in informal and formal ways to evaluate their teachers. It seems essential that these and other principles of adult education which are feminist at their root be expressed and maintained in the new educational settings.

More work needs to be done exploring and analyzing the changes in midwifery practices that have come about following legislation. Several midwives have suggested that the study reported here be repeated when adjustments to the changes have occurred and sufficient time has passed for reflection on the meaning of these changes. In the future it may be useful to look at literature which studies the nature and sequelae of 'change' in general and explore what happens to individuals and groups when they enter into situations which involve major changes. For example, many midwives noted the changes that government-funded midwifery care had brought. It might be interesting to explore changes experienced in the past by other health professionals as they moved from private billing to public funding, and report their perceptions of the effects of these changes on their relationships with clients.

We need studies comparing the safety and cost effectiveness of midwifery before and after legislation in Ontario to realistically assess whether legislated midwifery is superior to unlegislated midwifery. The outcomes of physicians' and registered midwives' care need to be compared as well. Statistics might be gathered, for example, on rates of neonatal and maternal morbidity and mortality, rates of operative and pharmacological interventions, psychosocial outcomes and client/patient satisfaction.

Among midwives interviewed only one midwife had a solo practice. A future study of the perceptions of other midwives in solo practices, especially those working in rural areas, may yield very different impressions. The group of midwives not included in this study, because they were excluded from midwifery practice pending further assessment, could be interviewed. Perceptions of these midwives might bring alternative perspectives to the findings in this study because legislation effectively stopped some of their practices permanently, and others, temporarily.

Another omission from this study were midwives who had practiced prelegislation in Ontario for fewer than five years. Some of these midwives had worked in a Ontario government pilot project[32] as 'nurse-midwives' in the hospital setting and two were interviewed outside of this study. As they have now moved into a new model which includes attendance at home births and continuity of care, it might be interesting to analyze their perceptions of the changes in their practice and compare them with those of midwives in the study. For example, I noted that these midwives perceived that their practices had moved further away from the medical model with legislation and that increased continuity with their clients had made their working lives more satisfying but less predictable.

One midwife interviewed for my study summarized some of the challenges that newly legalized midwifery presently faced:

> The biggest problem that I see right now is that we are just in the beginning years and we are all just catching up to what we are supposed to be doing, and we are all babies about it ourselves because integrated formalized professionalized midwifery is new. And I think that we are catching a huge amount of flack from both ends of the spectrum over this first year: whether it's physicians and nurses who believe that we are part of dismantling the healthcare system and/or that the government is just on a one track thing to knock out doctors and nurses and hospitals; or on the other hand from feminist scholars, sociologists, lay midwives, childbirth educators and community people who have very strong concerns that professionization is the first step towards institutionalized midwifery that will hold back people in the same way that medicine held them back. I mean, I think it is a very unconfident beginning and we just have to carry on with some belief that basically the model we've got is going to flower.

The struggle to legislate midwifery involved an enormous expenditure of time and resources. To what extent have these efforts made a difference in the wider political context which seems to determine so much? What circumstances would cause funding to the midwifery profession in Ontario to be curtailed or limited? What will happen in the future? Some midwives in the study remarked that midwifery clients in Ontario receive special care with adequate time for appointments with their caregivers, 24-hour accessibility, nurturing labour support, respect for their style and choices, and home visits. Some midwives worried that the Ontario healthcare system might in future consider that this care is excessive, and attempt to pare away the time and services midwives offer women or increase their work load. Cutbacks in caregiving services might necessitate efficiency and cost effectiveness, and the emotional component of care could be reduced to a series of easily measured tasks.[33] One midwife noted:

> I think if we move like the US to a more reactionary, restrictive, less social-service-oriented kind of government, we are really going to face a challenge. So that's why I feel so good about the regulations that we have in place, that they aren't at the superficial level or just that each practice has a good philosophy or something — they are actually right there so it's not so easy for economic or institutionalized forces to change the model.

The provincial government of Ontario has demonstrated its willingness for midwives to attend home births by passing the Midwifery Act; legislation has preserved the option of home birth. Current community attitudes towards home births seem to indicate that only a small percentage of childbearing women in the Ontario population may request home births. In my study, midwives repeatedly mentioned that the home was the crucial site where the philosophy and practice of midwifery could best be preserved. Over the coming few years, the number of clients requesting home births and the reasons for their choice might be studied. Will more women choose home births with midwives now or will home birth requests decrease since women can now have midwives as their primary caregivers at their hospital births? It seems essential that action be taken to encourage home births in Ontario. It may be interesting to review the studies on the safety, convenience and cost effectiveness of home birth. Lessons could be learned from the Netherlands with its incentives for women and midwives participating in home birth. Work could be done with the Ontario Ministry of Health to formulate ways of advertising home births so as to encourage more childbearing women to feel comfortable with the home-birth option.

Professional midwifery developed in response to powerful consumer interest in a model of care for childbearing women that was antithetical to the medical model. Ironically, the professionalism of midwifery in Ontario requires that the midwife engage in activities linking her closely to medical practitioners and to the medical model; this new allegiance some midwives enjoy and others don't. Some appreciate the new opportunities for dialogue and interaction with medical colleagues; others worry about cooption and the loss of identity.

Many of the concerns about the impact of legislation on the relationship with the client had to do with the midwife's not being able to be 'with the woman' appropriately. One aspect of care, the clinical, has expanded and other aspects of care, the hands-on supportive work and the attending to the emotional and social needs of the client, may have contracted. Many midwives' work involved an advocacy role and supporting women in labour; spending long hours providing comfort with massages, cool cloths, encouraging words and suggestions for how to work with the challenge of labour. Feeding the client's family, doing the laundry and cleaning up after a home birth were also common tasks. With the professionalization of midwifery, some of these tasks may fall away.

Questions about the present and future use of the labour supporter as an adjunct to midwifery care may be relevant here. Will 'hands-on' work be left for other caregivers with different status than that of the Ontario midwife? If the midwife reduces her 'hands-on' caring for her client, will she feel differently about her work and her client? How will the relationship alter? Or is this kind of caring more appropriately done by family and friends in any case? And is the advocacy role one that now more appropriately belongs to someone other than the midwife? What constitutes caring? What are the limits or boundaries to caring? What are the ramifications of closeness? Are caregivers drawn to their work not only to provide a service but also because of the emotional attachment? Does the context in which the caregiver works enable or prevent the provision of ideal care? What is the most useful and helpful kind of relationship for a woman to develop with her midwife and vice-versa? What variables in a midwife's life constitute a satisfying work relationship? One might consider: personality, economic status, class, race, religious stance, age, parity. What do clients need and want from their caregivers?

Two principles of Ontario midwifery are that care is woman-centred and that the woman makes decisions based on informed choices; the midwife shares what she knows with her client. With new educational and professional requirements, the midwives' knowledge base and education are becoming very different from that of their clients, and perhaps this sharing is evolving from one of a peer friendship in the past to one of a professional nature which may create boundaries. Will it be more difficult now for midwives to provide care in a nonauthoritarian manner and assume that the client is the expert with respect to her own care?

It may be interesting to note that Ontario midwives do not call the women with whom they work 'patients' but 'clients.' Perhaps in an attempt to distance themselves from medical professional language, which may imply that the childbearing woman is passive in a patriarchal model, midwives use language usually associated with the legal profession. While accenting the advocacy role and contractual nature of the relationship, this is a shift to the language of another powerful patriarchal profession and brings with it other associations and meanings such as status and class. Would it be more appropriate to call clients 'customers'?[34] Midwives have acknowledged that it has been impossible to find a word to appropriately express the relationship between the woman and her midwife.

We cannot assume, post midwifery legislation, that the midwife won't simply become the new authority over the woman as the locus of power shifts from the doctor to the midwife as primary caregiver. There is evidence[35] that midwives are not always kind, supportive or wise nor that they provide care that many would consider to be woman-centred. Whenever there is the possibility of someone being in a vulnerable place and needing the help of another, there is also the possibility of the abuse of power.

Particularly because midwifery has traditionally been a consumer-driven and woman-centred occupation, it seems essential to assess without delay consumers' perceptions of the changes since legislation, by interviewing clients who have experienced midwifery care both before and after legislation. It may be important to identify whether there are some correspondences between midwives' and clients' perceptions of the changes in the midwife-client relationship and other aspects of midwifery care. In addition, it seems crucial for midwives to remain in close contact with the diverse needs and concerns of the changing consumer body, to be flexible and continue to educate themselves about how these needs can be met, and finally, continually to raise questions and reflect on what is good care and honourable work. Have the consumer body's options been narrowed by the professional decisions legislation confirmed? Is there the room for multiple visions? Does this professionalism limit or enlarge the creativity of the public?'

FINAL THOUGHTS

Legalized midwifery is the realization of a dream of some consumers and midwives in Ontario. Legislation created a shake-up which provided in the ensuing months an opportunity for midwives to examine their work before the dust settled and they became accustomed to their new professional roles. Some mourn the passing of an old way and note that qualitatively, the experience of providing care is different. Others rejoice that midwifery is more accessible and feel more enabled by their new status in the community to serve the women with whom they work.

With legislation, new content has been placed in the container of the midwife's work; different aspects compete for her attention and priorities must be re-evaluated. Where does she need to put her attention now? What is comfortable for her? What is most respectful for her clients? What is going on inside the midwife herself as she tries to make sense of this new content?

Legalized midwifery is being born. How can midwives nurture this birthing? How can they gracefully acknowledge the changes that its birth brings? Like labour, the midwives' present situation forces them to engage. As with birthing, for some, the adjustment to the circumstances is smooth; for others, it is more difficult. But usually women's great effort and courage are summoned. And with the birth, there is a sense of achievement and the acknowledgment of great possibility.

ENDNOTES

1. The point of view taken in this work arises from my situation as a white, middle-class, privileged woman. Material for this Preface comes from my memory of events of the time; see also Mary Fynes, "The Legitimation of Midwifery in Ontario, 1960-1987," MSc Thesis, University of Toronto, 1994.
2. In the summer of 1963, I had the privilege of residing with a Native community for three months and was inspired by learning of the nature of Aboriginal midwives' work.
3. Jutta Mason, "Appendix on the History of Midwifery in Canada," in *Report of the Task Force on the Implementation of Midwifery in Ontario*, (Toronto: Ontario Government Publication, 1987) — notes that in spite of the medical propaganda of the time on the perils of nonmedical birth, the home birth statistics of neighbour women helpers were exemplary. She further points out that many of these "midwives" may have attended no more than 60 births in their lives.

4. In 1977, the executive director of the American College of Obstetricians and Gynecologists claimed that "home birth is child abuse." See Cassidy-Brin, G., F. Hornstein and C. Downer, *Woman-Centred Pregnancy and Birth*, The Federation of Feminist Women's Health Centres. (San Francisco: Cleis Press, 1984), 103.

5. An important action of a local childbirth education group, the Toronto Lamaze Childbirth Association, founded in 1975 by five women, was the creation of a survey of Toronto hospitals' obstetric policies embodied in the *Toronto Hospitals Policies and Procedures Book*. We sold this booklet, which had a profound effect on changing practices, at the Toronto Women's Bookstore. By using this booklet, one could choose one's hospital according to who was 'allowed' to be present, required procedures, and the practice around the separation of mother and child. Hospitals could compare their practices with others. The resulting competition between hospitals led some towards policies more supportive of women.

6. The program, mounted at McMaster Medical Centre in Hamilton and at St. Michael's Hospital in Toronto, in the early 1980s, responded to women's needs not to be experimented upon by medical students.

7. See Sheryl Nestel, "Race and Class in the Re-emergence of Midwifery in Canada: An Exploratory Essay," (unpublished paper, 1996) for an extensive exploration of the possible forces which led to the exclusion of foreign-trained midwives in this early group of practising midwives.

8. La Leche League, an international organization which supported continuous mothering through breastfeeding, Frederick Leboyer's book, *Birth Without Violence*, and the work of therapist R. D. Laing and his graphic film, *Birth*, filmed from the baby's point of view, were some of the influences that helped shift concern from the needs of the birthing woman to those of the baby.

9. The Maternity Centre in El Paso and others like it in Texas have seen, from 1978 until the present, a steady stream of lay midwives from Ontario seeking birthing experiences principally with Mexican women. Until the mid-1980s, when a registration examination was required, registration as a midwife or as an undertaker in this state required only that you sign your name in a book at the court house. The lack of decent publicly funded local maternity care for women led women to these centres for care that was inexpensive and generally more woman-centred. Although somewhat supervised, students took on great responsibility early in their training in caring for these women. This led to a dilemma for some students from Ontario who felt awkward about using these women's births to gain their experience. It raised issues around opportunism and possible exploitation of these Mexican women.

10. From 1976 until 1982, I attended home births as a lay midwife with 13 different doctors who were willing to offer this service to women under their care.

11. These principles reflected what consumers felt they were not able to receive through physician maternity care: appointments with physicians often lasted a few minutes and birthing options were often not respected or even discussed; home birth was not considered a safe alternative. Women wanted continuity in their care and were opposed to being attended at their births by physicians unknown to them. See Vicki Van Wagner, "With Woman: Community Midwifery in Ontario," (unpublished paper, 1991), who provides an examination of the community midwifery system extant in Ontario in 1991 and details the historical development of aspects of the midwifery model proposed for legislation.

12. Direct-entry midwifery education programs do not require the prerequisite of nursing training.
13. See T.G. Johnson, *Professions and Power* (London: Macmillan, 1972); and M. Larson, *The Rise of Professionalism: A Sociological Analysis* (Berkeley: University of California Press, 1977). They suggest that the main elements of professionalism are: skill based on theoretical knowledge, provision of training and education, a mechanism for testing competence of members, an organization to which members belong and adherence to a professional code of conduct. These elements were expressed in Ontario midwifery legislation. Again, see V. Van Wagner, ibid.
14. The Ontario Midwifery Education Programme was mounted in three sites: Laurentian University, McMaster University and Ryerson Polytechnic University. Students were first admitted in the fall of 1993.
15. Issues of equity and midwifery were carefully considered in the work of the Equity Committee of the Interim Regulatory Council on Midwifery between 1989 and 1992. The findings of this committee have been summarized in F. Shroff and A.R. Ford, *An Equity Reader for Midwifery Students*, (Toronto: Ryerson University, 1994). All midwives in the pre-registration program mounted by the Michener Institute in 1992 were required to attend a series of workshops on equity concerns.
16. How much was this exemption ruling simply a token gesture? The destruction of midwifery practices within most Aboriginal communities by the dominant culture with its dominant form of health care was practically complete. Many Aboriginal midwives currently do not have in place the practical supports for their work that other Ontario midwifery registrants have.
17. In the late 1980s the Ontario Medical Association had a plan to expand the role of the nurse under the direction of medicine to satisfy consumer requests for midwives. See M. Fynes, "The Legitimation of Midwifery in Ontario, 1960-1987," (MSc thesis, University of Toronto, 1994). K. Kaufman and M. Renfrew, "Midwives, Nurses and Clinical Excellence," in *Recent Advances in Nursing*, (UK: Longman Group, 1988), recommended that the interests of midwives, nurses and women would best be served in Ontario if regulation defined midwifery separately from nursing so that the tradition of midwifery might be reclaimed. E. Declerc, "The Transformation of American Midwifery: 1975 to 1988," *American Journal of Public Health*, vol. 82, no. 5 (1992), analyzed the growth of midwifery in the United States from 1975 to 1988 through birth certificate data. Results showed that the number of midwife-attended births increased from 0.9% to 3.4% of all births occurring. 93.2% of this increase was primarily due to hospital births attended by nurse-midwives. In almost no states did lay midwives attend hospital births and rarely did nurse-midwives attend home births. Thus the number of home births and the number of lay-midwives practising was increasing very slowly in comparison with the significant growth in nurse-midwife attended births. See also I. Bourgeault and M. Fynes, "Midwives in Canada and the U.S." (unpublished paper, 1994) for the differing ways in which integration of midwifery has occurred in the healthcare systems in Canada and the United States.
18. This study fulfilled a requirement for a MEd degree in Adult Education, 1995, Ontario Institute for Studies in Education, University of Toronto.
19. R. Weitz and D. Sullivan, "Licensed Lay Midwifery and Medical Models of Childbirth," in *Circles of Care: Work and Identity in Women's Lives*, Emily Abel and Margaret Nelson, eds, (State University of New York, 1990) —

noted that following midwifery licensure in Arizona, clients tended to give the midwife more power in the relationship and midwives attempted in various ways to keep the client in the active role; with the growing social acceptance of midwifery that accreditation brought, there was a marked increase in clientele seeking a more medical model. When midwifery was previously underground, the midwife and client had a more compatible value base.

20. See M. Waring, *If Women Counted: A New Feminist Economics* (San Francisco: Harare Press, 1990).
21. See B. Fischer, "Alice in the Human Services: A Feminist Analysis of Women in the Caring Professions," in *Circles of Care* (New York State University Press, 1990), who notes that women working as service professionals are often exploited, having little control over their work, and receiving relatively low pay, and that they have difficulty placing limits on their work. Also, H. Levine, "The Personal is Political" In *Feminism: From Pressure to Politics*, Miles and Finn, eds, (Montreal: Black Rose Books, 1989), 233-267, who reminds us of how women are programed by the culture to see themselves as nurturers of others and have long served as unpaid workers in the home and in the community.
22. I. Butter and B. Kay, "Self-Certification in Lay Midwives Organizations: a Vehicle for Professional Autonomy," *Social Science Medicine*, vol. 30 (1990), studied 32 lay-midwife groups in the United States and noted that even with licensing these groups had more in common with alternative women's organizations than with conservative health professional groups; their nonhierarchical structures promoted consensual decision-making, minimized status differences among members, and tolerated diverse philosophical and political views.
23. D. Young and L. Page, "External Review Report of the Ontario Midwifery Education Program," (1996).
24. The concept of control by monitoring or surveillance in maternity care elaborated by the Foucaudian, W. Arney, *Power and the Profession of Obstetrics* (Chicago, 1982), was first brought to my attention by Jutta Mason.
25. See the plea for the resolution of this dualism in feminist pedagogy explored by H. Lenskyj, "Commitment and Compromise: Feminist Pedagogy in the Classroom," In *Feminism and Education: A Canadian Perspective*, vol. 2 (Toronto: Centre for Women's Studies in Education, OISE, 1994).
26. I. Illich, "Disabling Professions," *Ideas in Progress Series* (London: Marion Boyears Publishing, 1977), holds that professionals disable and delude members of the public by deciding what their needs are and by developing solutions to their needs. Some midwives question the necessity of certain forms of midwifery care and wonder if midwifery care will become a new orthodoxy.
27. The Task Force on the Implementation of Midwifery in Ontario in the late 1980s studied midwifery particularly in England, in the Netherlands, in the US and in some Scandinavian countries, in search of an appropriate model for legislation.
28. This point was noted by Leslie Thielen-Wilson, editor for Women's Press.
29. R. DeVries, *Making Midwives Legal: Childbirth, Medicine and the Law* (Ohio: Ohio State University, 1996). He suggests that the social position of midwives varies according to many factors: geography, technology, structure of society, political, legal, economic, religious and educational aspects, as well as the culture and the values of the people served by the midwife.

30. I. Bourgeault, "Delivering Midwifery: An Examination of the Process and Outcome of the Incorporation of Midwifery in Ontario," (PhD Thesis, University of Toronto, 1996).
31. H. Monk, "Ontario Midwifery in Western Historical Perspective: From Radicals to Reactionaries in Ten Short Years" (unpublished paper, 1994), considers the legalization process to be reactionary and restrictive and provides a voice for the interests of Ontario practitioners who are currently denied registration as midwives in Ontario.
32. It might be also fruitful to explore more fully the influence the Ontario in-hospital nurse-midwifery project at McMaster Medical Centre had on midwifery legislation and on the Midwifery Education Programme.
33. See Abel and Nelson, *Circles of Care: Work and Identity in Women's Lives* (State University of New York, 1990), who note that all 'professionals' learn codes of behaviour which enable them to distance themselves from their clients and that the emotional component of care is often compromised for economic reasons.
34. A well-loved 'home birth' doctor in Toronto, Dr. John McCulloch, in the 1970s and 1980s, used to refer to those with whom he worked in this way.
35. See Nicky Leap and Billie Hunter, *The Midwife's Tale: An Oral History From Handywoman to Professional Midwife* (London: Scarlet Press, 1993).

REFERENCES

Abel, Emily, and Margaret Nelson. *Circles of Care: Work and Identity in Women's Lives.* New York: State University of New York, 1990.

Annandale, Ellen. "How Midwives Accomplish Natural Birth: Managing Risk and Balancing Expectation." *Social Problems* (1988).

Arney, William. *Power and the Profession of Obstetrics.* Chicago, 1982.

Bourgeault, Ivy Lynn. "Delivering Midwifery: An Examination of the Process and Outcome of the Incorporation of Midwifery in Ontario." PhD Thesis, University of Toronto, 1996.

Bourgeault, Ivy Lynn, and Mary Fynes, "Midwives in Canada and the U.S.," unpublished paper, 1995.

Butter, Irene, and Bonnie Kay. "Self-Certification in Lay Midwives Organizations: a Vehicle for Professional Autonomy." *Social Science Medicine*, vol. 30 (1990).

Cassidy-Brin, G., F. Hornstein and C. Downer. *Woman-Centred Pregnancy and Birth.* The Federation of Feminist Women's Health Centres. San Francisco: Cleis Press, 1984.

Culley, M., A. Diamond, L. Edwards, S. Lennox and C. Portugues. "The Politics of Nurturance." In *Gendered Subjects: The Dynamics of Feminist Teaching.* Massachusetts: Routledge and Kegan Paul, 1985.

Declerc, Eugene. "The Transformation of American Midwifery: 1975 to 1988." *American Journal of Public Health*, vol. 82, no. 5 (1992).

DeVries, Raymond. *Making Midwives Legal: Childbirth, Medicine and the Law.* Ohio: Ohio State University Press, 1996.

Durkheim, Emil. *Professional Ethics and Civic Morals.* London, 1957.

Fischer, Berenice. "Alice in the Human Services: A Feminist Analysis of Women in the Caring Professions." In *Circles of Care.* New York State University Press, 1990.

Foucault, Michel. *Discipline and Punish: Birth of the Prison.* London: Allen Lane, 1977.

Fynes, Mary. "The Legitimation of Midwifery in Ontario, 1960-1987." Master of
    Science Thesis, University of Toronto, 1994.
Illich, Ivan. "Disabling Professions," *Ideas in Progress Series*. London: Marion
    Boyears Publishing, 1977.
Johnson, T. J. *Professions and Power*. London: Macmillan, 1972.
Kaufman, Karyn, and Mary Renfrew Houston. "Midwives, Nurses and Clinical
    Excellence," In *Recent Advances in Nursing*, UK: Longman Group, 1988.
Larson, Magali. *The Rise of Professionalism: A Sociological Analysis*. Berkeley:
    University of California Press, 1977.
Leap, Nicky, and Billie Hunter. *The Midwife's Tale: An Oral History From
    Handywoman to Professional Midwife*. London: Scarlet Press, 1993.
Levine, Helen. "The Personal is Political" In *Feminism: From Pressure to
    Politics*, Miles and Finn, eds. Montreal: Black Rose Books, 1989.
Lenskyj, Helen. "Commitment and Compromise: Feminist Pedagogy in the
    Classroom." In *Feminism and Education: A Canadian Perspective*, vol. 2.
    Toronto: Centre for Women's Studies in Education, OISE, 1994.
Mason, Jutta. "Appendix on the History of Midwifery in Canada." In *Report of
    the Task Force on the Implementation of Midwifery in Ontario*, Toronto:
    Ontario Government Publication, 1987.
-----. "The Trouble With Licensing Midwives." In *Feminist Perspectives: 20*,
    Canadian Research Institute for the Advancement of Women, 1990.
Monk, Hilary. "Ontario Midwifery in Western Historical Perspective: From
    Radicals to Reactionaries in Ten Short Years," unpublished paper, 1994.
Nestel, Sheryl. "Race and Class in the Re-emergence of Midwifery in Canada:
    An Exploratory Essay," unpublished paper, 1996.
Ontario Ministry of Health. *Report of the Task Force on the Implementation of
    Midwifery in Ontario*. Toronto, 1987.
Reid, Margret. "Sisterhood and professionalism: a case study of the American
    Midwife." In *Women as Healers: Cross Cultural Perspective*. New
    Brunswick, NJ: Rutgers University Press, 1989.
Rich, Adrienne. "What Does a Woman Need to Know?" (Commencement
    address, Smith College, Northampton, Massachusetts, 1979). In *Blood, Bread
    and Poetry*. Norton, 1986.
Shroff, Farah, and Anne Rochon Ford. *An Equity Reader for Midwifery Students*.
    Toronto: Ontario Midwifery Program, Ryerson Polytechnic University, 1994.
Tyson, Holliday. "Outcomes of 1001 Midwife-Attended Home Births,
    1983-1988." *Birth* vol. 18, no. 1 (1991): 14-19.
Van Wagner, Vicki. "With Woman: Community Midwifery in Ontario,"
    unpublished paper, 1991.
Waring, Marilyn. *If Women Counted: A New Feminist Economics*. San Francisco:
    Harare Press, 1990.
Weitz, Rose. "English Midwives and the Association of Radical Midwives."
    Women and Health, vol. 12 (1987).
Weitz, Rose, and Deborah Sullivan. "Licensed Lay Midwifery and Medical
    Models of Childbirth." In *Circles of Care: Work and Identity in Women's
    Lives*. Emily Abel and Margaret Nelson, eds. State University of New York,
    1990.
Young, Diony, and Lesley Page. "External Review Report of the Ontario
    Midwifery Education Programme," 1996.

Prior Learning Assessment for Midwives and the TECMI-Coloured Dreamcoat

Farah M. Shroff,
with Amy Hlaing and Betty Wu-Lawrence[1]

In this chapter we discuss the world's only Prior Learning Assessment (PLA) for midwives — based in Ontario. We then discuss a small pilot project, called the Toronto East Cultural Mentorship Initiative (TECMI), aimed at supporting the successful completion of Chinese-speaking midwives through PLA.

The authors of this chapter have been involved in midwifery in various ways. Race, class and gender issues have been central to our work.

THE PRIOR LEARNING ASSESSMENT PROCESS — BACKGROUND[2]

In order for a midwife to practise legally in Ontario, s/he has to be registered by the College of Midwives of Ontario, the regulatory and governing body which issues licensure for practice. One major task of the College is to set standards and guidelines to assess competency for registered midwives to practise within the healthcare system. The College has the responsibility for not only registering midwives who are graduates of the Ontario Midwifery Education Programme but also assessing those who have had education, training and experience outside of Ontario.

Although there is a move toward baccalaureate-level midwifery education internationally, there are currently only a few baccalaureate midwifery programs in the world that would be considered equivalent to the Ontario program: a four-year university program which includes clinical training in normal birth procedures as well as rigorous training in diagnosis of a potentially high-risk pregnancy, emergency skills and other clinical skills, and academic courses in midwifery theory, social sciences and biological sciences. While recognizing that establishing educational equivalencies would be the most efficient and cost effective means of assessment, the College felt this process had the potential to be restrictive. Given the diversity of midwifery training and practice around the world, the College recognized that the educational equivalency assessment would limit the number of eligible candidates for registration.

The College moved to recognize knowledge and skills gained through both formal learning and experience in a variety of contexts as well as informal learning and experience. Therefore, rather than rely exclusively on educational equivalencies or a comprehensive registration examination as key instruments for registration, in 1994, the College established a prior learning and experience assessment process to determine the knowledge, skills and experience of applicants in order "to provide a fair and equitable access to the profession of midwifery for these many individuals, while protecting the public through an assessment to common standards."[3,4]

While PLA has been a highly political and thus difficult road, most critics concede that the College of Midwives could have followed the path of their counterparts in other professions and simply shut the door to foreign-trained professionals. Many foreign-trained doctors for example, pursue education in other fields as they have virtually no chance to become licensed in Canada. While the PLA process has been flawed in many respects, it is important to credit the College of Midwives for their courage to attempt the implementation of a process which has not been done before. While it could have been designed differently, its very existence is in some senses a victory for foreign-trained midwives.

STAGES OF THE PRIOR LEARNING ASSESSMENT PROCESS

Through the PLA process, foreign-trained midwives and midwives who are not currently registered but have relevant experience, are eligible to have their prior learning and experience assessed, evaluated and recognized. This process potentially allows them to bypass redundant learning and training which may delay them in practising as midwives.

First, orientation sessions are held around the province to inform those interested in the steps of the process. This process is open to those with formal and informal midwifery education, who meet basic clinical requirements, including having attended 40 births. Eligible candidates then proceed to a Midwives' Language Proficiency Test which has both a written and oral component. The two-stage test (oral and written) evaluates language competency in the English or French language. According to those directing the process, competency in either of these languages is needed for the midwife to function adequately in the profession. The test examines competency in professionally-related linguistic skills so candidates are asked to display their knowledge of English or French in a role-play situation that is very similar to the actual work they may have to perform as midwives.

The first time the test was administered, 45% of the candidates failed. Many of these candidates and others have raised serious concerns about the validity and rationale for such a test. Anglophones who were made to go through the English Language proficiency test were particularly upset at the cost of the procedure, but the College saw this as the only way of giving every candidate equal treatment.

Those who pass the test may go on to the next phase, which is the Portfolio Assessment. Candidates are asked to provide evidence of 1) clinical experience, 2) baccalaureate equivalency in the areas of social science, basic sciences, women's studies, research, health sciences, 3) their commitment to the Ontario model of midwifery practice (through an autobiography), and 4) their knowledge and skills in midwifery and obstetrics through a self-assessment and a referee's assessment of the Core Competencies for Midwifery Practice.

Candidates with formal training who pass the language test and provide a satisfactory portfolio are eligible to apply for registration at this stage. Most candidates go on to the next phase — Multifaceted Assessment — which involves written, oral and practical exams in those areas where equivalency is not demonstrated through the Portfolio Assessment.

All candidates who pass the PLA process must attend a ten-day intensive course called "Midwifery in Ontario" to orient them to the specifics of professional midwifery practice in Ontario. Those who complete the course and who have their baccalaureate equivalency can register as midwives and those who do not have this equivalency are required to take additional courses and/or be registered under supervision.

EVALUATING THE PROCESS

The College stresses that, although it believes it has created a fair and inclusive process, it continues to evaluate the process for relevance and effectiveness. The College admits that there are challenges in the development and administration of the PLA process.[5] The limited resources of the College as well as its small size[6] have implications for the support that it can provide to applicants. There is a scarcity of programs and facilities for 'upgrading' and 'retraining' candidates who are not successful; there are insufficient funds to subsidize assessment costs, and no profession-specific language programs available to candidates who require language training. Because there is such a small group of registered midwives in the province, most midwives are under a great deal of pressure to be on committees of the College of Midwives, the Association of Ontario Midwives, or to be involved in other related activities. Since registration came into effect, most registered midwives complain of unbearable stress in their lives. Some have had to take time off due to serious physical and emotional health problems. Because of this climate of near burn-out (which has persisted since 1993), it is very difficult to make major changes within various programs of the midwifery profession, regardless of the good will that exists within its members.

It may be too early to criticize the PLA process since it has only gone through one cycle. During the spring of 1997 an evaluation of PLA's first round is being conducted by an external team. Evaluators will be contacting those who completed the process and those who dropped out. If helpful recommendations are made by the evaluators, the second cycle of PLA should be an improvement over the first cycle. (For the second cycle it will be called "Prior Learning and Education Assessment," to emphasize the educational aspects of the assessment process.)

However, it is worth noting that concerns were raised during PLA's first run. Many PLA candidates complained that the process was very expensive ($2500, plus the costs of university courses, and the language test — approximately $300). The College of Midwives notes that PLA is much less expensive than the baccalaureate program, and that the government did not fund the College adequately for PLA so that candidates must pay for most of the cost of PLA's implementation. Clearly, working-class women would experience difficulty in paying for this process.

Many have also criticized the process as being ethnically biased. At one public orientation meeting of PLA, women of colour were vocal about their anger at the Euro-Canadian women who were directing the process. Critics note that, of the 71 midwives who graduated through the registration process in 1994, only one was not European-descended. Midwives of colour did begin the registration process but dropped out; some did so because the English language requirements were too demanding. Many people question the ethics of forcing people to leave a profession because they do not speak English as eloquently as someone for whom English is a mother tongue.

POLITICIZING ENGLISH LANGUAGE "PROFICIENCY"

The English proficiency test within PLA has been highly controversial. Advocates claim that it is critical for midwives to be able to communicate with doctors in excellent written and spoken English. Because midwifery is under strict scrutiny from the medical profession and other hospital staff, many such harsh decisions have been made by midwifery leadership. Advocates of the rigid standards for English language proficiency feel that it is unfair to send people into a hostile environment unless they are extremely competent; after all, they state, each midwife is an ambassador for the fledgling professional body. However, this rigidity could be interpreted as patronizing. The English proficiency test currently consists of an oral and written portion. It will be administered one more time in two parts and re-evaluated; if it is deemed that both parts are not necessary, only one part will be administered and this will result in both the College and the candidates saving money.

An ability to communicate in English is vital for all practising midwives in Ontario. However, many English tests, like this one, have been critiqued for demanding more than functional communication skills. Critics note that the politics of language domination have not been thoroughly addressed; for a profession that prides itself on its inclusivity, this is one area where there exists a contradiction between rhetoric and reality.

Marlene Nourbese Philip writes of the politics of the English language in "Discourse on the Logic of Language":[7]

> English is
> my father tongue.
> A father tongue is
> a foreign language,
>
> ...my father tongue
> is a foreign lan lan lang
> language
> l/anguish
> anguish
> a foreign anguish
> is english —
> another tongue

Philip notes that Africans under forced genocidal labour (slavery) were forced to speak English and that those caught speaking their mother languages had their tongues removed and hung on a high place for display. In Canada, First Nations children were punished for speaking their languages in missionary and residential schools. The wounds from these attacks on First Nations cultures will be hard to heal. In some nations, the few surviving elders who speak the native language are dying with the language. Given the legacies of colonization, progressive people should at the very least problematize their endorsement of English language domination.

Language is the foundation of culture. The province of Ontario represents a multitude of linguistic and cultural groups. Many of these, particularly those who originate from nations of the South, continue to face racism in Canadian health service delivery. One way (amongst many others) to combat this racism is for health professionals to be representative of various ethnic groups and speak many languages. By enforcing English linguistic domination, the midwifery profession's structures are potentially denying various ethnocultural groups the opportunity to access midwifery care.[8] In Canada, with the exception of a few places, one 'standard' form of English is spoken. People who speak other than this 'standard' Canadian English are often told that they have an 'accent.' This social construction of 'accent' denies the fact that all Canadians speak with an accent and that the status quo defines which accents are acceptable. Sadeghbeigi, in her study of university students for whom

English was not a mother tongue, found that 'accentism' was related to racism. She argues that clear communication is more important than speaking 'standard' English.

However, Scottish, Irish, American or other European-linked accents are generally accepted within the Canadian status quo while linguistic racists are generally intolerant of 'third world' standards of English. It is this latter category of English speakers who are often told they speak with a 'thick accent.'

Some midwifery leaders have stated that a midwife with a thick 'accent' who does not speak and write 'perfect' English would embarrass the profession; they purport that such (potential) midwives would create two standards within the profession. Critics of this position respond that thick accents do not necessarily signify poor communication capability and that native speakers of English from countries like India are unfairly discriminated against for their different 'accent.' They further note that the profession has the potential to embrace diversity and celebrate the gifts that a midwife who speaks multiple languages would bring to the fold. Moreover, the possibilities for reaching a broader clientele and connecting with various communities could increase with more ethnic and linguistic diversity. This potential has yet to be fulfilled, for approximately 4 of the 27 women who graduated from PLA in 1997 were women of colour. Discussions with PLA candidates revealed that some who did not make it through PLA found the process to be humiliating, stressful and insulting. They found that their experience was not validated and that they received no support for filling in the gaps in their knowledge. In its defence, College representatives stated that they had no resources to provide this support, but would have liked to do so.

ETHNORACIAL REPRESENTATION
At this early stage then, midwifery is less representative of ethnic diversity in Ontario than most other health professions. Medicine, nursing and other professional bodies, while not nearly adequately reflective of the province's population, are more ethnically diverse than is midwifery. It is possible that this will change in the coming decades, as more communities of colour learn about the existence and viability of midwifery as a profession. Minimal class diversity also exists among the current body of mainly middle-class midwives and students — race and class structures being intricately linked within capitalism and imperialism.

The problem of exclusion in midwifery was not alleviated by the decision of the state and professionalizing midwifery leaders to implement PLA by prioritizing the registration of women who had been in active practice in Ontario. This decision sowed the seeds for much discontent within the sector of midwives, largely women of colour from the South,[9] who felt that their needs as professionals, as well as the needs of the ethnocultural communities they would potentially serve, were not prioritized.

The decision to register only midwives who had been practising in Ontario resulted in exclusion of midwives who came from countries such as the Philippines, Jamaica, Hong Kong and other nations of the South, as few of these midwives had chosen to practise in the quasi-legal environment prior to legislation, for a variety of complex reasons, some of which are explored in Al-Jazairi and Patel's chapter in this volume. Advocates of the exclusionary decision state that many of these midwives of colour were trained in a colonial style of midwifery which is authoritarian and do not understand the feminist principles of woman-centred midwifery care. Even though most former colonies are now 'independent' (at least politically if not economically), they argue that institutions of colonial (mis)education, medical systems, religious institutions and so forth, persist.[10] Opponents state that this may be true for some women who have been trained in nations ravaged by colonial violence but it is not true for all such women. Despite initial colonial training, they argue, most midwives of colour (like women who have gone through patriarchal education *here*) *are* capable of making a shift to a woman-centered model of care (described in the introductory chapter of this book). The few stories of women from the South who have graduated from the Education Programme or the PLA process bear witness to this possibility.

Among those women of colour who have not been successful in applying to or completing the university program or PLA, are women who are not versed and/or comfortable with the ideals of feminism as they are expressed in the woman-centered midwifery model. Women who do not see themselves as autonomous care-providers with a broad scope of practice are more apt to immediately seek guidance from a medical doctor in case of the slightest difficulty. With the development of feminist thinking comes the development of women practitioners who feel strong enough to develop their clinical skills so that they may deal with a broader range of clinical issues. Psycho-social learning about women's issues, particularly if done in a comprehensive manner so as to incorporate the struggles of working-class peoples, lesbians, racialized peoples and others, may therefore be closely linked to clinical skills development.

The College states that it is committed to structuring an assessment process that would provide fair and equitable access to registration. It also expresses the desire to "make the services of qualified midwives more accessible to the women of Ontario, and to enrich the pool of midwives with a range of language skills and cultural backgrounds."[11] The PLA process provides foreign-trained midwives an opportunity for registration based on their formal and informal learning and experiences without the need to 'relearn' skills and experiences under the Ontario baccalaureate program.

The TECMI (Toronto East Cultural Mentorship Initiative) project capitalizes on PLA's creation of opportunity and attempts to facilitate registration of foreign trained midwives with the recognition that the need for perinatal services exists within English as a Second Language (ESL) communities.[12]

THE TECMI PILOT PROJECT

There are approximately 350,000 Chinese-speaking people in Metropolitan Toronto. Among them is a high number of unilingual Chinese-speaking women. Given this reality, Betty Wu-Lawrence, an executive member of the Chinese Canadian Nurses Association of Ontario (CCNA), in collaboration with others, recognized the need for easier access to perinatal health services as a major healthcare need for this population.

Women for whom English is not a mother tongue lack adequate midwifery care in East Toronto. Almost half the families (47%)[13] served by the local hospital of Metropolitan Toronto are non-English and non-French speaking. There is thus a need for collaboration between various service providers to improve access to perinatal services for the ESL community and a need for ESL professionals to work with existing agencies to provide culturally and linguistically appropriate services. The Toronto East Cultural Mentorship Initiative (TECMI) was created as a modest means of beginning to meet the needs of this population.

This pilot project (TECMI) was developed to establish an interagency collaboration model. The project's initial and current focus was to serve the Chinese-speaking population of Toronto.

TECMI PROJECT OBJECTIVES

Three main objectives were initially established:

a. To provide linguistically/culturally appropriate interpreter services in East Toronto, East York and Scarborough areas for women who seek out midwives as their preferred caregivers during childbirth.

b. To provide resource assistance for the ESL candidates who apply for the Prior Learning Assessment (PLA) administered by the College of Midwives.

c. To establish an interagency, community-based, professional development model for the holistic pursuit of perinatal health care via effective integration and coordination of community resources.

With these objectives in mind, the project organizers sought midwives who were not currently registered and who were competent in both Chinese and English languages to assist them to become registered and capable of adequately serving the Chinese-speaking population in Metropolitan Toronto.

The TECMI project is designed to enable midwifery-skilled candidates who speak languages other than English to successfully complete the PLA process and to provide them with other valuable contacts and support within the community they wish to serve.

INITIATING THE TECMI PROJECT

The Chinese Canadian Nurses' Association (CCNA) of Ontario, City of Toronto Department of Public Health, Toronto East General Hospital and Riverdale Community Midwives are the four organizations working in partnership for this mentorship program. The primary individuals who have contributed to this initiative include: Christabel Chu, consultant for the CCNA; Shaheen Uddin, volunteer researcher for the CCNA; Betty Wu-Lawrence of the City of Toronto Department of Public Health; Wendy Goodman and Colin Goodfellow of Toronto East General Hospital; and Mary Sharpe of Riverdale Community Midwives.

The responsibilities of TECMI committee members are: to liaise with the agencies they represent; to achieve project objectives through specific plans, resource acquisitions, resource allocation and utilization etc; to gather information about community demographic and resource data about midwifery professional development; and research fiscal, human and material resources available to enhance the TECMI project.

To provide culturally sensitive perinatal care to the Chinese-speaking population, the TECMI project organizers sought out Chinese-speaking, foreign-trained midwives who were not yet registered for practice in Ontario. To recruit eligible participants, information about the project was publicized through CCNA and through local Chinese newspapers. As well, information meetings were held to discuss the PLA process and the roles of the partners of the initiative. Applicants were given and required to pass a language proficiency test. Of all the applicants, four passed the language test and two were selected and separately interviewed by each of the four partners.

Next, each partner of the project endeavoured to mentor the two candidates. With the understanding that they were foreign-trained midwives with Chinese-speaking (Cantonese mainly) ability, one major task of the project was to assist these candidates in the PLA process (considered to be stringent and detailed) in order for them to become registered and competent to practise within Ontario.

One of the roles the Toronto East General Hospital undertook was to provide financial assistance to the two candidates. Bursaries of $5000 were presented to each of the two candidates by the hospital to support them through the PLA process. The candidates had to be Canadian citizens or have landed immigrant status, be Ontario residents and be accepted in the PLA process, in order to receive the bursary. The bursary was awarded to the candidates with the agreement that upon becoming registered, the candidate would provide linguistic and culturally sensitive midwifery services to the

Southeast Metropolitan Toronto communities for two calendar years with primary privileges at the Toronto East General Hospital.

The candidates were also to receive cultural and membership support from the CCNA which may have meant filling knowledge gaps on aspects of practice and teaching them how to practise within Ontario. Professional peer support was to be given by the Riverdale Community Midwives which was to include on-site visits and observations at the clinics with exchanges on the fine points of midwifery practice within the Toronto environment.

The Department of Public Health was to liaise with different community groups to provide mentorship training to midwives on aspects of community perinatal services. The Toronto East General Hospital was to provide training about the institutional aspects of perinatal services. The components of the mentorship program provided by each partner were important aspects of the project as the candidates were to learn not only about the challenges of practising midwifery in Toronto but also learn of the support available. Although equipped with good clinical skills, the foreign-trained midwives needed to make adjustments and gain cultural familiarity with the 'Ontario model.'[14]

OUTCOME

The TECMI project commenced in 1993 and was to be ongoing until the two candidates become registered. As of spring 1997 one candidate has been registered; the other candidate failed one of the major examinations and did not feel that she would reapply to become a registered midwife through either PLA or the university program.

It appears that even with the best of intentions, TECMI functioned more as a bursary program than a comprehensive mentorship or social support program. Neither candidate ended up spending much time with any of the partners outside of organized meetings, due to a variety of factors. The biggest hurdle appeared to be the hectic pace of life and resulting lack of time on everyone's part. The midwifery practice was additionally under an obligation to meet the high-level practicum needs of university midwifery students and was thus unable to provide TECMI candidates with access to birthing women under their care. Other partners had similar constraints. While it is possible that the other TECMI candidate will change her mind and reapply to become a registered midwife, at this point, the pilot project is half successful.

The project hopes to demonstrate that high quality perinatal service can be provided by a midwife with language skills other than English. The need for these services is tremendous in the Metropolitan Toronto setting given the city's great cultural diversity.

STATE REGULATION AND THE TECMI PROJECT

With recent legislation of midwifery practice, foreign-trained midwives now have the potential to practise midwifery in a legal environment. State regulation potentially breaks the barrier of the 'informal network'[15] that foreign-trained midwives frequently face. Legislation may not assure equity for foreign-trained midwives, particularly women of colour, but without it, many midwives of colour feel unsafe to practise their art and science in a new country. Many do not feel that they could risk their legal lives and face costly court cases, so they refrain from practising midwifery.

Without legislation, it would be difficult to recognize and validate the midwifery needs of demographic stakeholders such as ESL communities. Since midwifery is now publicly funded, and since stakeholders are in some cases determined by demography, legislation makes it more possible to take action on the needs of consumers. Legislation of midwifery begins to ensure that services provided by midwives are universal and adequately serve *any* resident who wishes to access midwifery services.

TECMI did not exist in pre-legislation days. TECMI's existence is based on the assumption that over 300,000 Chinese-speaking individuals in Toronto need and will utilize perinatal services provided to them by Chinese-speaking midwives. While this assumption may not necessarily be true for all members of the community, only a small percentage of them could be served in any case by one or two midwives. With state legitimization, hospitals and city departments of health are more comfortable in making partnerships with midwives and midwifery initiatives.

In addition, legislation also enables midwives to reach out to different groups of women in Ontario as the services are covered by the state. Women may thus access midwifery services without having to pay extra dollars.[16] Many women of colour, immigrant and refugee women may have a family/cultural history of midwives providing prenatal and postnatal services. As many may be working in 'pink collar' jobs without health benefits or may not be working at all, legislation and funding of midwifery provide a better opportunity for them to seek midwifery services. TECMI aims to provide easier access for women wishing to receive midwifery care.

Besides benefits of legislation, negative implications exist for many trained midwives, including foreign-trained midwives who may not use the title "midwife" as of January 1, 1994, without risking legal action. Those who were serving specific communities are no longer able to do so. Legislation disqualifies these midwives from practising legally in Ontario, although their specific communities may require their language and culturally appropriate skills. One major implication of midwifery legislation is the potential loss of a wealth of knowledge on different midwifery skills when foreign-trained midwives find it difficult to become registered in Ontario.[15] The work of projects like TECMI addresses this problem by aiding these midwives to become registered in order for their knowledge and work to be integrated into the delivery of health care to ethnically diverse women (and other women).

FUTURE DIRECTIONS

For many women, being able to communicate their needs and have them acted upon is a central aspect of a positive childbirth experience. During pregnancy women seek information, advice and practical help which enables them to make informed choices.[18] It is thereby essential that women are able to communicate effectively with their caregivers during their pregnancy and childbirth.

During pregnancy and childbirth, when women of varying cultural and ethnic backgrounds seek professional health care, they come with varied cultural beliefs and health practices. Women's expectations of childbirth are formulated by all their life experiences, education, upbringing, culture and belief systems.[19] Rice warns, "Without a knowledge of these cultural differences, misunderstanding between healthcare professionals and clients can occur during important occasions as childbirth."[20] A study by Narang and Murphy found that antenatal care was not meeting the needs of pregnant Asian women due to a lack of common language and the inadequate provisions of written and spoken information.[21] The Women's Health Bureau of the Ontario Ministry of Health reported language difference as the biggest obstacle to health care; in other words, a refugee or immigrant woman whose first language is not English may not receive adequate care.[22]

The onus of communication must be shared between provider and recipient. It is often believed that misunderstandings arise out of ESL women's lack of English skills. This 'blaming the victim' approach denies that good communication requires *both* parties to listen well and to speak in a manner in which they can be understood. One suggestion Rice makes to improve care of perinatal women is to employ bilingual health workers so that access by non-English-speaking women to birthing services can be improved by eliminating misunderstanding and mismanagement during prenatal care and childbirth. TECMI was one small initiative in this area.

Related to the issue of language barriers is racism. There is a need for anti-racism training for midwives which will show them how power manifests itself in racialized ways within caregiving situations. The Ontario Ministry of Health urges that immediate solutions be found to register and train foreign-trained health professionals, as women of colour and refugee and immigrant women are underrepresented in health service organizations. Ministry support for the integration of foreign-trained health professionals to serve the multicultural society of Ontario shows that the ministry is willing to take on the responsibility in providing quality care for all, and that ensuring the right to adequate and appropriate health care is no longer just the burden of the citizen.

Within many countries around the world (e.g. New Zealand, Australia, the USA) there is a growing recognition of the need to educate and employ midwives of underrepresented communities to provide ethno-specific midwifery services.[23] The Ontario Midwifery Education Programme, recognizing that the province is multilingual and multicultural, is 'labouring' towards more effective and culturally appropriate midwifery care. This is being accomplished largely through a first-year compulsory course which focuses on the potential for anti-racist midwifery care, described in Shroff's chapter in this volume. In the ideal Canada, First Nations peoples would have sovereignty over the land. French and English would not be official languages; instead MicMac, Cree, Slavey, Haida and other Nations' languages would be the official languages of the land. Until such a time, it is imperative for progressive peoples to question and challenge English- and French-language domination and its outgrowth — accentism.

Depending on the success of the TECMI pilot project with the two candidates who are Chinese-speaking, there is a vision to fund and initiate other pilot projects involving midwives who have language abilities other than English. As of spring 1997 no decision had been made about continuing the initiative or not.

The long-term reality is that many Chinese-speaking Canadian women and mothers, like most other Canadian women and mothers, are not aware of the accessibility and advantage of using midwives rather than obstetricians. Even when registered Chinese-speaking midwives will be available to Chinese-speaking Canadian women, they, like other Canadian women, may not utilize them. Women today may be unaware of the care potential of midwives (e.g. midwives providing prenatal and postnatal visits at home), and may make choices about perinatal caregivers out of fear of a possible crisis at birth.[24] Thus, women may feel that utilizing a physician may be better and safer than using a nonphysician. Additionally, the high status of physicians in most working-class communities and communities of colour leads most families to encourage their 'bright' children to study medicine. Midwifery does not bring similar status or income as does medicine.

TECMI is one limited project that has been partly successful on a small scale but there is still a need to expand the linguistic and racial diversity within the midwifery profession and among the clients of midwives.

Along with the pilot project to mentor midwives of colour, adequate prenatal education for ESL women is essential to build their confidence in midwives and to provide them with adequate information to make autonomous choices. Much societal education is still needed for most women to trust a nonphysician. The future of midwifery for midwives of colour and for birthing women of colour lies in providing them with access to information about their choices and in dispelling the fear which resides within clients, their families and Canadian society. By addressing the lack of diversity among midwives, the Toronto East Cultural Mentorship Initiative is taking a small step in this direction.

ENDNOTES

1. Betty Wu-Lawrence's contribution to this chapter was focused on the TECMI section.
2. Some of the information in this section is from a paper by E. Allemang, J. Rogers and V. Van Wagner, "The Ontario Prior Learning and Experience Assessment" (unpublished mimeograph, 1996), and we would like to thank them for providing us with further clarification of its contents.
3. College of Midwives of Ontario, *Annual Report* (Toronto, 1995), 14.
4. In 1994, the structure of the process was completed and the first applicants began assessment. The first orientation session was attended by more than 400 applicants. It was offered in five sites throughout the province through in-person and teleconference sessions. The number of applicants who remained after four stages of the PLA process (i.e. Orientation and Application, Midwives' Language Proficiency Test, Portfolio Assessment, and Multifaceted Assessment) was 35. As of September 1996, these remaining applicants were anxiously awaiting their results from Stage III of the Multifaceted Assessment. As of the spring of 1997, 27 women had completed the PLA process and approximately half of them are close to registration, while most of the others were completing Baccalaureate equivalency. At least one of the TECMI-sponsored candidates has registered.
5. Applicants were informed when they began the process in 1994 that the entire process would take a year. When this did not occur due to various reasons, including administrative and staff changes, many of the applicants became frustrated.
6. Most of the PLA exams have been developed by only three midwives (two from Ontario).
7. Marlene Nourbese Philip, *She Tries her Tongue: Her Silence Softly Breaks* (Charlottetown: Ragweed Press, 1989).
8. Currently, many other women are also being denied midwifery care, as most practices are turning away hundreds of women each year. Midwives may choose their clients based on a number of informal criteria; for example, returning clients may be a major priority for some midwives, as may be women who choose to have a home birth or a vaginal birth after a Cesarean. However, while groups are not singled out to be denied midwifery care, language accessibility remains an important issue.
9. The South is defined here as countries largely in the southern hemisphere that were former colonies of European nations.
10. Chinweizu, "The Re-Education of a Colonized Consciousness," in *The West and the Rest of Us* (New York: Random House, 1974); Fanon, *The Wretched of the Earth*, trans. Constance Farrington (USA: Grove, 1963).
    To illustrate, in modern day life in many nations of the South, these institutions continue the colonizing mission of the European nation which implanted them. Children are tested on poetry by English poets, for example, which describes dandelions in spring. These tests are marked in England and mailed back to the school. Dandelions do not exist in most nations of the South and neither does spring. While many flowers and different seasons exist and have been amply written about in the poetry of the South, the messages conveyed by the exclusive use of the English language and poetry, and sending the tests

to colonial/imperial headquarters, is that South languages, poetry, and teachers are inferior to those of the English.

11. E. Allemang, J. Rogers and V. Van Wagner, "The Ontario Prior Learning and Experience Assessment," (unpublished mimeograph, 1996).

12. The term ESL has been criticized because English may be a third, fourth, or fifth language for some people learning English. Some prefer to use the term English as a Foreign Language (EFL). For some, English may be neither a foreign nor a mother tongue. This may be the case for someone from India for example, where Hindi and English are the official languages. Neither ESL nor EFL is an adequate term but the former is more commonly used, and so we use it here.

13. This data was obtained from the Toronto Board of Education, 1995.

14. The Ontario Model reflects the tenets of choice of birth place, informed decision-making and continuity of care.

15. Without formal regulation there are no set rules or a registration process for which unregistered foreign-trained midwives may appeal to become registered. Without state regulation the registration process can be an inconsistent, unpredictable, unreliable and sometimes unfair process depending on who holds the power to grant registration. With regulation, unfair practices persist but they are generally more difficult to perpetuate on a large scale.

16. C. Lusson, "Obstacles to Social Change: The Legalization of Midwifery in Ontario," Master's thesis, Trent University, 1994.

17. Midwifery legislation has not only potentially harmed midwives originally from the South, but those who are Euro-Canadian women who received training in Texas, England or elsewhere. The group of Euro-Canadian women who have been left out of the legislative process have been vocal about their opposition to legislation and have written critical pieces in magazines such as *The Compleat Mother*. Professionalizing midwifery leadership has been criticized as being elitist, and reactionary, and creating a fiefdom which they alone control.

18. J. Munns and E. Galsworthy, "Expectations of Pregnancy and Birth in First-time Mothers," *British Journal of Midwifery* vol. 3, no. 4 (1995): 231-36.

19. A. Powell, "Class and Ethnicity," *British Journal of Midwifery* vol. 3, no. 3 (1995): 162-7.

20. P.L. Rice, "My Forty Days: Childbearing Experiences of Non-English Speaking Background Women," (The Vietnamese Antenatal/Postnatal Support Project, Australia, 1993): 1.

21. I. Narang and S. Murphy, "Assessment of the Antenatal Care for Asian Women," *British Journal of Midwifery* vol. 2, no. 4 (1994): 169-73.

22. Ministry of Health, "Immigrant, Refugee and Racial Minority Women and Health Care Needs" (Toronto: Queens Printer for Ontario, 1993).

23. S. Kitzinger, "Change in Midwifery: A Cross-cultural View," *Modern Midwife* (May/June 1993): 4-5.

24. See: "Deliverance: In January, An Infant Died at the Hands of a So-called Midwife. Will New Regulations Prevent Future Such Tragedies?" *Ottawa Magazine*, September 1994, 16-20; "Home Birth, Death Linked: Medical Officers Seek Inquest after Baby Dies," *Winnipeg Free Press*, November 19, 1994, A1; "NS Criticizes Support for Home Deliveries," *Medical Post*, April 15, 1996, 38; "Winnipeg Home Birth Death Revives Midwifery Debate," *Globe and Mail*, May 26, 1990, D2.

REFERENCES

Allemang, E., J. Rogers and V. Van Wagner. "The Ontario Prior Learning and Experience Assessment." Mimeograph, 1996.

Chinweizu. *The West and the Rest of Us.* New York: Random House, 1974.

College of Midwives of Ontario. *Annual Report.* (2195 Yonge Street, Toronto, ON, M4S 2B2) Toronto, 1995.

Fanon, Frantz. *The Wretched of the Earth.* USA: Grove, 1963.

Kitzinger, S. "Change in Midwifery: A Cross-cultural View," *Modern Midwife* (May/June 1993): 4-5.

Lusson, C. "Obstacles to Social Change: The Legalization of Midwifery in Ontario." Master's thesis, Trent University, 1994.

Ministry of Health. "Immigrant, Refugee and Racial Minority Women and Health Care Needs." Toronto: Queens Printer for Ontario, 1993.

Munns, J., and E. Galsworthy. "Expectations of Pregnancy and Birth in First-time Mothers," *British Journal of Midwifery* vol. 3, no. 4 (1995): 231-6.

Narang, I., and S. Murphy. "Assessment of the Antenatal Care for Asian Women," *British Journal of Midwifery* vol. 2, no. 4 (1994): 169-73.

Oakley, Ann, and Susanne Houd. *Helpers in Childbirth: Midwifery Today.* New York: Hemisphere Publication, 1990.

Philip, Marlene Nourbese. *She Tries her Tongue: Her Silence Softly Breaks.* Charlottetown: Ragweed Press, 1989.

Powell, A. "Class and Ethnicity," *British Journal of Midwifery* vol. 3, no. 3 (1995): 162-7.

Rice, P.L. "My Forty Days: Childbearing Experiences of Non-English Speaking Background Women." The Vietnamese Antenatal/Postnatal Support Project, Australia, 1993.

Sadeghbeygi, Farangis. "Silence is Full of Meanings." Master's thesis, Ontario Institute for Studies in Education/University of Toronto, 1996.

Wa'thiong'o, Ngugi. *Decolonizing the Mind: The Politics of Language in African Literature.* USA: Heinemann, 1981.

All Petals of the Flower

Celebrating the Diversity of Ontario's Birthing Women within First-Year Midwifery Curriculum

Farah M. Shroff

PREAMBLE

One of the promises of state-regulated midwifery is increased access to midwifery education and midwifery services for all women; prior to state regulation, midwives and their clients represented a small segment of the Ontario population and were not reflective of the demographics within the province. This chapter focuses on diversity issues for midwifery clientele.

Diversity issues have been raised within the Ontario Midwifery Education Programme — recently rated as a world leader in midwifery education by an external team of evaluators from England and the U.S.A. The Education Programme is based on feminist ideals and students are taught a broad range of science, clinical, and social science courses in an attempt to create practitioners with a broad range of training. Students follow women clients immediately as they begin their studies.

The Ontario Midwifery Education Programme is based at McMaster, Laurentian and Ryerson Polytechnic universities. Students learn in small group tutorials based on the McMaster "problem-based learning" model in which students work in small tutorial groups with a discussion facilitator. Many of their classes are taught using distance education technology. Laurentian University has a program for bilingual (French- and English-speaking) students. First Nations students are also encouraged as five spaces are reserved for them each year. Classes began in September 1993 at all universities, with five-year pilot funding from the Ontario government. The Bachelor of Health Sciences degree that is conferred upon successful graduates takes three years to complete, in an academic year of eleven months (in contrast to the usual eight-month year). At Ryerson Polytechnic University, virtually all students are enrolled with part-time status. McMaster and Laurentian students are all enrolled on a full-time basis (making it impossible for them to hold other work during their studies). By the end of the century, the program will shift to a four-year curriculum and students and faculty will have full four-month summers away from the program.

Students are selected on the basis of their desire to be a midwife, ability to function in a high-level academic setting, their previous experiences which show commitment, social justice ideals, and an understanding of the woman-centred model (described in the introductory chapter). An external reviewer of the program commented that the academic standards are closer to a Master's level than an undergraduate Bachelor of Health Science (which is currently offered to successful graduates). Only students who cope well under (at times intense) pressure and who have access to significant financial resources succeed in the program. Students are required to own a vehicle (to get to births at whatever time they may arise), respond to a pager (dropping whatever they are doing in order to get to a birth), juggle studies and follow women clients, as well as still nurturing relationships with partners, children and others. Even for those students whose lives are relatively privileged vis-à-vis race, class, sexual orientation, ability, age and so forth, a great deal of stress enters their lives as a result of the requirements of this program. Only part-time students are able to work at the same time as they are studying. The others rely on savings, family/community support, and loans — usually from the Ontario government.

Class and racial diversity in enrolment, up to the fourth year of the Education Programme's existence, does not reflect current Ontario demographics. Students are chosen largely on their desire to become a midwife and their ability to complete a highly demanding program. Greater racial diversity is hoped to be achieved within the applicant pool to the Prior Learning Assessment process (discussed in Shroff, with Hlaing and Wu-Lawrence's chapter).

One first-year course, "Social and Cultural Dimensions of Health," is focused on social power and the imperative for midwives to work toward and embrace diversity within their clients. The course overview states:[1]

> This course is designed to introduce student midwives to social analysis, related both directly and indirectly, to midwifery issues. Using a multidisciplinary perspective, the integrated analysis of 'race,'[2] class and gender will be applied to topics relevant to midwifery in Ontario. Students are encouraged to develop critical approaches to social phenomena AND to develop constructive, solution-oriented approaches. Cooperative learning techniques and verbal participation will be emphasized.
>
> The course consists of a few major segments. Following an introductory workshop and preparation for distance education is *an introduction to social analysis and to the integrated analysis of 'race,' class, gender*. Then comes a section on *working 'with woman'* in the diverse cultural communities of Ontario. Next is a module on *'the big picture'* issues related to social analysis and

midwifery. The course ends with more discussion about midwifery practice within diversity.

Course Goals:

    a)   To introduce students to analyses of social phenomena, particularly as they relate to midwifery issues. The course's primary foci include a critical analysis of social issues, an anti-racist approach to the study of culture and a 'beyond iconoclasm' (solution-oriented) approach to the study of social problems.

    b)   To incorporate macro, meso and micro analyses and where possible apply these to the future practice of midwifery students.

    c)   To foster the development of midwifery students so that they may provide competent, respectful and compassionate care to the women of Ontario.

The following pages reflect beginning attempts to assist midwifery students in their efforts to provide appropriate care for marginalized women. "Diversity Dynamics: A Practical Primer for Midwifery Students" is partially a result of the resources available within the context of state regulated midwifery. It remains to be seen whether or not this primer and the course within which it is taught have been effective tools to sensitize midwifery students to the needs of women who are disenfranchised within Ontario/Canadian culture. It appears that the bulk of midwifery clientele come from communities other than those mentioned in the Primer. However, it is possible that diversity will increase as Ontario midwifery becomes more known within broader-based circles.

The rest of this chapter is the fifth edition of the text of "Diversity Dynamics: A Practical Primer for Midwifery Students" by Farah M. Shroff. Readers are welcome to use this primer in educational settings and elsewhere with written permission from the author.[3]

DIVERSITY DYNAMICS: A PRACTICAL PRIMER FOR MIDWIFERY STUDENTS

Preface

This Primer's eight sections covers a selection of groups in Ontario/Canadian society who have been politically and/or socially marginalized. Marginalization may have been under colonialism, imperialism or other structural forces, or on the basis of class, sexual orientation, age, ability, ethnicity, skin colour, religion, or other historical and current categories of difference. Recognizing that structural forces, beyond patriarchy, impact upon women's perinatal needs, the following pages provide a brief contextual overview and practical suggestions for midwives who hope to provide appropriate care for these groups of women.

Clearly, this is a limited collection. The section titled "Recently Arrived Immigrant and Refugee Women," for example, is a vast classification which encompasses women from many parts of the globe and whose differences may be greater than their commonalities; they have been defined here based upon a shared experience of, and resistance to, European colonialism. Otherwise, socially, culturally and linguistically, they may be very different. Francophones and Mennonites, two subpopulations of Euro-Canadian women, have been chosen. Although they may have geographically similar roots with the dominant culture, these minorities have varying access to power in this society. All of the above communities have immigrated to Canada for varying reasons. The Primer thus begins with the original inhabitants of this land: First Nations peoples.

An array of other cultural minorities who experience discrimination in this society has also been presented here. This list is not exhaustive. Teenagers, lesbians, women with disabilities, and women in prison may all face social, attitudinal, financial, legal and other barriers when they become pregnant. Within each of these groups, many variations exist, either due to personal preferences or due to internal hierarchies. Additionally, any one woman may be affected by more than one of the categories discussed here. To illustrate, a lesbian mother may also be a Mennonite or a woman in prison may be Aboriginal. The experiences of the groups discussed here are thus not discrete. Rather, various forms of marginalization are intricately interconnected. This Primer has been written within an anti-oppression framework based on anti-racist feminist principles.

Within capitalism, implicit in the study of racism and sexism (and a separate category unto itself), is the importance of class. These forms of oppression tend to operate in tandem; poverty is often a result of institutionalized racist and sexist violence. Indeed, many women of colour are sweeping the floors of Euro-North America, and are maintained at a working-class level by the racism and sexism of educational institutions, the job market, and virtually every powerful institution in this society.[4]

Audre Lorde[5] states that "[i]nstitutionalized rejection of difference is an absolute necessity in a profit economy which needs outsiders as surplus people." She defines racism as the belief in the inherent superiority of one race over others and thereby the right to dominance. She similarly defines classism, sexism, heterosexism, ageism, and elitism. Of racism, sexism, heterosexism and homophobia, Lorde asserts: "the above forms of human blindness stem from the same root — an inability to recognize the notion of difference as a dynamic human force, one which is enriching rather than threatening to the defined self, when there are shared goals."[6]

In my view, third-wave feminist theory[7] (this term is virtually synonymous with the integrated analysis of race, class and gender) is grounded within everyday struggles of oppressed peoples and this makes it relevant to people living outside the academy. By theorizing, in a multidisciplinary fashion, the intersections of three major social variables — race, class and gender — third-wave feminist theory provides a more 'whole' picture of social reality than other recent bodies of theory. In the past few decades, disciplines have tended to become narrowly concentrated on the study of one social variable. Anthropologists have conceptualized culture, and to some extent ethnicity and *race*; sociologists have theorized *class*; women's studies scholars, more recently, have theorized *gender*. Third-wave feminist theory paints a composite picture of these variables. I visualize this as an image which is brought into fuller view by the use of mirrors on three sides.[8]

The integrated analysis of race, class, gender (R.C.G.) is not a 'complete' study of social reality because it does not include sexual identity, age, ability, childhood traumas, mother tongue, and various other categories. Audre Lorde, who identifies herself as a black lesbian warrior poet, brilliantly analyzes race, class, gender *and* sexual identity in her work. Very few theorists are able to deal with this kind of complexity. Another major addition to race, class, gender theory is the analysis of ecology, or the environment. Vandana Shiva[9] is probably the most accomplished theorist in this endeavour.

Race, class, gender theorists have been criticized for trying to do too much, to achieve the impossible and juggle too many balls in the air. Clearly, the enterprise of trying to study three social variables and their intersections is difficult, but critical theorists and activists have recognized the need to widen their lens. This emerging field of theory is one possible solution to the problems with dissected and atomized scholarship. It will take a generation or more of race, class, gender theory to know whether or not the challenge of providing a fuller picture of the social world has been accomplished. As yet, there is no treatise on race, class, gender theory. This discussion does not attempt to create a grand theory of race, class, gender analysis (as this is not its purpose) but to offer a general overview of this emerging field, concretized within midwifery work.

Several theorists use this type of analysis. They include Himani Bannerji, Noga Gayle, Tania Das Gupta, Patricia Hill Collins, bell hooks, Audre Lorde, Swasti Mitter, Patricia Monture-Angus, Roxana Ng,[10] and others. Himani Bannerji[11] discusses the need for new compositions of social theory, and explains how she and students of colour experienced the urgency of this project:

> Neither sociology (not even the conventional marxist variety) nor feminism (not even marxist feminism) spoke to our lives, our experience, histories and knowledges of the world. The existing literature, the conventional paradigms — of both left and 'bourgeois' sociology/feminism, or radical ones — had little or tangential application for us.

In this Primer, I attempt to apply this emerging and expanded theory to midwifery's scope of practice and the woman-centred model of care.

Patricia Hill Collins' *Black Feminist Thought*[12] is one of the only works which creates a body of race, class, gender theory. Focusing on American women of African descent, she aims to show the intellectual and social contributions of black women to the advancement of theory and social justice concerns. With a historical perspective, she cites examples of black feminist intellectuals who profoundly understood the meanings of oppression and activism. Reclaiming the black feminist intellectual tradition, Hill Collins leads the way for women of colour from other communities to examine their traditions, most of which have been suppressed.

Himani Bannerji's address at the University of British Columbia's 1995 Conference titled "Race, Gender and the Construction of Canada" examined historical and contemporary aspects of the Canadian social landscape, exposing the (neo)colonialist, racist, capitalist and patriarchal relations of ruling. She highlighted the First Nations struggle for sovereignty, and the anti-racist struggle of all immigrants of colour. The way in which she integrated diverse women's issues throughout made this powerful address a major addition to R.C.G. theory in Canada, and its publication boosts the development of this emerging field. At the same conference, various other papers were delivered by notable R.C.G. theorists. Tania Das Gupta discussed immigrant women's organizing in Canada, and the differences between multiculturalism and anti-racism. She noted that official policies of multiculturalism neglect power differences between races and discussed the importance of anti-racist consciousness for immigrant women of colour. She also spoke about the dangers of appropriation of anti-racist discourse by the state, noting that the force behind community based organizing efforts for social transformation may be lessened when the language of racism is taken up and trivialized by the state. Enakshi Dua's paper at the same conference discussed the racist and sexist immigration policies of the Canadian state toward Hindu women in the 1800s and early 1900s. Carefully documenting public debates about the need for South Asian cheap labour and the vehement Euro-Canadian resistance to the long-term presence of South Asian people in this country, Dua too made a significant contribution to R.C.G. theory.

These contributions add to the essays in *Race, Class, Gender: Bonds and Barriers*,[13] which for long has been one of the only Canadian readers on the subject. In this collection, women and men, mostly sociologists, write about the dangers of: genocide against First Nations peoples, nationalism, racism, sexism, slavery and other forms of oppression.

George Dei has provided a clear guiding pathway for the application of R.C.G. theory. He prefers not to dwell on the need for grand theoretical bedrocks and states that an anti-racist discursive framework, for the field of education, centres on the need for *equity* (dealing with the qualitative value of justice in the delivery of education), *inclusivity* (power-sharing by school administrators and educators with students and parents), and *representation* (having a multiplicity of perspectives entrenched as part of mainstream academic knowledge). Dei notes that an anti-racism discursive framework acknowledges the reality of racism and other forms of social oppression including but not limited to class, gender and sexual orientation. He asserts:

> Anti-racism moves beyond acknowledgment of the material conditions that structure social inequality to question White power and privilege and its accompanying rationale for dominance... It questions the marginalization of certain voices in society and the delegitimation of the knowledge and experience of subordinate groups.[14]

Dei's examination of the Canadian educational system could aptly be applied to the medical system. He questions the role of the educational system in producing and reproducing racial, gender and class-based inequalities in society. He calls for a more inclusive educational system which is responsive to diverse community's needs. By challenging definitions of valid knowledge, and how such knowledge should be produced and distributed nationally and internationally, an anti-racist political project "is oppositional to established social, economic, and political interests and forces. The public school system, as a state-sanctioned institutional structure, has historically served the material, political, and ideological interests of the state and the social formation of the *status quo*."[15] These ideas have great import for midwifery education. To date, no large-scale sociological study has applied Dei's anti-racism discursive framework to the medical system in Canada.

The Primer is an attempt to dismiss stereotypes of cultural communities and social groups. Some broad themes have been outlined which may or may not apply to all women who identify themselves as members of a particular group.

The complexities and uniqueness of each birthing woman's experience may best be understood through an exploration of the variety of factors which impact upon her life. Sensitized midwifery practices have the potential to contribute to positive experiences of pregnancy, childbirth and childraising, for all women. Woman-centred care ideally embraces the diversity of womanhood in all its forms.

An Introduction to the Information in this Primer

Written materials about marginalized groups specifically in relation to midwifery are not abundant. It is based on a number of sources. The primary source is a series of consultations carried out with various groups across Ontario by the Equity Committee of the Interim Regulatory Council on Midwifery (IRCM) between 1989 and 1992 as recorded by Ann Rochon-Ford. These consultations yielded a large body of reports which are available through the offices of the College of Midwives (see list in Appendix A). This reader represents a distillation of those reports, along with information taken from two other sources:

- existing written and audio-visual material and;
- presentations by guest speakers at a series of workshops for students of the Michener Pre-registration Program for Currently Practising Midwives in 1993.

When quotations appear in the text without a specific source, they have been taken from either individuals who were consulted throughout the work of the IRCM or one of the guest speakers from the Michener workshops. Where this is not the case, the source of the quotation is cited. Individual names have not been used for reasons of confidentiality.

A lesbian mother who spoke to the class of the Michener Pre-registration Program for Currently Practising Midwives, emphasized the importance when addressing equity issues, of not trying to "fit people into a little box." Within all groups of people, there is variation and there are differences amongst all individuals. When speaking in general terms about any group of people, this distinction should always be kept in mind.

This Primer does not attempt to address *all* groups who may require particular attention or have unique needs in relation to midwifery. Missing, for example, is a discussion of low-income women and women with mental disabilities. By covering the groups it does cover, it is hoped that the reader will cultivate an open mind and a habit of asking questions when working with clients whose backgrounds and culture may be different from their own.

Specifically, to begin anti-oppression work, the most powerful starting point is the self. Midwives must ask themselves about their own power and privilege — and lack thereof — in this society. This self-reflection and self-location ought to encompass at least the following points (but is by no means a full list of issues):

- What social class do I belong to? Has this changed, even for temporary periods in my life? If so, how have these changes impacted on me? Have I ever lived in poverty?
- What is my race? Does my skin colour give me privilege in this society or does it make me a possible target of racism?
- What is my ethnicity? In the society in which I live, how does this play itself out?
- What is my sex/gender? What are the benefits and disadvantages of my gender/sex?
- What is my sexual orientation? Do I enjoy the privilege of everyday assumptions of heterosexuality or am I constantly targeted by heterosexism?

- What is my age? Do I get told that I am "too old" or "too young" on a regular basis?
- Am I able-bodied or do I live with a physical or mental disability of some sort? Does able-ism affect me in a conscious manner?
- Am I from a rural or urban setting? How does this impact on my identity and the way others view me?
- What is my first language? If it is neither English nor French, have I been told I have a thick accent?
- Which country was I born in? Am I constantly reminded of my status as an immigrant?
- Am I of mixed racial heritage? Has this created identity conflict?
- Was my childhood affected by abuse of any kind (incest, family alcoholism, violence etc)? Do I live with the memories of being abused or seeing abuse in my childhood?
- Have I been beaten, raped or violated at any point in my life? Do I live with the pain of past or current violence?
- Do I consider myself to be overweight? Do I live with fat oppression? Do I have an eating disorder?
- Have I been institutionalized (in a mental-illness facility, jail or other such place)? Am I on medication of any type for depression or other mental health issues?

Virtually all women experience some power and some oppression. Some strands of feminism have encouraged us to see ourselves as victims. Third-wave feminism encourages women to see the places in which we have strength, to be honest about our privilege and to examine how privilege can create blindspots. Taking action in the spaces where we have privilege can be very powerful; it may involve risks. Being willing to take risks is essential to anti-oppression work. Heterosexual women, for example, may argue/lobby/demand for the rights of lesbians. They may get labelled as lesbians in the process or may lose friends, jobs or more.

Middle-/upper-class, European-descended, able-bodied, heterosexual, urban, university-educated — these are some of the categories of privilege. Without being dogmatic about social justice issues, third-wave feminism is about taking responsibility for change in the places we have privilege. This could be interpreted as somewhat suicidal because successful efforts may eliminate the power that people have: if we smash capitalism it means that we probably will cease to enjoy certain class benefits.

What are each of us willing to give up? Sometimes social change does not mean that each of us have to give up something, but large-scale movements for justice generally involve a redistribution of resources from the 'haves' to the 'have-nots.'

This Primer encourages midwives to engage with questions of power in their professional practice. How accessible is their practice to diverse groups of birthing women? How open are they to learning about the needs of women they have never worked with? Are they willing to change the location of their practice or the way they practice?

A Nigerian proverb states, "treat every person you meet as your teacher." Humility, compassion, respect, well-honed listening skills — these are qualities of people who are willing to examine themselves and work with others in partnership.

Having undertaken a thorough self-reflective process of the type described above, midwives may choose to do integrated anti-racism training which focuses on the dynamics of intercultural contact. Mistrust and apprehension often characterizes contact between cultures. The negative dynamics of this contact have generally been built up over centuries of oppressive relations of ruling. Working-class peoples, First Nations peoples, immigrants from nations of the South, lesbians, bisexuals, transgendered persons, gay men, and others have been at the brunt of untold horrors which have by no means ended. All these communities have histories of resistance and activism against their oppressors; they are not 'victims' in the passive sense of the concept and thus do not require pity or other patronizing communication. Rather, respectful attitudes toward people who have undergone histories of violent oppression are crucial to positive relationships with others. Understanding a general overview of these power dynamics is thus critical.

Having undertaken a self-location and anti-racism training, midwives may then be prepared for the kind of culture-specific education offered in this text. In the course "Social and Cultural Dimensions of Health," in which this reader is used, students go through all of these steps. They are required, by the end of the course, to submit an assignment which describes and analyzes their social location; then they describe and analyze a community that is different than their own community, and one that has endured racism. In the last part of the assignment students describe transcultural and anti-racism approaches to midwifery practice, pulling the threads of the first parts of their assignment through to the working reality which they will hopefully be putting together. Students are encouraged to make this as practical as possible. If they know that they will be working in communities in which large populations of South Asian Canadians live, then their submission flows something like this: self-location (what kinds of power, privilege and oppression do I face in my life?); analysis of a cultural community other than my own which has faced racism (including colonialism, imperialism, racism and resistance to these forms of oppression); and anti-racism/transcultural approaches to midwifery (how will I as a future midwife create an accessible and innovative midwifery practice within the cultural community I have described?).

In the four years that I have designed and taught this course, I have found that some students experience most difficulty with the self-location exercise. The difficulty of this self-examination comes for some because they have been taught to be 'colour blind' and not see 'race' or they have bought into the notion that Canada is a classless society and they have never been prepared to look at their middle-class privilege. Sometimes students choose to do more than examine the categories of race, class and gender. They delve into their childhood or other parts of their lives which are painful and go through emotional journeys which are usually helpful in the long-run but difficult in the short-run. (These kinds of internal-searching projects go well beyond the scope of this course and may involve the assistance of counsellors and other trained people.) Seeing ourselves as powerful is difficult, particularly if it means owning the reality of our own behaviour and unconscious forms of privilege. Taking for granted that the 'new world' provides for everyone makes it difficult to look at the enormous trauma of being 'othered' in Canadian society, and genocide of First Nations peoples.

Early in the course we read the novel *Obasan* by Joy Kogawa[16] and listen to an interview with Roy Miki, a central figure in the Japanese-Canadian Redress Movement. The novel is a 'fictional' account of a young Japanese-Canadian girl whose family is interned in British Columbia during the war in the 1940s. Most students have never heard of this internment of Canadian citizens and often get angry. Some think back to stories they have heard within their own family and recognize the compliance that their own kin had in this atrocity. They then look at their current lives and see things they may not have noticed before: street people, killings of young African-Canadian men by police officers, and more. By the end of the course, some students are thankful that they have heard 'a true Canadian history' and some are still experiencing difficulty with a university course requiring them to do heart and head learning of this sort.

The third part of the assignment, anti-racism/transcultural approaches to midwifery practices (or celebrating diversity), tends to be a highly productive exercise that students sometimes do in groups. They submit creative projects; submissions have included: a video with various women of colour speaking about their midwifery needs and how these can be met; a professionally produced pamphlet about a group practice in an ethnically diverse neighbourhood, translated into several languages; a graphic lay-out of an accessible midwifery practice for women with various disabilities and other needs.

"Diversity Dynamics: A Practical Primer for Midwifery Students" has thus been used in an eight-month university course where students are exposed to a great deal of literature, audio-visual material, speakers, and class lectures/workshops which paint a comprehensive picture of race, class, gender issues in Canadian society and how midwives may use this knowledge to continue in a midwifery tradition of working with marginalized communities.

The next sections represent beginning attempts to examine practical ways for midwives to work in various cultural communities.

Aboriginal Women

Between 1989 and 1992, the Equity Committee of the IRCM had the honour of being welcomed to several First Nations communities throughout Ontario to talk with people about midwifery. They visited and met with community members in Sioux Lookout, Moose Factory, Moosonee, Attawapiskat, Akwesasne, Six Nations, Walpole Island, as well as in Timmins, Thunder Bay and Toronto, and on Manitoulin Island. Their consultations took a number of forms: community meetings, meetings with people who work at different Native organizations, and sometimes informal conversations with local people in less formal settings. They learned more than can be recorded in this brief space, but there were many recurring themes which have been summarized here.

In the course of the three-year period in which they visited different communities and met with Aboriginal people, an unprecedented move took place when the provincial government moved to grant exemption from the Registered Health Professions Act (RHPA) to Aboriginal midwives and healers. What this means is that Aboriginal midwives and healers can practice without being accountable to a regulatory body such as the College of Midwives. This move came about as a result of lobbying on the part of a few key Aboriginal organizations and echoed the sentiments of many Aboriginal people with whom the Equity Committee spoke. The Interim Regulatory Council on Midwifery applauded this measure.

The oldest tradition of midwifery practice in this province is unquestionably that of the First peoples, whose cultures and traditions vary a great deal, with many commonalties binding them together. Childbirth customs and the tradition of midwifery vary greatly in Ontario's Native communities. As Brenda Thomas notes in her research on the topic recently carried out for the Ontario Native Women's Association:

> What may be appropriate childbearing practice in Cree, Ojibway or Navajo territory, may be strictly forbidden or inappropriate for an Algonquin or Iroquois community. There seems to be some across the board concerns within Aboriginal communities in relationship to childbearing care.[17]

The practice of midwifery in Aboriginal communities has been until very recently an integral part of the culture. Midwives for centuries in Aboriginal cultures have passed their role and their practice on to succeeding generations through apprenticeship and through the wisdom of their elders. Their roles have extended beyond that of care throughout the prenatal, intrapartum and postpartum period to include the roles of teacher, herbalist, nurturer, dietician, and in some communities, incorporating the teaching of parenting and other reproductive care for women. The traditional midwife[18] also had a very special relationship to those babies she delivered throughout her lifetime. It is only in very recent history — in the past three decades — with intrusion of Western European medical practitioners into Aboriginal communities, that this tradition has begun to erode.

How Aboriginal women deliver their babies in most parts of Ontario has changed radically since approximately the 1950s.[19] For centuries, women delivered babies amongst their own people — in their home community, out in the bush, or on the trapline, with the aid of a midwife. The Equity Committee learned that usually this was a woman — although there were some men — who had felt a calling to do this from a younger age or who had been chosen to do this by elders or an older midwife in the community. It was not uncommon for the midwife to be the baby's grandmother, aunt, or another relative. She had acquired her knowledge by watching others do the same. She had knowledge of healing plants and proper diet for all phases of pregnancy and for mother and baby in the postpartum period. She knew the traditional customs and ceremonies performed at the time of birth by her people, including, in most communities, a welcoming ceremony, a ceremony for burial of the placenta and a naming ceremony. She had a special status in the community and was widely respected for her knowledge. Some of these women, although much older now, are still living and were interviewed for the Ontario Native Women's Association and Equay-wuk Women's Group for a report compiled for the Aboriginal Health Office.[20]

Since the 1940s and 1950s, women living in remote communities in northern Ontario must leave their communities roughly two weeks before their due date and fly to the nearest community where Medical Services[21] offers maternity care. In north-western Ontario, this is the Sioux Lookout Zone Hospital; in the James Bay region, this is the Moose Factory General Hospital. Women wait in a hostel or a designated ward near or in the hospital until they go into labour or are induced if they go beyond a certain date. If all goes well, the woman is able to return to her community after the delivery. The woman can be away from her family and community for as little as two weeks or as long as several months. The Equity Committee was told that some women deliberately stayed behind, either lying about their due dates, missing the plane or going into hiding to avoid being flown out. The Equity Committee heard of one woman in her ninth month of pregnancy, who had been brought down to Sioux Lookout from Pikangikum and wanted so badly to be back home to have her baby, that she managed to get part-way back on a skidoo. The distance was several hundred miles.

The system of evacuation, which many people feel was imposed on them without consultation, has had considerable negative effects on communities.

The Equity Committee was told that separation from families causes pain and may contribute to family violence. Fathers and siblings missed the opportunity of making a connection to a new family member from the beginning. One community member in Sioux Lookout commented that he felt birth was an important part of bringing the family and community closer. A young woman at Akwesasne, who had recently been able to give birth at home with an Aboriginal midwife following Mohawk customs, told us that the process not only brought her closer to her husband, but it had been a part of healing her family "which has been divided like the blockades at Oka."

One participant at a community meeting in Thunder Bay commented: "At a time when there is so much sadness in Aboriginal communities, one of the few joys we have — a baby being born in the community — has been taken away from us." The impact of colonialism and the destruction of Aboriginal cultural traditions and approaches to healing were illustrated by a staff member of a Aboriginal-run health service in Thunder Bay. He told us of how his mother was once visited in her home by a doctor from Medical Services at a time when she had hung some healing herbs to dry. The doctor pulled the herbs off the wall, threw them in the fire and said, "We're here to provide your medical services now."

He spoke of the "waves of mistrust and discouragement" which Aboriginal people in the north have experienced over the years. Trust has eroded because of bad feelings and discouragement which has built up between Medical Services and Aboriginal people; he said that trust would have to be rebuilt before his people will buy into any more government programs. He said that Medical Services has shown either no regard or ill regard for traditional midwives, and as a consequence, Aboriginal people have come to fear sanctions if they want to deliver in their communities. An Aboriginal staff member at the Sioux Lookout Zone Hospital added:

> People are now dependent. They see white nurses and doctors as people to respect. It was almost a brainwashing. They gradually put aside their own knowledge. It has eroded their traditions and culture.

The research conducted in northwestern Ontario by Carol Terry and Laura Calm Wind for Equay-wuk Women's Group of Sioux Lookout speaks, on page iv, of the loss to the community this way:

> It has been said that when the mothers began leaving the communities to have their babies, the joy and experience of giving life in the communities left with them. Today, the Nishnawbe-Aski people constantly hear and experience the tragedies of suicides. With the future possibility of birthing in our own communities, some balance of life will return.

In the research conducted for Equay-wuk by Brenda Thomas, 19 formerly active traditional midwives in seven communities in the Sioux Lookout Zone were interviewed. All of them indicated that "they would have remained active in their role were it not for the intervention of the Euro-Canadian medical system/establishment."[22] The loss of midwives in Aboriginal communities has meant the disappearance of a source of valuable health information not just for pregnant women but for community members in general. They add in their report that "the elderly Nishnawbe-Aski midwives have instructed the authors to pass on the message that they are willing to share their knowledge and experience of traditional midwifery practices with other First Nations people before it passes on with them."[23]

The Equity Committee was told that the reason given to Aboriginal people (by officials from Medical Services and the Department of Indian and Northern Affairs) for the change in practice from midwife-assisted deliveries in the community to the system of evacuation currently in place is "to improve perinatal and maternal outcomes." Importantly, the Equity Committee was told by a number of people with whom they met that the improvement of perinatal and maternal outcomes in women who are flown out versus women who deliver in their home communities has not been clearly established. This point was reinforced in the literature. The policy of evacuation was ostensibly intended to improve the quality of life for Aboriginal people and yet this has not yet been adequately studied in Ontario, nor elsewhere in Canada, to the best of our knowledge. In fact, many people with whom the Equity Committee spoke, both Aboriginal community members and non-Aboriginal healthcare providers felt that low-risk women would do *better* if prenatal care and nutrition counselling were provided by a community-based midwife, and if they could stay in their communities to give birth. One of the recommendations of the report by Terry and Calm Wind is that "NAN (Nishnawbe-Aski Nation) women be given the choice to give birth in their traditional home lands/communities without reprisal."[24]

Irene Beardy, a traditional midwife from Bearskin Lake, spoke with us about the importance "of the need to fit the new ways with the old ways." She pointed out that we must consider how some traditional advice or practices may no longer be relevant for young women having babies today. For example, a young woman who is sedentary and eats poorly will not be as strong for childbirth as the woman who was constantly active out on the traplines and eating traditional foods. She felt that midwifery, if brought back to Aboriginal communities today, would best include a mix of traditional health practices and some of what has been learned from Western medicine. She summarized her comments on this when she said:

> We had our own way. It was suited to the lifestyle of the past. Now we have new ways which need to include modern medicine. Midwives have to be taught modern skills. There is a need for education and teaching families in the community, especially about parenting.

She expressed concern about the use of drugs and medication used in pregnancy, and that these were bad for Aboriginal people. She said: "We used to sing and nurture women. We had the best system. Now we need to fit in the new ways with the old ways."

This opinion was shared by the midwives interviewed by Terry and Calm Wind for Equay-wuk. They suggest that this marrying of the old and the new would "ensure future safe birthing and deliveries." More specifically, they said:

> For the peace of mind of many concerned individuals, Equay-wuk, along with the encouragement of NAN midwives, recommends that the practices of the Aboriginal culture and Euro-Canadian practices regarding modern midwifery be integrated.

The Equity Committee was told by many with whom they met that there is strong need for a serious evaluation of the process of evacuation from Aboriginal communities in the north. It is recognized that women identified as being at high risk do need to get to a centre where additional services are available to them; however, this does not necessarily mean that all women need to be flown out of their communities to give birth. In every community the Equity Committee visited, the sentiment was repeated over and over again that low-risk women should have the option of giving birth in their home communities, in familiar surroundings with familiar caregivers.

The possibility of birthing centres staffed by trained community members would be a very appealing option to many communities. Interest in this option has already taken hold in Six Nations in the south and Fort Albany in the north, where plans for such centres are in their early stages. At such centres, a woman would receive prenatal care with appropriate nutrition counselling, would deliver her baby with a known midwife, and would be able to return to the centre for postnatal care or have the midwife visit her in her home. The model at Povungnituk on the east coast of Hudson's Bay in Québec has been looked at by a number of Aboriginal communities recently as one where the holistic models of care and obstetrical models of care have been well-integrated.

Women in most southern communities must leave their reserve to deliver in hospitals elsewhere, although the distance from community to hospital is rarely as great as it is in the north. On Walpole Island in Lake St. Clair, for example, when a bridge was built (in the past three decades) to connect the island to the mainland, the practice of babies being delivered on the island with midwives declined rapidly. Women could quickly be taken over to the hospital in Wallaceburg, a short drive away. A number of women described the attitudes of some of the healthcare workers in this hospital and spoke of the racism they dealt with when they were there as patients. As one community leader commented, "They built a bridge but it didn't bridge the gap."

The Equity Committee also learned of more variance of customs in the south, primarily due to a broader range of different communities. Whereas all communities the Equity Committee met with in the north were either Ojibway or Cree, in the south the Equity Committee met with people from Ojibway, Cree, Iroquois and Mohawk communities. The threat of assimilation, although great in the north, sometimes appeared more immediate on southern reserves especially those next door to large urban centres.

In addition to their visits to a number of First Nations communities, the Equity Committee also met with a number of urban Aboriginal people. Similar to those on reserves, they also spoke of experiences of racism, a history of residential schooling and a gradual loss of their cultures. However, urban Aboriginal peoples may have experiences that vary greatly from those who live on reserves. The lack of community in the cities often leads to a sense of desperation for those Aboriginal people who have left their reserves to live in large cities. Nonetheless, the many efforts that have been made over the years through the Friendship Centre movement[25] and by a growing number of urban Aboriginal organizations, have come a long way in helping to create a sense of community for Aboriginal people living off-reserve. The Anishnabwe Health Centre in Toronto, an Aboriginal-run health service for Toronto's Aboriginal population, has worked hard at bringing the values of Aboriginal healing and spirituality to the running of their centre.

With the inclusion of an exemption clause for Aboriginal midwives and healers in the Regulated Health Professions Act, it remains for the Aboriginal population of Ontario to define if and how they will bring traditional midwifery back to their communities. This being stated, the exemption clause leaves many gaps and has been critiqued by Aboriginal people for not *actively* supporting and funding self-determined Aboriginal midwifery services. It is clear from the sentiments of many of the people with whom the Equity Committee met that self determination is vital to their survival as Aboriginal people.

Recently Arrived Immigrant and Refugee Women

Although the experiences of women refugees are often quite different from those of women who have chosen to immigrate to Canada for other reasons, the Equity Committee put these two groups together because they did not consult with them separately. Each refugee woman's experience is unique. However, a refugee woman and an immigrant woman may have significant commonalities. They may both have come from the South, be women of colour and thus possibly subject to racist practices in Canada. Like all women, they may struggle with patriarchal and misogynist violence in its many forms. Additionally, midwifery may be the norm in the countries from which many refugee and immigrant women originate.

These common experiences between immigrant and refugee women are the focus of this chapter. (For further reading on refugee women, see references at the end of this chapter.) Melida Jiminez, an Ontario midwife, writes:

> To be an immigrant woman and to have a baby in Canada is a stressful experience. We are discriminated against because we are poor, because our skin colour is different, because our faces are shaped differently, because our customs and language are different. Many people have stereotyped us as passive, subservient, ignorant Third World women.
>
> Because we do not speak English, we are forced to be silent — to accept the rules; to accept the methods doctors use during the birth; to be without power. Because of the language barrier we can't say no or ask questions. Because of the environment we are afraid to challenge what the doctors are saying and doing to us. We become the objects of medical intervention.[26]

The Equity Committee's meetings with immigrant and refugee women, and those who work with them in different settings in Ontario, were often charged with strong emotions about the sexism, classism, racism and other forms of oppression they experienced during pregnancy and childbirth at the hands of the Ontario healthcare system. Women from many parts of the world were represented in these discussions: Africa, Latin America, Southeast Asia and the Caribbean. Sentiments like those expressed by Melida Jimenez above were heard repeatedly.

Every woman's experience is her own. It is affected by many factors including: the country from which she comes; whether she has had to leave her country under duress and come here as a refugee or whether she has left it willingly; whether she has papers to be in Canada; her social class, both here and in the country from where she emigrated; the status of women in her culture; the role of midwifery in her country of origin; the colour of her skin; her religious beliefs; her knowledge of English; and the length of time she has been in Canada. However, it was significant that there was a good deal of consistency in what the Equity Committee heard. The concerns the Committee heard from immigrant women of one ethnocultural group were often echoed by women of another; the concerns of immigrant women in Toronto were echoed by immigrant women in Ottawa.

The women with whom the Committee spoke expressed a high degree of dissatisfaction with the way they themselves or others they know have been treated in the medical system, particularly in hospitals. Women spoke of the cultural bias in prenatal classes and in the written information distributed to them during their pregnancies. The issue was not just language. The Equity Committee was told over and over again: *it is cultural appropriateness*. One example which illustrated this point very well related to working with pregnant women from Iran and Vietnam. Emphasis on exercise in a prenatal class may be viewed quite differently by pregnant women from these two communities. A woman having recently immigrated from Vietnam, for example, might see exercise during prenatal stages as perfectly normal. Exercise would be an essential part of a healthy pregnancy right up to the time of delivery. On the other hand, the Equity Committee learned from a Jamaican midwife that in some circles in Jamaica, exercise — bending and stretching in particular — is not encouraged because it is believed to tie up the umbilical cord. The Equity Committee heard that in Iran women are generally encouraged to eat large amounts of food. Differences such as these are many. The women with whom the Equity Committee spoke encouraged midwives to learn about different customs from the clients themselves or their family members or friends.

Language barriers are a major problem for many immigrant and refugee women seeking maternity care. The Equity Committee was told that some will avoid seeking out care because they have already had the experience of not being understood by their doctor or other healthcare providers. One woman who works with immigrant and refugee women in Ottawa commented that she has seen how nurses and doctors "assume because she doesn't speak any English, they can do what they want to her." Few services offer materials printed in other languages to help women understand the system, although some feel this is changing slowly in larger centres with larger communities of new immigrants.

An Egyptian woman from Ottawa who works with immigrant people stressed that new immigrants often find large institutions intimidating. She noted that many immigrants come from small communities and may feel more comfortable with "health clinics rather then huge hospitals and one caregiver rather than several experts." In many cultures, people only go to a healthcare worker if they are very ill. Because pregnancy in many countries is seen as a natural part of life rather than an illness, many women do not seek out prenatal care from a healthcare provider. Pregnancy and birth are often not associated with doctors and medical care. She also added that in some cultures, men are not involved in birth. The cultural norm may be that the female relatives in the woman's extended family are involved in the birth. Birth is seen as women's business in a number of cultures and women may seek female midwives as caregivers.

Attitudes towards midwifery and place of birth varied amongst those women with whom the Equity Committee spoke. The Committee was told that women who come from countries where midwifery is a strong and important part of their culture are often quite surprised to learn that midwives are not incorporated into provincial medical systems. In meetings in both Toronto and Ottawa, participants felt that choice of birth place would be important to many immigrant women. Many would have had home births in their country of origin and would feel most comfortable giving birth at home. For others, the idea of a home birth may also be entirely out of the question if a woman is living in crowded quarters with various family members; in such cases, the Equity Committee was told that the woman may also welcome the break from the family that the hospital stay provides.

It is often hard for women new to this country to be separated from the support of their families while in hospital. On the other hand, within every culture, some people feel the need to be 'modern' and that part of being modern is having an obstetrician and a hospital birth, thereby rejecting more traditional practices like midwifery. Similarly, some people feel strongly that they are entitled to what other Canadians have; since the majority of Canadians are having hospital births with obstetricians, they come to see this as the norm and something they, too, should have. For some, the Equity Committee was told, a doctor's presence at your birth represented social mobility and, therefore, was highly desirable.

A Jamaican midwife with whom the Equity Committee met said she felt that people from her culture coming to Canada had a strong and growing faith in the Canadian medical system. She said that many of them were keen on technology because they have come to believe that "the old ways are the wrong ways." She saw this as a form of "self-colonization," meaning that those who came here from colonized cultures have absorbed the negative ideas that Western European (neo)colonialism instilled about their culture (e.g. midwifery is backwards and high technology births represent the right way to do things). She spoke of the need to "de-colonize" members of the Jamaican community, so that they do not lose their faith in doing things in a more natural way.

The women with whom the Equity Committee met warmly welcomed the idea of having a birthing centre for immigrant and refugee women which would be staffed by midwives of various cultural groups. Some mentioned that it would be particularly important for women without immigration papers to be welcomed at such a centre. A nurse-midwife from the Caribbean who works with refugees and new immigrants in the Guelph area, said that women have told her they felt tremendously frustrated about not being able to speak their own language when they were having their baby. One woman she knew completely forgot how to speak English when she was delivering. She said the whispering that most nurses and doctors do in the delivery room made the situation even more alienating for her. The nurse-midwife told of another woman who had recently lost her husband, who said, that when she was in labour, "my 4-year-old daughter gave me more comfort than the nurses and doctors did." A birthing centre where women's cultural and language differences would be closely attended to was perceived as a useful starting point to begin to deal with the alienation in childbirth of which many immigrant and refugee women speak.

In addition to the linguistic and cultural barriers which make it difficult for many immigrant women to use mainstream services, there can be major legal and financial barriers, particularly for refugee women. Melida Jimenez commented about the group without health insurance cards, "They fall through the cracks, and the cracks are getting bigger and bigger."

In Ontario over the past ten years, many people have immigrated from countries where the practice of female circumcision or (female genital mutilation)[27] is still prevalent. A nurse and midwife from Somalia told us that in her country, a woman often weeps when she gives birth to a daughter because she knows what pain her daughter will have to go through with circumcision, usually performed in her country between the ages of 5 and 8 years old. She told us, "There are certain things you don't even have words to express." Women who come to Canada from countries where this practice is carried out often go through even more pain and humiliation when they face unbelieving and judgmental healthcare workers. They often go from doctor to doctor until they find one who has some understanding of how to work with them during pregnancy; one who will not make her feel, as the Equity Committee was told, "like a freak." In one woman's experience, she felt that when she expressed her concerns to her obstetrician about the delivery of her baby as a circumcised woman, these concerns were not taken seriously and that she "had to put a lid on" talking about it.

One woman who worked extensively with refugee women, said that when they have had to leave their homeland because of oppressive political regimes it is not unusual for them to be cautious and possibly fearful of institutions such as the medical system, and authority figures such as doctors. Women who are survivors of torture or violence/persecution based on their gender, ethnicity, race, religion, may have psycho-social healthcare needs.

The Equity Committee was told that, for a wide variety of complex psycho-social reasons, a refugee woman or an immigrant woman who is concerned about her immigration status may consent to a treatment or particular advice even though she does not necessarily agree with it. A Caribbean-Canadian nurse from Ottawa pointed out that it is frequently immigrant women who are the victims of unnecessary procedures and surgery.

Some refugee women who have spent many years of their lives in refugee camps may have no family structures and therefore no traditions passed on to them. A Guelph-area nurse-midwife remarked that this causes terrible isolation.

The experiences and expectations of new Canadians are as varied as the countries, cultures and religious backgrounds from which they come. For many, their experiences to date have been marked with the constant struggle to be heard by medical providers, let alone to be treated with respect. For some, the loneliness and isolation of being new to this country is heightened when they go through the experience of pregnancy and childbirth in the obstetrical system. The Equity Committee was told that some immigrant and refugee women are hesitant to talk about their own cultures because they are so anxious to fit into this one.

Sensitized midwifery practice with recently arrived immigrant and refugee women thus requires understanding the complexities of immigration, racism, ethnic and linguistic discrimination, and the various forms of difficulties this large and diverse group of women may face. Good listening skills and compassion facilitate this kind of understanding. Midwives of all social groups ought to be capable of listening to women's self-defined needs and offer woman-centred care to women of all ethnicities.

Ontario Mennonite Families

Although the Mennonite population in Ontario is relatively small in number — an estimated 250,000 — this community has a longstanding relationship with midwifery in this province. For this reason, and because they have specific needs in relation to childbirth, they have been included in this Primer.

There are more than a dozen different Mennonite groups in Ontario and, while their practices and customs may vary considerably, they share a common history and many common beliefs. Their origins date back to 16th century Europe, when they were also known as Anabaptist Mennonites. A Christian sect with a strong commitment to the daily life practice of their beliefs, they were heavily persecuted and frequently forced to flee their communities. This led them to become isolated and insular groups who cut themselves off from the rest of the world for the preservation of their religion and beliefs.

Today, Mennonites in Ontario are concentrated in rural areas of southwestern Ontario, although Mennonites can be found throughout the province in both rural and urban settings. Old Order Mennonites, a term used to describe the most traditional of Mennonites, form closely-knit communities united by their common beliefs. A pamphlet available to visitors of the (Mennonite) Meeting Place in St. Jacobs, Ontario reads:

> Mennonites believe that they have been called to take the Jesus-way in all of life. They believe that faith needs to be expressed daily and radically. As reconcilers of Christ, they are committed to non-violence and are ready to accept unjust suffering in order to follow Christ faithfully. For centuries they have refused to take part in military service.

The Equity Committee learned from a trip to St. Jacob's Ontario that Old Order Mennonite families in Ontario constitute a small but very strong community, with many concentrated in southwestern Ontario, particularly in the region around Kitchener-Waterloo. Some families are without hydro and many are without telephones. The practices of this one group have particular implications for the delivery of midwifery services in the southwestern Ontario region. Their religious beliefs dictate that they do not accept anything from the government, since they believe the government may in turn ask them to fight in wars in which they do not believe. This means that they do not have OHIP (Ontario Health Insurance Plan) numbers[28] and usually insist on paying directly for healthcare services.

The Mennonite presence in the Kitchener-Waterloo region has somewhat influenced societal attitudes and practices regarding childbirth. Mennonite philosophy places a high degree of respect for what is natural and in doing things naturally, along with a certain disdain for modern technology. This philosophy is parallel in some respects to the woman-centred model of midwifery care although the social context in which the two philosophies were formed varies significantly.

The Equity Committee was repeatedly told by Mennonites themselves and the healthcare providers who work with them, that Old Order Mennonites tend to be very private about birth[29] and like to be able to control who is in the surroundings. These factors led naturally to the development of a birthing home in St. Jacobs (near Kitchener-Waterloo) which has been in operation since 1984. The familiarity with home birth and midwifery in the Kitchener-Waterloo region has also been largely enhanced by the work of one particular midwife, Elsie Cressman, a Mennonite herself.

Clients of the St. Jacobs Family Birthing Home are a mixture of Mennonites and a predominance of non-Mennonite couples seeking alternatives. The Equity Committee was told that Mennonites are "bound to their doctors" and would not dream of confronting or arguing with them. There was a time when all Mennonites gave birth in their homes with the help of doctors. But when doctors stopped coming to their homes, they obeyed the doctor, and went into hospital even though as one Birthing Home Board member put it, "the experience was mortifying for them." Because the Mennonite community is very private about birth, there is a great deal of appeal in the idea of giving birth without having to go into a large public place such as a hospital. The idea of a birthing home also appeals to them because it is helpful to be able to get away from their families to have the baby. One Board member commented, "It's not just a case of believing everything should be natural; they [the Mennonites] do what they do to *not* be involved in the world." In this regard they differ from other marginalized communities who often seek to be accepted and to have the advantages of mainstream culture.

The Equity Committee of the IRCM had the unique opportunity of being able to meet with an Old Order Mennonite family. The mother willingly spoke about the Mennonite community and her reasons for choosing a midwife and home births. Her husband talked about being comfortable assisting at his wife's births. Both spoke of the importance of keeping the issue of birth and pregnancy very private and quiet, that talking about it would detract from its sacredness. The father felt that learning about these things too early was the reason for a lot of the problems in the world today, to which the mother added, "That's just the way we are."

Particular health risks of the Old Order Mennonite population include lack of access to prenatal services (sometimes for cultural reasons, sometimes due to transportation problems), nutritional inadequacies, both prenatally and in the general population, and disorders found to be more common in this population, such as maple syrup urine disease (a problem of protein absorption which can be fatal) and certain eye problems. Severe health problems may arise in Old Order Mennonite families as a result of a tendency to leave any condition be until it gets very serious.

The Mennonite community's birthing needs are diverse. Like with other communities, midwives may serve them best by dismissing stereotypes and judgements, and learning what they can from literature, other midwives, and the clients themselves.

Francophone Women

With more than half-a-million Francophones living in Ontario, this province has the largest concentration of French-speaking Canadians living outside of Québec. In recognition of the historic importance of French-speaking people in this province,[30] and of the state-regulated linguistic duality of this country, the provincial government has enacted legislation (the *French Language Services Act of 1986*) which guarantees access to French language services in Ontario government offices in or servicing a designated area[31] of the province. Section 5. (1) of the *Act* states:

> A person has the right, in accordance with this Act to communicate in French and to receive available services in French from any head or central office of a government agency or institution of the legislature that is designated by the regulations, and has the same right in respect of any other office of such agency or institution that is located in or serves an area designated in the schedule.

As noted in background material[32] about the *French Language Services Act of 1986*, and significant to the profession of midwifery, government services are delivered not only by government ministries and their branches but by community agencies and their institutions in the fields of health and social services. In practical terms, this could mean that a hospital, birth centre or community health centre located in a designated area, may wish to actively recruit a Francophone midwife in order to better serve Francophones in their community.

Consultations with Francophone women by the Equity Committee took place in Ottawa (1990) and Sudbury (1992), two centres with significant Francophone populations. Approximately 20% of the population in Ottawa is Francophone. There is also a large population of midwifery consumers in Ottawa and the surrounding area. Surprisingly, as the Equity Committee found in research done in advance of their visit, there were no native-speaking Francophone midwives in the area, nor Francophone chapters of the (then Midwifery Task Force of Ontario), the Midwifery Consumers Network of Ontario, or the Association of Midwives. Francophone women who wished to have midwifery services in French could access one of a few French-speaking midwives in the area but, as one of the women the Equity Committee spoke with put it, "it's just not the same." She felt that even though someone may be able to speak to you in your mother tongue, that doesn't mean they necessarily understand the cultural context in which you live or all the subtle nuances of your language.

Sudbury, like Ottawa, at the time the Equity Committee met with women there in 1992, had no native-speaking Francophone midwives.[33] Approximately one-third of Sudbury's population is Francophone, with an even slightly higher percentage when the surrounding region is included. Since 1988, and as a result of the *French Language Services Act*, a committee of the Manitoulin-Sudbury District Health Council has been coordinating the French-language services in collaboration with health agencies in the area. The availability of services should include: bilingual signs, French-language documents, a bilingual human-resources plan, and identification of Francophone personnel. Jocelyne Maxwell of the Manitoulin-Sudbury District Health Council points out that one of the main objectives of making French language health services available is that "people live in French on a daily basis, speak their language, live in their culture and this is what they have done all their lives."[34]

The Equity Committee learned from the women they met that the implementation of such services is happening with varying degrees of success in different agencies. Some pointed out considerable resistance and ignorance on the part of staff and administration in some areas. The Equity Committee was told that the number of Francophone personnel who work on labour and delivery wards in Sudbury hospitals was minimal, and that the likelihood of getting a French-speaking nurse when you are having your baby was very low. One woman commented, "You have a better chance of winning the lottery!"

So, although the theory behind the availability of French language health services sounds good, its application leaves something to be desired for some Francophones in Ontario. As one woman commented during a break in the group discussion in Sudbury, "What's the point of them putting up bilingual signs in the hospital, and then hearing them talk behind your back about 'those French'?"

Most of the issues raised by the Francophone women in both Ottawa and Sudbury were not any different from the concerns expressed by most Anglophone women the Equity Committee had met with in different parts of the province. The only distinction made was the lack of services in French, or, more specifically, the lack of Francophone midwives and other health personnel. Like other non-English-speaking women, Francophone women spoke of the importance of being able to communicate in their mother tongue when going through pregnancy, labour and delivery.

Women spoke most readily about language but this was not the whole issue. Like women who are more recent immigrants, the issue of cultural appropriateness was also raised. This was much more difficult to articulate in a group who have had such a long history of assimilation into Ontario's predominantly English world. For decades, Franco-Ontarians have worked hard to carve out an identity which is both distinct from English Ontario, and more than just a mirror image of French Québec. *The French Language Services Act*, and the growth of French-only school boards, community colleges, universities, literacy programs, health and social services are all a reflection of a strong will to preserve a language and a culture which could easily perish without such an infrastructure.

Some women also speculated on cultural differences between Euro-Canadian Anglophones and Euro-Canadian Francophones which may affect their desire for midwifery services. A Francophone nurse working in a community health centre in Ottawa commented that she thought Francophones seemed more attracted to holistic therapies and health professionals than Anglophones. While this was a purely speculative comment, recent surveys have found that Francophones are more inclined to use holistic health care than some other Canadians.[35] Dr. Yves Lamontagne, director of the psychiatric research centre at Louis-H. Lafontaine Hospital in Montréal, commented at a recent symposium of the Corporation Professionnelle des Médecins du Québec: "Anglosaxons are more practical, while Latins are more exuberant. They are more likely to try different things."[36] Comments like this must be viewed with caution since they can paint stereotypes and may not assist Francophones in gaining more rights. It could be argued just as persuasively that it is the struggles which French Canadians have had to keep their language and culture alive in Canada which have made them more ready to pursue nonconformist options. Some of the women with whom the Equity Committee met enjoyed speculating on these differences, but it is important to point out that they were mostly speculations and have yet to be researched adequately.

Francophones in Ontario have fought for a recognition of their right to French-language services as a reflection of the linguistic plurality of this province and country. Other linguistic groups may choose to do the same.

Lesbian Mothers

Some have spoken of a 'baby boom' amongst lesbians since the late 1980s, with a growing number of lesbians having children. Some are having them in the context of a lesbian relationship, others on their own. One of the biggest issues facing lesbians who choose to have children is the heterosexist attitudes which they often face. Heterosexism[37] is the belief that heterosexuals are superior to 'queers' — lesbians, gays, bisexuals and transexuals. Heterosexism permeates virtually every aspect of Canadian culture: language, guiding practices of all gatekeeping institutions, and social interactions. Lesbians describe the sense of 'invisibility' they often experience in their dealings with healthcare providers. The Equity Committee was told that most care-providers presume that lesbians are heterosexual. In a society which is barely recognizing the rights of gay men and lesbians, assumptions of heterosexuality are usually automatic. One lesbian described attending her first prenatal class with a number of heterosexual couples as "the first real taste of how invisible you feel as a pregnant lesbian." One lesbian mother who had her two children in the context of a heterosexual marriage, noted the harsh difference between how her community — the families, the people she works with and comes in contact with every day — celebrated these births because they were an affirmation of family and marriage, and how the community does *not* celebrate her lesbian friends having children.

Lesbian mothers with whom the Equity Committee spoke described what they viewed as a persistent myth: that lesbians would not make good parents and that it is unhealthy for children to be raised by two women. One speaker referred to a growing body of research which shows that lesbians make no better or worse parents overall than heterosexual women and that children raised by a lesbian couple are not hurt in any way by the experience. Far more education of the public is needed before these ideas receive widespread mainstream acceptance, as witnessed by a number of court cases in the United States recently where lesbians have had their children removed from their care. One lesbian mother said she felt that attitudes towards homosexuality is "the last bastion of acceptable prejudices."

On the issue of coming out,[38] one woman emphasized that midwives should check with their lesbian clients about whether they want them to be public about their sexual orientation, such as whether to refer to it in their records. If it is in her charts, the information could be used against her. Lesbian mothers, for example, have been denied immigration on the basis of their sexual orientation. Lesbian mothers have often experienced heterosexism in renting homes, gaining child custody, and from within the school system when their children are known to have two mothers.[39]

Lesbians can become pregnant through a variety of ways. A lesbian may choose to have intercourse with a man or she may use donor insemination. For the latter, she can go to a fertility clinic if she lives in an area where there is one and where they are willing to inseminate lesbians — some are not. In a fertility clinic, she would be inseminated by a physician using previously frozen sperm. Lesbians going this route may also be put on fertility drugs such as Clomid, regardless of whether they are having fertility problems. In a clinic, the donor will likely be anonymous. California has an 'identity-release' system whereby information on the donor is available to the woman or her child should she or they choose to access it.

Lesbians who wish to have more control over the procedure, or who wish to have less contact with the medical profession or who do not have easy access to a fertility clinic, may use self-insemination, also referred to as 'alternative insemination.' In this case, the woman must find the donor herself or have a friend find a donor for her. The donor may be known or unknown. When the donor is known (e.g. a family member of her partner), an arrangement is usually worked out in the form of a contract or letter of agreement. This agreement outlines issues of financial responsibility and any relationship the donor may or may not have with the child. When the donor is unknown, a third-party intermediary (sometimes referred to in the lesbian community as a 'sperm runner') is necessary. If a midwife has any involvement with this process, it may be in the form of teaching a woman how to chart her ovulatory cycle in order to determine her fertile time, or in actually doing the insemination or teaching the woman how to do the insemination. A number of lesbian mothers the Equity Committee spoke with indicated that they hoped more midwives would play a greater role in the future in helping them to get pregnant.

The issue of donors who are HIV (Human Immuno Virus) positive has become one of growing concern in the lesbian community and amongst physicians who provide donor insemination. It is largely for this reason that all Ontario clinics now only use frozen (vs. fresh) sperm. Some women using a known or anonymous donor will require that the donor have appropriate testing where the sperm is quarantined for six months and then retested.

One lesbian mother who had her baby in a hospital described the role which the midwife played as being one of a "cultural interpreter"; she knew she could count on her midwife to defend her choice to have her female partner with her during the delivery and get the hospital staff to acknowledge her partner as one of the child's parents. Where the choice is available, lesbians having babies frequently choose home birth because it is a way to get away from what some lesbians describe as "the heterosexist environment in hospitals." They were very drawn to the woman-centred approach which midwifery offers.

The Equity Committee learned that among some lesbian couples, when a decision is made to have a child, there is considerable discussion about which one will get pregnant — sometimes easily answered or determined, sometimes not — and around what the role of the 'nonbiological' partner will be. One lesbian mother noted that this can lead to tensions during the pregnancy to which a midwife should be sensitive.

Lesbians have advocated for prenatal classes which are inclusive of lesbians. A midwifery practice which has a number of lesbians pregnant at any given time could also offer a lesbians-only prenatal class. In such groups, lesbians would be able to discuss more freely such issues as difficulties in getting pregnant, coming out to family members and the role of the 'nonbiological' or 'nonlactating' partner.

As parents, lesbians have worked out different arrangements. In some cases, both women see themselves as the mothers or parents, while some nonbiological mothers identify themselves as 'co-parents.' It is important for midwives to check this out with both partners before making any assumptions. Other arrangements exist where the biological father, although not sexually involved or living with the mother, acts as a parent to the child, with all the necessary responsibilities of a parent. This may be the case where the woman who, within the context of a lesbian relationship, worked out an arrangement with a man to be not only the biological father but also the child's parent, or where the woman originally had the child in the context of a heterosexual relationship and then left that relationship for a lesbian relationship.

Clearly, because the issue of lesbians having babies in increasing numbers appears to be a relatively new phenomenon, it is important for midwives to realize that there are no officially prescribed answers to the questions which may arise when they work with lesbian clients. Lesbian mothers are continually being asked questions in what one described as "new territory we're carving out here." The lesbian mothers, like many other mothers with whom the Equity Committee met, repeatedly asked that midwives be reminded that they should assume nothing when working with a couple, and should look to the couple for guidance.

Teen Mothers

In a discussion held by the Equity Committee in 1992 with a number of health and social-service providers who work with teen mothers in Toronto, one physician commented that "teens are the perfect group to use midwives." Having worked with teen mothers and midwives she has seen positive relationships between a teen and her midwife and she believes midwives can serve as good female role models for teen mothers. She feels that teens benefit from having a female caregiver as they will often relax and be more open about their lives and bodies. Over the years that she has worked with teen mothers she has observed that they are often treated poorly by institutionally based care-providers and assumed to be "irresponsible or stupid for being pregnant."

A nurse who works in a centre for teen mothers felt that "teens are not respected or allowed to participate in their care." In her words, teens are "always told, never asked." She added that lack of informed choice and respectful treatment is especially hard on pregnant teens, whose self-esteem is often already low. She feels they can suffer "long-term emotional scarring" as a result of this kind of treatment. All agreed that healthcare workers sometimes treat teens badly as a "form of punishment" for being pregnant. Concerns were raised that under the current system of care teens may receive second-class care, as they are often sent to clinics where they see a different physician every visit and rarely know the person who attends their birth. This fragmentation of care is especially harmful to teens who need continuity and personalized care.

Teenaged women who are pregnant and have children often experience a high degree of social isolation. One caregiver noted that "there is no place for them" in North American society's culture of childbirth. Many teen mothers do not have supportive partners or family support and are very alone and frightened. In order to do well in their pregnancy, childbirth and early motherhood, the Equity Committee was told, teens need a supportive and accepting environment. One adult woman who had been a teen mother a number of years ago stressed the need to talk about fears of the birth process, especially the pain of labour.

The group also discussed the problem of teens being characterized as high risk. They have observed that teens tend to be referred to obstetricians and high-risk clinics. The physician in the group referred to a study done at McMaster University, which showed that pregnancy outcome of teens were no different than those of adults if they receive prenatal care. She argued that risk status is different for a 12- or 13-year-old who is still growing and whose menstrual cycle is not yet established than that for a healthy 16-year-old. All observed that teens have very high rates of intervention in their births — particularly episiotomies, epidurals and Cesarean sections. These procedures may not always be necessary.

The group noted that there is a great deal of variance in how different cultural groups treat pregnant teens. In many cultures, such as those of some Caribbean countries, teen pregnancy is generally quite acceptable. A nurse from the Caribbean who works with teens also noted that when the teen's mother is a single parent and struggling to support her family, it may cause stress between the mother and daughter.

There may be rivalry about who is in charge in cultures where grandmothers take a great deal of responsibility for childrearing. In other cultures, for example in some traditional Chinese families, there is often a reluctance to discuss the pregnancy and denial of the teen's situation. All stressed the need for caregivers to be sensitive to cultural variations and customs about birth and baby care. For example, many Greek families believe that mothers and babies should not leave the house for one month. Some Caribbean families may tend not to want their children to be touched a lot or to be with too many people in the first weeks after birth.

A nurse with the Hospital for Sick Children who has had extensive experience working with street youth explained that for many teenage women, having a child is "their only way out." When they are pregnant, the government has money and a place for them. Young women who live on the streets may hope to "make themselves better by having someone they love." However, she added, most street youth are very wary of institutions and may need advocates. They are very concerned about losing their babies — "They are afraid of the system and the system is afraid of them." She feels that street youth need a constant person with whom they can make a connection, and even if it is only for the duration of the pregnancy and postpartum period, midwives can make a considerable difference by providing that connection.

On the question of place of birth, the Equity Committee learned that most will choose not to give birth at home, largely because of fears about pain, and because some teens do not have a home, or want to escape from home. Many teens want to go to the hospital hoping that they will receive care. Although one nurse observed that most teens are afraid of big institutions, they often trust them and believe they will be looked after. She also believes that teens often seek to do what they see the adult women around them doing: "go to a hospital, have an epidural, breastfeed for three days and then stop."

When the Equity Committee had the opportunity to speak to some teen mothers who had been clients of the midwives in the Midwives Collective of Toronto, many of the points made by the care-providers above were confirmed. They felt that it was very important to them to know their midwives and to trust them to "stick up for them." They expressed considerable fear about their baby being taken away from them, having been frightened by stories that they heard from friends, parents and, in one case, a social worker. A teenaged mother who spoke to a group of midwives in Ottawa said that she keeps her baby close to her at all times because her first one was taken away from her by the Children's Aid Society.

A teen mother from Toronto who spoke to a group of midwives there said that, in addition to having the same anxieties as any other new mother would have, she had the additional burden of society thinking she is not capable of being a mother. She also pointed out that in the existing climate where midwifery is seen as somewhat marginalized, it is sometimes difficult or even out of the question for a teen to choose the option of midwifery since "she just wants to be accepted, to do the most normal thing."

Teens, like many first-time mothers, also need a lot of support in order to assess the beginnings of labour. Midwives in Toronto who have worked with teens reported that care of teens tends to involve more home visits prenatally and postnatally. The midwives felt that home visits are an important way for the midwife to make a link to the teen's social situation. They stressed the importance of midwives learning to respect and trust the teen, even "if she comes from a world the midwife is not familiar with." Teens often have trouble attending regularly scheduled prenatal visits and often need support to work out problems that arise in caring for their newborns.

They may not be as skilled as some adults in differentiating between the minor problems that arise in pregnancy and postpartum, and problems which require assessment by a midwife or physician. On the other hand, the Equity Committee was told that teen mothers often have the physical energy which would be the envy of many first-time older mothers!

Working with teens, the Equity Committee was told, may require that the midwife be connected with other social agencies which may be involved in providing support services. Several of the midwives stressed that this may become very important as the midwife's involvement is ending and other supports need to take over. In working with the other agencies, however, the midwife may often find herself drawn into playing a role that extends beyond her usual scope of practice, involving education, counselling and support long past the early postpartum period. Many teens need the most support when the baby becomes more active and demanding from six months to one year of age.

One midwife described the attitude healthcare workers tend to have toward teens as a "double-edged sword." Teens are simultaneously told they must learn to take responsibility for their lives and their babies, yet are undermined by the assumption that they cannot succeed, and not allowed to make decisions for themselves. She pointed out that this needs to be recognized and counteracted in order to work well with a teen client.

In summary, the following were some of the key themes which the Equity Committee heard repeated by teen mothers and caregivers working with them:

1) continuity of care and the development of trust is essential;
2) midwifery services with teens should be integrated with other services for teens in order to make the services accessible and to facilitate good communication between caregivers;
3) perinatal home visits are an important part of midwifery care for teens and should include modelling and teaching aspects of baby care and parenting;
4) visits should be on a flexible schedule;
5) pre- and postnatal care should focus on individual education and counselling and informal group classes geared specifically to teens, allowing peer support and interaction; and
6) support for breastfeeding is important.

Women with Disabilities

Canada's disabled population is made up of a wide range of people. Some are born with their disabilities and others acquire disabilities as they age, either genetically, from accidents, viruses or other sources. People with disabilities are not all in wheel chairs. They may have mental, hearing, sight, limb, or other disabilities.

In discussions with disabled people, the question of accessibility is often revised. But accessibility does not just mean having wheelchair ramps for those using wheelchairs and sign-language interpreters for the deaf. Issues of physical access are relatively easy to point out and, when the will and the resources are present, they are easily rectified. As one woman who has been active with the women with disabilities movement for a number of years said, it is *attitudes* toward people with disabilities which are much more problematic and harder to correct — as is the case with most forms of systemic oppression.

Women with disabilities told the Equity Committee that often some healthcare providers make them feel they were foolish to be having a child. Many healthcare providers feel uncomfortable around pregnant women with disabilities. Women with disabilities often hear insensitive comments about their ability to raise a child from healthcare providers. One woman with whom the Equity Committee spoke, who is in her 50s and has a rare metabolic disorder, remarked that in her younger days (the 1950s and 60s), "it was even a no-no to get married." She added that, "On the whole, as soon as our doctors found out we were pregnant, they said we should have an abortion." She recalled one nurse in the hospital where she delivered her child calling out, "Have fun," in a sarcastic tone as the woman left the hospital with one of her babies in her arms. To counteract these kinds of attitudes, she became friends with a group of women with a similar disability, and they supported each other throughout the years they were bearing and raising children.

Another woman with polio, having learned from her doctor that she was pregnant, was told that she had been booked for an abortion, without having been consulted. She felt that the alienation caused by actions like these could lead disabled women to refrain from seeking out prenatal care. This same woman went on to have her baby. When the baby was born, the doctor held him up to her proclaiming, "his legs are fine." Polio is not a hereditary condition. Another woman with a form of muscular dystrophy recalled that when she had her first child, "I had to wait awhile before someone said 'congratulations.'"

Societal discomfort with pregnant women with disabilities can stem from an ingrained belief that disabled people are not and should not be sexually active. The Equity Committee learned that this is particularly true for women with mobility impairments and women in institutions.[40] Many disabled adults have commented that their parents had difficulty accepting their sexuality. One woman felt that she was never spoken to about sexuality as an adolescent because her parents feared it would raise her expectations that she might some day be sexually active. Because there is an expectation that women with disabilities are not sexually active, they are not expected to get pregnant. When they do become pregnant, there is often shock and outrage expressed by their caregivers. And yet women with disabilities told us over and over again that pregnancy, birth and lactation can be extremely important and validating experiences in the life of disabled women.

The Equity Committee was told that negative stereotypes of disabled women who are contemplating pregnancy, or are pregnant or with children, are based on a belief in the dominant culture that disabled people should not reproduce. This notion is further based on other discriminatory beliefs such as: more disabled people are not needed in society; people with disabilities are not sexual beings and should not be allowed to engage in sexual activity; and disabled people are incapable of doing a good job raising their own children.

Although it is difficult to gauge how common these beliefs are, women with disabilities reminded us that the widespread acceptance and use of prenatal diagnostic techniques (ultrasound, amniocentesis, chorionic villi sampling, etc) provides some indication of the lack of acceptance of disabled people in our society. This issue is one which has been struggled with for a number of years by advocacy groups for those with disabilities. Some women with disabilities feel strongly that prenatal diagnostic techniques only perpetuate intolerance of people with disabilities in our society, and making them so widely available is a way of saying to disabled people, "You are worthless. Your life is not valued. People with your disability can be done away with." As one physically disabled woman who chose not to have any testing stated, "We either accept disabled people in our society or we don't." On the other hand, some women with disabilities feel the availability of such techniques is important to them because they know better than anyone else what it means to grow up disabled in an unsympathetic society. And so they would rather not bring children into the world who have to go through what they did.[41]

Women with disabilities have the same concerns and worries as nondisabled pregnant women, but have additional concerns related to their disability. Because every disability and every woman with a particular disability is unique, it is important for women to have the kind of care which will pay close attention to their needs. Women with disabilities usually know more about their disability than caregivers working with them and appreciate being respected for that knowledge. Women who have had their disability since childhood are usually quite familiar with all the particulars of their history and which drugs and procedures are recommended or contraindicated for them. As one woman with a form of muscular dystrophy who was mistakenly almost given Valium during labour told us, "The consequences of certain interventions may be annoying for nondisabled women (e.g. giving Valium post-surgically), but can be life-threatening for a disabled woman."

A resounding message from the women with whom the Equity Committee spoke is that women with disabilities expect and deserve to be treated with dignity. It is an all too common experience for women with disabilities to have spent a good part of their childhood being paraded in front of doctors and medical residents and having to partake in humiliating exercises with their caregivers in the name of medical education. One woman with a rare disability for whom this was the case when she was growing up in Toronto in the 1950s and 1960s, said, "The worst part is that you're supposed to be grateful for all they're doing for you, and the way you're expected to say thank you is by prostituting yourself — acting as a guinea pig and providing teaching material for medical students." It should not be surprising, with all they might have been through, that some women with disabilities may be reluctant to seek out care when they need it or to be trusting of their caregivers as adults.

Deaf and hard-of-hearing women have particular problems in dealing with the health and social service system when they are pregnant. Access to sign language interpreter services is very limited in most places in Ontario. For the most part, hospitals, public health departments or health units do not offer this service to deaf clients nor do they pay for private interpreters.[42] The Equity Committee was told that the result of having no sign language interpretation for deaf and hearing impaired clients quite simply is that there is little or no communication, that they are left out, and they must rely on other deaf people and written material to get information. There is a prevailing myth that all deaf people can read lips; however, the Equity Committee learned that lip-reading is a particular skill and not everyone can do it. Nonetheless, whether reading lips or not, deaf people tend to observe facial expression more carefully than hearing people. The Equity Committee was told that the common practice that healthcare providers have of turning away and speaking in hushed tones when a woman is in labour may be well-intentioned; however, it may only cause worry for a deaf woman who does not have a sign-language interpreter, since she relies on seeing facial expression to get a sense of what is going on.

One of the cornerstones of the practice of midwifery is the notion of 'normal,' meaning that pregnancy is a normal part of most women's lives and does not usually require treatment in the same way as illness. Women with disabilities told us how the idea of 'normal' may actually leave them out. Long conditioned to believe that they are 'abnormal,' women with disabilities may exclude themselves from midwifery care, assuming their pregnancies will automatically be classified as high risk. Discussions in Ontario are revealing that midwives can play a critical role in the care of women with disabilities. Many women with disabilities told us that support and advocacy which is so often missing in some high-risk care (and is characteristic of midwifery care) would be a tremendous help for some disabled women. A midwife who has come to know a woman and the details of her disability could be an important bridge between the woman and her other caregivers. For example, the continuity of care and the personalized attention which a midwife provides can be invaluable in helping a woman to establish breastfeeding, an activity which takes on particular importance for some disabled women. A woman with a disability who is not high risk could be made to feel more confident and reassured through a midwife's care. Women the Equity Committee spoke with felt strongly that more work is needed in publicizing to women with disabilities the availability of midwifery as an option. Pamphlets produced by the Health and Disabled Women Project of DAWN (DisAbled Women's Network) Ontario (see references at end) are one way the message is getting out. Women with disabilities often do not have access to information from mainstream sources because of inaccessible services, buildings and events, and lack of materials in Braille, large print or on tape. Materials should be made available in alternate formats; in addition to the above, materials available in clear language would be accessible to a larger population, disabled and otherwise. The availability of midwives with sign-language interpretation skills should be publicized.[43] Information should be disseminated to DAWN, the Canadian Hearing Society and other associations for the deaf, the CNIB (Canadian National Institute for the Blind) (in Braille or tape), schools for the deaf, other disability-specific associations, and the Disability Network (a television program). Independent Living Centres found in most major cities in Ontario are also important resources for people with disabilities and a good place to publicize information.

Women in Prison

When the Equity Committee began its work in 1989, member Jesse Russell pointed out that one group of women who is often left out of consultations is women in prisons. It was agreed that the Equity Committee should find out more about women who have babies when they are prisoners and what this might mean for midwifery. The Equity Committee decided to visit Prison for Women (P4W) in Kingston, the only federal prison for women in Canada at that time.

Most of the 100 women from across Canada who are presently in this prison were 'lifers.' The facility is old and in a decaying state; plans are underway to decentralize the prison system for women and to house female inmates in their home province. Grand Valley Institution for Women is the decentralized site for Ontario inmates. This Kitchener facility opened in January 1997.

The Equity Committee met with two nurses on staff and six inmates, one of whom was Chair of the Inmates Committee. There appeared to be a sense of ease between the nurses and the inmates and dialogue between them appeared uninhibited. One of the nurses had been there 20 years, the other 12 years. Most of the women were in their 30s and facing 25-year sentences with possible reviews in 15 years. The vast majority of women in P4W at any given time were in their 20s and 30s, with a very small number in their late teens and over 40. The majority, therefore, were in their childbearing years. Historically, about one-third of all inmates at any given time have been Aboriginal women; the Equity Committee was told that this has changed in recent years, with the percentage of Aboriginal women being somewhat less.

Although many women at P4W were still in their childbearing years, few babies were born to women there. The Equity Committee was told that on average, about one inmate a year becomes pregnant and has a baby. Some women come in pregnant; others get pregnant during visits or while out on passes, usually for longer periods of time. Many of the 'lifers' were married. One of the women who spoke to us had four children living in northern Manitoba and was unable to see them with any regularity because of the distance.

Currently, women at P4W have to give up their baby at three to five days of age. In some cases, the woman's family takes the baby and raises her or him; however, the family may live far away. Women giving birth who do not have families have to give their child up to foster care. The Equity Committee was told that adequate psychological counselling was not available to prisoners when they had to go through the hardship of giving up a baby. The majority of women in prison who were sexually active with a male partner were practising birth control because they knew the pain caused by giving up the baby.

Since the visit to P4W, the Committee learned that one Aboriginal woman who knew she would have to give up her baby was able to keep her baby for a week after delivery. Healthcare staff at P4W who phoned around trying to get help in the form of donated formula or diapers found that "social agencies won't touch inmates."

Two of the prison physicians do deliveries but these take place at the local hospital, the Kingston General. Ultrasounds and other procedures are also done outside the prison at MDS (Medical Diagnostic Services) labs. The Equity Committee was told that going outside for services is a difficult and humiliating experience for the women. National policies are dictated by Correctional Services Canada as to how services are to be delivered to prisoners in hospitals. As one woman said, "They treat us like pieces of shit because we come in handcuffs and shackles." The Equity Committee was told that the prison policy is that shackles are restricted to maximum-security cases, but the Kingston General Hospital policy requires handcuffs, shackles and two guards for *everyone* from the prison. Many of the women are embarrassed to go into the hospital with escorts or guards and some refuse to go outside for medical treatment because of the guards and shackles. The prison almost lost access to outside hospitals because of the alleged behaviour of some inmates and concern for the safety of hospital staff. Staff and inmates with whom the Equity Committee spoke felt that these policies appear to be based mostly on the behaviour of male prisoners. The Equity Committee was told, however, that a woman in labour once stole the keys to the narcotics cupboard at the hospital.

Policies now dictate that in the delivery room, handcuffs are kept on the prisoner and two guards remain but the shackles are removed. The woman may be handcuffed to the table. One of the women said she once had to give a urine sample in a large bowl because they would not remove her shackles during the procedure. She found this very difficult as well as embarrassing. Cuffs, shackles and guards are removed only if the hospitalized person is anaesthetized.

Some women felt that better facilities for delivering babies inside the prison would eliminate the need for transfer, cuffs, shackles and guards. They spoke of the possibility of the proposed new decentralized facilities being designed to accommodate not only deliveries but living arrangements for the mother and baby for an extended period of time following the birth, for example three to five years. This is possible in some prisons in the United States. Writing of the experience of running a parenting class in a prison for women in New York state, Jean Harris observed, "If you know a woman is going to be a child's main caregiver, and you know she may not have experienced much mothering during her own childhood, it is logical to take advantage of the time she is required to be in prison to help develop parenting skills along with the job skills to enable her to support the child."[44]

Although the women present supported the idea of a woman being able to keep her baby for a longer period of time than is currently possible, concern was expressed about possible harm coming to the baby either from other inmates or from being raised in a prison environment. One woman said, "Reality is reality! Some women are here for having killed their kids. Some women are child molesters." She said that there would need to be a screening process, perhaps a screening committee, to decide about management problems, health problems, and the security risks involved.

Women spoke of what it felt like to be 30 years old and facing a life sentence. One of the women asked if she was going to be deprived of the experience of being a mother because she had a hard life and found herself in prison. One woman spoke of the need to bring "humanness (children and family) into the prison." She added, "It's not so much what they (certain prison officials) do to your body; it's what they do to your soul, your spirit, your mind."

The issue of their lives being controlled was a recurring theme throughout the discussion, whether about nonsmoking areas, the availability of condoms and dental dams, opportunities to continue one's education or to receive fair payment and credit for work done. The women with whom the Equity Committee spoke felt very strongly that there was distinct discrimination between the opportunities available to male inmates in comparison to female inmates. One woman said, "Correctional Services says, 'We're here to assist you,' and all we get is training to be a hairdresser." This is in contrast with male prisoners at the Kingston Prison who can leave with qualifications to enter various trades.

Although the discussion the Equity Committee had with a group of inmates at P4W strayed away from midwifery at times, it was clear that midwives could play an important role in providing care to women in prison. As part of the healthcare team, midwives could do much to humanize the system, particularly regarding maternal and child care, if only by reducing the need for all women to go outside of the prison to deliver their babies in cuffs and shackles, surrounded by strangers. Models from prisons in the U.S. may pave the way for a more humane approach to childbearing for incarcerated women. The move to decentralization may also prove to present an opportunity where the current practices are re-evaluated. The women the Equity Committee spoke with were optimistic on both of these points.

THOUGHTS TO TAKE FURTHER

This Primer has explored some ways in which midwives may celebrate and embrace diversity among birthing women by providing some practical suggestions for comprehensive woman-centred care. The ideas here are a beginning in this field.

Unity in diversity is a central theme in the thought of many cultures of the world. Stoney Chief John Snow writes:

> Another theory among us is that in creating so much diversity in nature the Great Spirit revealed..., love for diversity: the diversity of peoples, cultures, and languages, of animals large and small, birds of all colours, fish of all sizes, plant life so numerous, rocks as huge as the mountains and as small as the sands of the seas.[45]

Indian philosopher Swami Vivekananda stated that, "The end and aim of all science is to find the unity, the One out of which the manifold is being manufactured, that One existing as many."[46] He also observed, "As rain falling upon a mountain flows in various streams down the sides of the mountain, so all the energies which you see here are from that one Unit."[47]

ENDNOTES

1. Farah Shroff, "Social and Cultural Dimensions of Health," Ryerson Midwifery Course, 1996.
2. The term 'race' will often be used in quotation marks in this course, as it is a social construct which is often confused as a biologically defined category. It is used here because there is a growing body of thought called "'race'/class/gender" studies, and because racism will be examined in this course. More adequate terminology does not exist.
3. The first edition of "Diversity Dynamics" was published in 1994. © Farah M. Shroff, PhD. All rights reserved. No part of "Diversity Dynamics: A Practical

Primer for Mifwifery Students" may be reproduced in any form without permission in writing from Farah M. Shroff, except for brief passages quoted for review purposes. Farah M. Shroff, 3530 West 15th Ave., Vancouver, B.C., V6T 1X7, Canada, ph/fax (604) 736-7523. The author would like to acknowledge the work of Ann Rochon-Ford in preparing text which was used to draft this Primer in 1993. Significant changes have been made since then.

4. Tanya Das Gupta, 1996.
5. Audre Lorde, 1984, 115.
6. Ibid., 45.
7. First-wave feminism is the beginning of the very recent feminist movement in North America, and refers to the movement which was reflected in Betty Friedan's *The Feminine Mystique* (1963), when mostly middle-class women of European descent recognized their gender oppression. Major goals at the time were to fight for women's admission into exclusively male clubs and to remove the upper age limit for work done typically by women, such as flight attendants. In the 1980s, the second wave was set off by more activist and community-based women who fought for such things as abortion rights, pay equity, and women's access to trades and professions. The third wave is the feminism of diversity and has been set off in the 1990s by women of colour, working-class women, women with disabilities, and lesbians, who saw a need to expand the feminist circle to embrace more women's lives and experiences. Race/class/gender (or feminist anti-racist) theory is part of this newest movement.
8. That does not mean, however, that I am restricting myself to this theoretical basis, as I borrow from a variety of schools of thought.
9. Vanadana Shiva, 1993a, 1993b, 1988.
10. Himani Bannerji, 1993, 1991; Noga Gayle, 1992; Tania Das Gupta, 1994; Patricia Hill Collins, 1992, 1990; bell hooks, 1994, 1984; Audre Lorde, 1984; Swasti Mitter, 1986; Patricia Monture-Angus, 1995; Roxana Ng, 1988, 1981.
11. Himani Bannerji, 1991, 73.
12. Patricia Hill Collins, *Black Feminist Thought*, 1990.
13. Jesse Vorst et al, eds, *Race, Class, Gender: Bonds and Barriers*, 1991.
14. George Dei, 1995, 180.
15. Ibid., 181.
16. Joy Kogawa, *Obasan*, 1981.
17. Brenda L. Thomas, "Report on Tradional Aboriginal Midwifery in Ontario, Phase 1," Ontario Native Women's Association research paper (Toronto: Aboriginal Health Office of the Ontario Ministry of Health, 1993), 9. Navajo communities are not found in Canada, but Thomas draws comparisons with some of their customs in her research.
18. There is no universally agreed upon definition of "traditional midwifery," but Thomas in her work for the Ontario Native Women's Association and Terry and Calm Wind in their work for Equay-wuk Women's Group (referred to below) each provide a definition. Thomas notes, "It includes both midwives who concentrate on the spiritual and cultural aspects of the role and midwives who concentrate on the more technical aspects of care during the reproductive cycle... All traditional Aboriginal midwives hold the view that midwifery is a calling rather than a professional occupation." Terry and Calm Wind add, "...the practice of traditional midwifery was holistic, harmonious and sacred. The midwife upheld fundamental moral and ethical value systems that reflected the philosophy of life held by the Nishnawbe people. The midwife's spiritual and cultural understanding of humanity's place in creation

and the appropriate behaviour required to support the harmonious and holistic existence within the family circle, community and environment shaped all aspects of her work as a midwife."

19. I use the expression 'roughly' because the change has not been consistent from one region to the next or from one nation to the next. Change has come much more recently in more remote parts of the province such as Nishnawbe-Aski Nation, the area which runs from the Manitoba border to the Quebec border within the Hudson and James Bay Watershed. First Nations which are closer to large urban centres, such as Akwesasne and Walpole Island, have been dealing with assimilation into the Western way of birthing for a longer period of time. One is less likely in southern Ontario to meet someone in their thirties who was brought into the world with the aid of a traditional midwife; in the north, the Equity Committee met women in this age group who said things like, "I was born in the bush [with a midwife] and that made me strong," "A midwife is like your mother; she follows you throughout your life," and "I was delivered by grandmother; that makes me special."

20. Laura Calm Wind and Carol Terry, op. cit. and Brenda L. Thomas, op. cit. contain a wealth of information for anyone wanting to learn more about traditional midwifery in Aboriginal communities.

21. Medical Services Branch of Health and Welfare Canada is the branch of the federal government responsible for the delivery of services to Aboriginal people in Canada.

22. L. Calm Wind and C. Terry, op. cit.

23. Ibid.

24. Ibid., 19.

25. Friendship Centres are found off-reserve in cities and towns where there are a number of Aboriginal people.

26. Melida Jimenez, "Teniendo a Mi Hija (Having my Baby)," *Healthsharing Magazine* (Fall 1991).

27. Female circumcision, also known as female genital mutilation, is practised on girls and young women in many African and Middle Eastern countries, in parts of Indonesia, Malaysia, Pakistan and India, and in countries to which people from these countries immigrate. It is usually performed on girls when they are seven or eight years old (i.e. before puberty), although some African communities perform it on much younger girls and others on young adult women. It is usually performed by midwives, traditional birth attendants, or an older woman in the family/community who is experienced in the practice; in more urban and modern settings, doctors also perform the operation.

    There are different types of female circumcision with varying degrees of mutilation to the female sex organs. The least drastic type (clitoridectomy) is comparable to male circumcision in that it consists of removing the clitoral prepuce circumferentially. A more invasive form (sunna) involves removing the entire clitoris often along with part or all of the labia minora. Another particularly invasive type of circumcision is known as infibulation or "pharaonic circumcision" and involves the same procedure as above with the addition of the removal of the labia majora. In this latter form of circumcision, the raw edges of the wounds are sewn together at the time of removal leaving only a small opening for urination and menstrual fluid. A wide range of health problems can and often do result from all forms of female circumcision but most from infibulation.

THE NEW MIDWIFERY

28. For some community members, numbers are associated with evil and the anti-Christ.
29. The Equity Committee heard that it is common for other children in the family not to know that their mother is pregnant. One midwife who works with the Mennonite community told of arriving at the home of her client to do a prenatal visit only to be told she couldn't come in until the hired hand had finished his lunch — no indications of the woman's pregnancy must be visible to outsiders.
30. The preamble to the *French Language Services Act of 1986*, 2, elaborates this point: "Whereas the French language is an historic and honoured language in Ontario and recognized by the Constitution as an official language in Canada; and whereas in Ontario the French language is recognized as an official language in the courts and in education; and whereas the Legislative Assembly recognizes the contribution of the cultural heritage of the French-speaking population and wishes to preserve it for future generations."
31. Designated areas, of which there are 22 in Ontario, are areas where the French-speaking population is greater than 5,000 or 10% of the total population.
32. The Office of Francophone Affairs in the Ontario government, which is responsible for implementation of the Act, along with the Office of French Language Health Services in the Ministry of Health, offer a wide range of material explaining the *French Language Services Act* and its implications for health and social services.
33. This changed in 1994/95 with the French-speaking stream of the midwifery baccalaureate program at Laurentian which brought Francophone midwives to Sudbury.
34. Jocelyne Maxwell, "Your Health in Your Region: Sudbury," *To Your Health* vol. 1, no. 2 (Fall 1992), 3.
35. Carl Berger, *Canada Health Monitor Survey* (Toronto: Price Waterhouse, 1995).
36. "The Attraction is Real for Quebecers," *Medical Post*, September 15, 1992.
37. Use of the term 'homophobia' has been critiqued because it can be seen to legitimate discrimination by labelling it as a fear ('phobia') on a par with other fears like 'agoraphobia.' It is for this reason that the term 'heterosexism' has been used here.
38. The term 'coming out' is used to refer to the act of declaring oneself as 'queer.'
39. For similar reasons, the Equity Committee was advised that it was a good idea to counsel lesbians who were becoming parents to draw up wills.
40. There has been a common practice of administering the drug Depo Provera to young women with physical and mental disabilities living in institutions. This every-three-months injection not only stops them from having periods (considered to be an advantage for caregivers who no longer have to deal with the hygiene problems of menstruation) but also prevents them from getting pregnant if they are sexually active. One of the side effects in women who have been given Depo Provera for extended periods of time is that it can ultimately render them infertile even after they have gone off of the drug. There has been a great deal of controversy over the use of Depo Provera in the past ten years, since it has not been formally approved for use as a contraceptive in Canada though it may be approved in the future. Some activists for the disabled have argued that it is a violation of human rights to continue to use it on disabled girls and women.

41. The issues surrounding prenatal diagnostic techniques and what they mean for people with disabilities are complex and are not meant to be reduced to simplistic solutions by this account. Further reading about this issue is available from the resources listed at the end of this primer.
42. In some countries, deaf women are not able to become midwives because of their inability to hear a fetal heartbeat, although there is new technology which would allow them to do this. In Ontario, this would be considered grounds for discrimination, and the "Entry to Practice Regulations" for the College of Midwives specifically contain a clause which stipulates that ability to speak and write in English or French is an exemptible requirement to allow access for deaf and hard-of-hearing women.
43. The Transitional Council of the College of Midwives used to ask this question of applicants to the College, in the hope of building up a database of midwives with these skills. However, the Council found that the questionnaires had become lengthy and unwieldy and stopped this practice. Currently, the College of Midwives does not ask this of their applicants but it may revisit this issue in the future (Jane Kilthei, personal communication, College of Midwives).
44. Jean Harris, "The Babies of Bedford," *New York Times Magazine* (1993).
45. Chief John Snow, *These Mountains are our Sacred Places: The Story of the Stoney People* (Toronto: Samuel Stephens, 1977), 17.
46. Swami Vivekananda, *Conquering the Internal Nature: Raja Yoga* (Calcutta: Advaita Ashrama Publication Department, 1990), 13.
47. Swami Vivekananda, *The Yoga of Knowledge: Jnana Yoga* (Calcutta: Advaita Ashrama Publication Department, 1989), 185.

REFERENCES

General

Bannerji, Himani. Keynote Address at the University of British Columbia Conference, "Race, Gender and the Construction of Canada, " Vancouver, B.C., October 1995.

------. "But Who Speaks for Us? Experience and Agency in Conventional Feminist Paradigms. " In *Unsettling Relations: The University as a Site of Feminist Struggles*, by Himani Bannerji et al. Toronto: Women's Press, 1991.

Berger, Carl. *Canada Health Monitor Survey.* Toronto: Price Waterhouse, 1995.

Collins, Patricia Hill. *Black Feminist Thought.* Harper Collins, 1990.

Das Gupta, Tania. "Political Economy of Gender, Race and Class: Looking at South Asian Immigrant Women in Canada, " *Ethnic Studies*, vol. 26, no. 1: 59-73.

Dei, George. "Taking Inclusive Education Seriously, " *Canadian Journal of Black and African Education*, vol. 1, no. 1 (1996).

Gayle, Noga. "Black Women's Reality and Feminism: An Exploration of Race and Gender." In *Anatomy of Gender: Women's Struggle for the Body,* Dawn Currie and Valerie Raoul, eds. Ottawa: Carleton University Press, 1992.

Harris, Jean. "The Babies of Bedford," *New York Times Magazine* (1993).

hooks, bell. *Feminist Theory: From Margin to Center.* Boston: South End Press, 1984.

Lorde, Audre. *Sister Outsider.* Freedom, CA: The Crossing Press, 1984.

Maxwell, J. "Your Health in your Region," *To Your Health* vol. 1, no. 2 (1992).

Mitter, Swasti. *Common Fate, Common Bond: Women in the Global Economy.* London: Pluto, 1986.

Monture-Angus, Patricia. *Thunder in My Soul: A Mohawk Woman Speaks.* Halifax: Fernwood Publishing, 1995.

Ng, Roxana. *The Politics of Community Services: Immigrant Women, Class and State.* Toronto: Garamond, 1988.

Snow, Chief John. *These Mountains are our Sacred Places: The Story of the Stoney People.* Toronto: Samuel Stephens, 1977.

Vivekananda, Swami. *The Yoga of Knowledge: Jnana Yoga.* Calcutta: Advaita Ashrama Publication Department, 1989.

------. *Conquering the Internal Nature: Raja Yoga.* Calcutta: Advaita Ashrama Publication Department, 1990.

Vorst, Jesse, et al, eds. *Race, Class, Gender: Bonds and Barriers,* revised edition. Toronto: Garamond, 1991.

Aboriginal Women

Written materials

Akwesasne to Wunnumin Lake: Profiles of Aboriginal Communities in Ontario, Toronto: Ontario Native Affairs Secretariat and Ministry of Citizenship, January, 1992.

Calm Wind, Laura, and Carol Terry. "Nishnawbe-Aski Nation Traditional Midwifery Practices," Equay-wuk Women's Group, Sioux Lookout, Ontario; a research paper prepared by and available from the Aboriginal health Office of the Ontario Ministry of Health, August 1993.

Crnkovich, Mary, ed. *Gossip: A Spoken History of Women in the North* Ottawa: Canadian Arctic Resources Committee, 1990.

Kalnins, Ilze V., Carol S. Farkas, Carol Howell, Reva Jewell and Sheila Sorrell. "Explanatory Models of Health During Pregnancy of Native Women and Non-Native Health Care Providers in Toronto," (March 1990), unpublished paper available from the Native Women's Resource Centre, 245 Gerrard St. East, Toronto, M5A 2G1 or Department of Behavioral Science, McMurrich Building, University of Toronto, Toronto, M5S 1A8.

Malloch, Lesley. "Indian Medicine, Indian Health," *Canadian Woman Studies* vol. 10, no. 2 & 3 (Fall/Winter 1989), 105-112.

"Ontario Native Women: Health and Midwifery." Package of materials prepared by the Equity Committee of the Interim Regulatory Council on Midwifery, 1991. This can be obtained from the College of Midwives of Ontario, 2195 Yonge Street, Toronto, Ontario. Ph: (416) 327-0874; fax: (416) 327-8219.

Thomas, B.L. "Report on traditional Aboriginal midwifery in Ontario, Phase I," Ontario Native Women's Association; a research paper prepared by and available from the Aboriginal Health Office of the Ontario Ministry of Health, September, 1993.

Webber, Gail, and Ruth Wilson. "Childbirth in the North: A Qualitative Study in the Moose Factory Zone," *Canadian Family Physician* vol. 39 (April 1993), 781-8.

Audio-visual Resources

Ikajurti (The Helper): Midwifery in the Canadian Arctic, a one-hour video produced by Pauktuutit (The Inuit Women's Association) and the Inuit Broadcasting Corporation ; available through Pauktuutit (address below)

Further Information

The Inuit Women's Association (Pauktuutit)
200 Elgin St., Suite 804
Ottawa, Ontario K2P 1L5
ph: (613) 238-3977

The Ontario Native Women's Association
172 North May St.
Thunder Bay, Ontario P7C 3N8
ph: (807) 623-3442

Equay-wuk Women's Group
PO Box 1781
Sioux Lookout, Ontario P0V 2T0
ph: (807) 737-2214

Aboriginal Health Office (Ontario Ministry of Health)
700 Bay St., 24th floor
Toronto, Ontario M5G 1Z6
ph: (416) 314-5513

Recently Arrived Immigrant and Refugee Women

Written Materials

Asma, El Dareer. *Women, Why Do You Weep? Circumcision and Its
    Consequences*. London: Zed Press, 1982.
Indra, Doreen. "Gender: A Key Dimension of the Refugee Experience," *Refuge:
    Canada's Periodical on Refugees* vol. 6, no. 3 (February, 1987), 3-4.
Kelly, Ninette. "Refugee Women and Health." In *Working with Refugee Women:
    A Practical Guide*, proceedings from the International Consultation on
    Refugee Women, Geneva, 1988. Geneva: United Nations High Commissioner
    for Refugees, 1989.
Omer-Hashi, Kowser. "Female Genital Mutilation," *Treating the Female Patient*
    vol. 7, no. 2 (May, 1993), 12-13.
Romero-Cachinero, Mary Carmen. "Refugee Women in Canada: The Lingering
    Effects of Persecution, War and Torture," *Refuge: Canada's Periodical on
    Refugees* vol. 6, no. 3 (February, 1987), 6-7.
Spencer-Nimmons, Noreen, and Chow-Ying Wong. "Refugee Women: Canadian
    Concerns, Canadian Considerations," paper delivered at the International
    Symposium, "The Refugee Crisis: British and Canadian Responses." January
    1989. Available from the Centre for Refugee Studies at York University,
    North York, Ontario.
Waxler-Morrison, Nancy, Joan Anderson and Elizabeth Richardson. *Cross
    Cultural Caring: A Handbook for Health Professionals in Western Canada*.
    Vancouver: University of British Columbia Press, 1990.
Women's Health Bureau. "Immigrant, Refugee and Racial Minority Women and
    Health Care Needs: Report of Community Consultations." Ontario Ministry
    of Health, 1992.

Audio-visual Materials

"Silent Tears: An Educational Programme about Female Circumcision," produced
by Tower Hamlets Health Promotion Service in conjunction with the
London Black Women's Health Action Project, available along with a
package of information materials from the Toronto Women's Health Network,
ph: (416) 482-6591.

Further Information

Immigrant Women's Health Centre
489 College St., Suite 200
Toronto, Ontario M6G 1A5
ph: (416) 323-9986

New Experiences for Refugee Women
815 Danforth Ave., Suite 406
Toronto, Ontario M4J 1L2
ph: (416) 469-0196

Canadian Centre for Victims of Torture
40 Westmoreland Ave.
Toronto, Ontario M6H 2Z7
ph: (416) 516-2977

Multicultural Health Coordinator (Maria Herrera)
City of Toronto Dept. of Public Health
Health Policy and Advocacy Section
277 Victoria St., 6th floor
Toronto, Ontario M5B 1W1

Ontario Coalition of Visible Minority Women
579 St. Clair Ave. West, Suite 203
Toronto, Ontario M6C 1A3
ph: (416) 651-5071

Women's Health in Women's Hands: A Community Health Centre for Women
2 Carlton Street, Suite 500
Toronto, Ontario M5B 1J3
ph: (416) 593-7655

Ontario Mennonite Families

A large body of knowledge (both written and amongst staff) is available through
the St. Jacobs Family Birthing Home, located at the Woolwich Community
Health Centre, 10 Parkside Dr., St. Jacobs, Ontario, N0B 2N0.

Francophone Women

Written Materials

To Your Health: A Newsletter About French Language Health Services in Ontario/
À Votre Santé: Un bulletin d'information sur les services de santé en français
en Ontario, available from the Ontario Ministry of Health.

Répertoire des resources pour les Franco-Ontariennes, Ontario Women's Directorate, 1993. (This contains information on groups, associations and centres in the community that offer French-language services in areas such as health, education and help for victims of violence.)

Lesbian Mothers

Written materials

Clay, James W. "Working with Lesbian and Gay Parents and their Children," *Young Children* (March 1990), 31-5.

Donor Insemination: An Overview. Ottawa: Royal Commission on New Reproductive Technologies, 1992.

Handscombe, Gillian E., and Jackie Forster. *Rocking the Cradle: Lesbian Mothers: A Challenge in Family Living.* London: P. Owen, 1981.

Martin, April. *The Lesbian and Gay Parenting Handbook: Creating and Raising Our Families.* New York: Harper Collins, 1993.

McClure, Regan, and Anne Vespry, eds. *Lesbian Health Guide.* Toronto: Queer Press, 1994.

Pies, Cherry. *Considering Parenthood: A Workbook for Lesbians.* San Francisco: Spinsters/Aunt Lute, 1985.

Pollack, Sarah, and Jeanne Vaughn, eds. *Politics of the Heart: A Lesbian Parenting Anthology.* Ithaca, New York: Firebrand Books, 1987.

Rohrbaugh, Joanna Bunker. "Choosing Children: Psychological Issues in Lesbian Parenting," *Women and Therapy* vol. 8, no. 1/2 (1989), 51-64.

Schulenberg, J. *Gay Parenting: A Complete Guide for Gay Men and Lesbians With Children.* Garden City, New York: Anchor Press, 1985.

For Children

Newman, Lesléa. *Heather Has Two Mommies*, Diana Souza, illust. Boston: Alyson Publications, 1989.

Severance, J. *Lots of Mommies.* Chapel Hill, NC: Lollipop Power Press, 1983.

Valentine, Johnny. *The Father Machine.* Boston: Alyson Publications, 1989.

Teen Mothers

Written Materials

Letourneau, Laurie. "Midwifery and the Care of Childbearing Adolescents: A Review of the Literature." Prepared for the Division of Adolescent Medicine at the Hospital for Sick Children and the Midwives Collective of Toronto, August 1988. Available from the Midwives Collective of Toronto or the College of Midwives.

Simkin, Penny. *Cami Has a Baby.* Seattle: Pennypress Inc., 1100 23rd Avenue East, Seattle, Washington, 98112 (comic-book style format geared to teens).

Audio-visual resources

"Playing for Keeps," produced by Studio D of the National Film Board of Canada, 1990. Directed by Lyn Wright and produced by Silva Basmajian.

Other Resources

Jessie's Centre for Teenagers
205 Parliament St.
Toronto, Ontario M5A 2Z4
ph: (416) 365-1888

This service centre for pregnant or parenting teenagers up to 18 years of age
provides:
- pregnancy counselling
- individual and group support
- health services
- nursery drop-in
- housing assistance
- school upgrading

Women with Disabilities

Written materials (including materials on tape and produced in Braille)

Abilities. Quarterly publication of the Canadian Abilities Foundation, Box 527,
Station P, Toronto, Ontario, M5S 2T1.

Campion, Mukti Jain. *The Baby Challenge: A Handbook on Pregnancy for
Women with a Physical Disability.* London and New York:
Tavistock/Routledge, 1990.

Hall, Jennifer. "Jane: The Care of a Deaf Woman," *Midwives Chronicle and
Nursing Notes* (September 1991), 251-2.

"The Happiest Time of Your Life?" *Soundbarrier* no. 43 (December, 1990),
10-11.

Health and Disabled Women Project of the DisAbled Women's Network (DAWN)
of Ontario. Pamphlets, brochures and booklets available:
"I want to be a mother; I have a disability; What are my choices?" (pamphlet)
"Women With Disabilities: A Guide for Health Care Professionals" (booklet)
"You and Your Doctor: Partners in Care" (pamphlet)
"Women With Disabilities talk About Sexuality" (pamphlet)
"Access Checklist" (brochure)

Lippman, Abby. "Prenatal diagnosis: Reproductive Choice? Reproductive
Control?" in *The Future of Human Reproduction*, Christine Overall, ed.
Toronto: Women's Press, 1989.

"Nursing the Hearing-impaired Patient," *Canadian Nurse* (March 1989), 34-36.

"Pregnant and diabetic?" A question and answer fact sheet about pregnancy and
diabetes. Available from the Canadian Diabetic Association, National Office,
123 Edward St., Suite 601, Toronto, Ontario, M5G 1E2.

Ridington, Jillian. *The Only Parent in the Neighbourhood: Mothering and Women
with Disabilities*, DAWN Canada Position Paper 3, March 1989.

Rogers, Judith, and Molleen Matsumura. *Mother to Be: A Guide to Pregnancy
and Birth for Women with Disabilities.* New York: Demos Publications, 1991.
156 Fifth Ave., New York, New York, 10010.

*Table Manners: A Guide to the Pelvic Examination for Disabled Women and
Health Care Providers.* Alameda, San Francisco: Planned Parenthood, 1982.
815 Eddy St., Suite 300, San Francisco, California, 94109.

Through the Looking Glass. A newsletter for disabled parents, 801 Peralta Avenue, Berkeley, California, 94707.

Word Choices: A Lexicon of Preferred Terms for Disability Issues. Toronto: Office for Disability Issues, Ministry of Citizenship, 1989. Available through Ontario Government Publications Office, Toronto.

Audio-visual resources

"Toward Intimacy," a film about women with disabilities and sexuality, produced by the National Film Board, available for rental or purchase through your local office of the National Film Board.

The Health and Disabled Women Project (Ontario) has also compiled a video of clippings on the issue of parenting and disability, mostly from television news features.

Other Resources

DisAbled Women's Network (DAWN) Ontario
P.O. Box 781, Station B
Sudbury, Ontario P3E 4S1
ph: (705) 671-0825
fax: (705) 671-0829
TTY: (705) 671-0825
Outside Toronto, call toll-free: 1-800-561-4727

Birth Signs
(childbirth education classes for deaf and hard-of-hearing women)
c/o Lainie Magidsohn
93 Arlington Ave.
Toronto, Ontario M6G 3L2
ph: (416) 657-8160 (Voice and TDD)

Childbearing and Parenting Program for Women with Disabilities
    or Chronic Illness
c/o Elaine Carty, School of Nursing
University of British Columbia
2211 Wesbrook Mall, #206
Vancouver, British Columbia V6T 2B5

Women in Prison

Written Materials

Harris, Jean. "The Babies of Bedford (It's wrong to separate infants from their imprisoned mothers. An insider's account)," *New York Times Magazine*, 1993.

Task Force Report on Federally-Sentenced Females, Correctional Services Canada, 1991. This report involved the participation of a number of outside organizations including Native organizations and the Elizabeth Frye Society. It led to the decision to close P4W and decentralize the prison system for women in Canada.

Audio-visual Resources

"To Heal the Spirit." A film about Native women in the prison system and the attempts they are making to make change through Native spiritual processes.

Available on loan from the Ontario Regional Office of Correctional Services Canada, Kingston, ph: (613) 545-8107.

"P4W." A film on life inside the Prison for Women, produced by Studio D of the National Film Board. Distributed by Kinetic Inc., Toronto, ph: (416) 963-5979. There have been mixed reactions over the years about this film, in part because it was done by women "from the outside." As one of the nurses who has worked there for over 20 years commented, "It didn't win any friends amongst people inside." Nonetheless, for anyone who has never been inside P4W, the film does document important aspects of daily life there.

Opinions of Certified and Lay Midwives About Midwifery in Quebec:
Perspectives for the Future of Their Profession

Marie Hatem-Asmar
Régis Blais

INTRODUCTION

Canada is the last industrialized country to legally recognize the profession of midwives. Ontario is so far the only province that has fully legalized this practice. Several other provinces have begun the process of recognizing midwifery.[1] Quebec has chosen to first experiment with the practice of midwives for a few years before deciding whether to legalize this profession.

On an international level, the World Health Organisation provides a single definition of a midwife.[2] In practice though, there are different types of midwives, the two most common being the certified nurse-midwife and the midwife by direct entry (i.e. from whom a nursing degree or any other qualifications are not required as a prerequisite). These categories of midwives must be differentiated in terms of various criteria such as their duties, the required level of competence, and the degree of initiative and judgement.[3]

A third group is comprised of lay midwives who appeared, outside of Aboriginal communities, during the second half of this century on the North American continent.[4] The lay midwife practises the profession on a house-call basis and has diverse training not affiliated with any formal program offered at an educational institution. Therefore, this training is not accredited, but consists of substantial clinical experience acquired through apprenticeship.[5] In developing countries, especially in rural areas, this category of midwives corresponds more or less to "traditional midwives" as defined by the World Health Organisation. The similarity between lay midwives and traditional midwives is mainly in the apprenticeship model of training to be a midwife and the style of practice outside the organized health system. The differences between the two categories lie in the level of education and in what motivated their existence. Whereas traditional midwives often do not have any formal education, lay midwives have at least a high school degree. While lay midwifery emerged as a response to women's requests for more humanized maternity care, especially in the United States and in Canada, traditional midwives have always evolved parallel to traditional medicine in many developing countries, as well as in North American Aboriginal communities.

The existence of different types of midwives raises the question as to whether their philosophy of care, the services they provide, and the outcome of their care, differs. In the event that these differences are considerable, the question arises of whether the various types of midwives who wish to practise in Canada, and particularly in Quebec, can build a unified and credible profession.

TYPES OF MIDWIVES AND THEIR CHARACTERISTICS

Studies comparing the different types of midwives based on empirical data are rare. Most of the writing on this subject is descriptive, anecdotal or extrapolatory in nature. Nevertheless, the existing literature suggests the elements that characterize the professional midwife, certified nurse-midwife and lay midwife, as well as their interprofessional relationships. These are socioprofessional characteristics, philosophy of care, relations with the clientele, practice setting, services provided, training, integration within a multidisciplinary team, and legalization or certification.

Socioprofessional Characteristics of Midwives

In the United States, lay midwives are generally younger, interested in education, interested in standards of care and have newer practices when compared to certified nurse-midwives.[6] On the other hand, the certified nurse-midwives have less recent training, are more experienced, and support alternative methods of birth even though they do not practise these methods. This view is shared by various authors.[7]

Philosophy of Care and Relationship with the Clientele

The lay midwives' philosophy comes from their commitment to women, their approach towards holistic care and their belief that pregnancy, labour and delivery are natural, healthy events.[8] This philosophy is similar to that of the certified nurse-midwives; these midwives expect the birth process to proceed normally, but they remain particularly alert to any possible anomaly.[9] In addition, the certified nurse-midwives attach more importance to prevention and education. The lay midwives are known for the provision of alternative care, essentially for controlling pain during delivery,[10] and are considered 'champions' of the demedicalization of care.[11]

The *raison d'être* of lay midwives is their global orientation towards the protection of a woman's right to benefit from alternative methods of birth.[12] They are the product of the feminist movement that claims that women have a right to control and decide what happens to their bodies.[13] Thus, lay midwives tend to be more articulate and more politically oriented than certified nurse-midwives,[14] and identify more with women's health organisations than with other professional healthcare organizations.[15] The certified nurse-midwives are known to be both sensitive and attentive to the needs, demands and preferences of their clients and to respect their autonomy. This double constraint forces them to seek an equilibrium between care administered in an authoritative manner and that administered in a more flexible manner. This aspect is especially important in situations where birth occurs outside the hospital.[16]

Training, Practice Setting and Services Provided

Lay midwives do not necessarily possess medically based or nursing based training. Unlike certified nurse-midwives and professional midwives, lay midwives do not have nationally established standards of training or norms of professional practice.[17] Certified nurse-midwives are trained in two disciplines, nursing and midwifery. Some authors believe that the direct-entry program is preferable in training midwives to be independent.[18] Lay midwives fear that by becoming nurses they will lose their independence with respect to the healthcare system and medical hierarchy, and that they will become more medically oriented.[19] Amongst themselves, midwives generally agree on the level of training required. Nevertheless, the legislation requiring a master's degree to practice midwifery in the United States has disturbed the cohesiveness among midwives, since many of them consider a bachelor's degree sufficient.[20]

In the United States, unlike certified nurse-midwives, the lay midwives and the professional midwives are separate from the medical community.[21] Lay midwives practise almost exclusively at home and rarely in birth centres; certified nurse-midwives practise mostly in hospitals and birth centres; and professional midwives practise exclusively at home.[22] In Europe, professional midwives practice both in the hospital, and at home, but the popularity of each setting varies from country to country.[23] In developing countries, where there are midwifery services, professional midwives practice mainly in urban areas and tertiary hospitals. In rural areas, traditional midwives provide maternity services at home.

In principle, all midwives provide antepartum, intrapartum and postpartum care, but the specific services may vary by jurisdiction and by type of midwives. Rooks[24] considers that lay midwives, who practise outside the medical system, are free to do what they want, and have developed a style of care similar to certified nurse-midwives. In the United States, lay midwives and professional midwives are responsible for the prenatal care of about 3% of all pregnant women who consult birthing centres, while certified nurse-midwives take charge of 81% of these women.[25] The major difference between the percentages of certified and lay midwives in birthing centres is due to the fact that lay midwives mainly attend home deliveries and prefer not to be involved with institutional services, like birthing centres.

LEGALIZATION, CERTIFICATION AND ORGANIZATION OF THE PROFESSION

The question of certification is a sensitive issue among midwives. Lay midwives often practice in an illegal context. They prefer direct government legalization to certification by a professional body (e.g. College of Physicians) which is unfamiliar and different from them.[26] They consider self-certification a very important mechanism in their self-promotion and self-management. In fact, they use self-certification to 'officialize' their competence, and that permits them to negotiate the regulations of their profession with the governmental authorities.[27] Lay midwives would like to join forces with the certified nurse-midwives. They have formed the Midwives Alliance of North America (MANA), to establish standards of practice and obtain recognition by the American College of Nurse Midwives (ACNM). This would facilitate their recognition by the International Confederation of Midwives (ICM).[28] However, the ACNM is still hesitant about recognizing lay midwives.[29] This hesitancy on the part of the ACNM has created tension among the different types of midwives and has led feminist support groups of lay midwives to consider certified nurse-midwives to be false midwives[30] and an elite group that discriminate against lay midwives in a manner similar to obstetricians.[31]

THE SITUATION OF MIDWIVES IN QUEBEC

In the province of Quebec, instead of openly legalizing the profession of midwife, the government adopted a law[32] to try out midwifery in eight pilot projects before deciding to generalize the practice. Since there are no formal education programs yet, the candidates who have come forward to practice as midwives in the pilot projects have various profiles. Those who are lay midwives are for the most part Quebecois, trained according to the norms of their association, l'Alliance Québécoise des Sages-femmes Praticiennes (AQSFP). The others are either professional midwives or certified nurse-midwives who are generally not Quebecois, who have obtained their degrees outside Quebec and are members of l'Association des Sages-femmes du Québec (ASFQ).

As part of the process of recognizing the profession in Quebec, questions have often been raised about the differences between certified midwives (certified nurse-midwives or professional midwives) and lay midwives. The selection of the midwives who were candidates for the pilot projects has not focused on these differences. Instead, the admission criteria were: past clinical experience, results of theoretical and clinical exams and additional recommended clinical training. Consequently, although all the midwives who are participating in the Quebec pilot projects have demonstrated that they have the competence required, they nonetheless come from different backgrounds.

Considering all that is known about the differences that exist among midwives, it seems relevant to ask to what extent accredited midwives in Quebec represent a single professional profile. If they don't, the midwifery profession may risk undergoing an identity crisis related to the conflict that would arise among the different groups of midwives, each of them trying to impose their specific way of seeing the profession.

Most of the studies which we consulted described midwives' practice characteristics and opinions with respect to the group to which they belonged as defined by their training (certified nurse-midwives, professional midwives or lay midwives). Other factors such as sociodemographic or professional characteristics that may influence midwives' practice and opinions, were rarely examined.

A SURVEY OF QUEBEC MIDWIVES

To attempt to fill this gap, a survey of maternity care-providers practising in Quebec was conducted in 1991, including 92 midwives who were members of the two Quebec midwives' associations (AQSFP and ASFQ).[33] Data were collected using a self-administered questionnaire. Seventy midwives returned their completed questionnaires for a response rate of 76%. The first objective of the study was to compare the professional background and opinions of the different types of midwives, according to them being certified (nurse-midwives or professional midwives) or not (lay midwives). The second objective was to determine if midwives' opinions are associated with certain professional and personal characteristics other than their certification.

Quebec's Midwives Professional Profile

Of the 70 respondent midwives, 27 were lay midwives and 43 were certified midwives. For all items, significant differences were observed (Table 1). The majority of lay midwives were trained in Canada, while the majority of certified midwives were trained elsewhere (France, Switzerland, United Kingdom, North Africa, Middle East, etc.). All of the lay midwives were trained from 1980 onwards, but more than two-thirds of certified midwives were trained prior to 1980. Half of the lay midwives were trained in nursing, as compared to three-fourths of the certified midwives. Only 15% of lay midwives have practised outside Quebec, while almost all of them practise as midwives in Quebec.[34] The situation is almost reversed for the certified midwives. Among the AQSFP, only one member had formal training with a midwifery degree, while all members of the ASFQ were certified midwives. Finally, the two groups of midwives differ in terms of age: lay midwives were younger than their counterparts.

TABLE 1: Professional profile of respondents

Variables		Lay midwives		Certified midwives		
		No.	%	No.	%	p*
Duration of training:	12 months	2	8	5	12	
	12-24 months	1	4	20	46	0.000
	24 months	22	88	18	42	
Place of training:	Canada	18	72	10	23	
	elsewhere	7	28	33	77	0.000
Year of training:	1959-1969	-	-	17	40	
	1970-1979	-	-	13	30	0.000
	1980-1989	11	50	13	30	
	1990-1991	11	50	-	-	
Nursing training:	yes	13	48	31	72	
	no	14	52	12	28	0.043
Midwifery practice outside Quebec:	yes	4	15	37	86	
	no	21	85	6	14	0.000
Current midwifery practice:	yes	25	93	13	30	
	no	1	7	30	70	0.000
Midwife association of affiliation:	AQSFP	27	100	1	2	
	ASFQ	-	-	42	98	0.000

* A "p" value smaller than 0.05 indicates that differences between the two groups are statistically significant (that is, they can be judged as real differences and not due to chance alone).

Opinions of the Different Types of Midwives, According to Their Training

It seems that lay midwives and certified midwives largely share the same philosophy of care. Indeed, they had similar client-centred and noninterventionist attitudes and agreed on a full range of services that midwives should be allowed to provide. The similarities in the philosophy of care are consistent with what was found in the literature, although, to our knowledge, there are hardly any empirical studies that have made systematic comparisons between the different groups of midwives.

They largely agreed on the organizational aspects of their profession: the status that midwives should hold and the close collaboration that should take place with the other maternity care-providers (Table 2).

Midwives also agreed on the practice settings for prenatal and postnatal care. However, compared to certified midwives, lay midwives were slightly more in favour of prenatal and postnatal care being provided in private offices, independent birthing centres, and at the client's home (Table 3). Their opinions were very similar for other places of prenatal and postnatal care. The two groups of midwives seemed to disagree more on where they could carry out deliveries. The lay midwives were more in favour of deliveries at home or in independent birthing centres, whereas certified midwives showed no preference for any of the birthing places studied (home, birthing centre, hospital).

Concerning the future training of midwives, differences in points of view between lay midwives and certified midwives, already noted in the literature,[35] emerged. There was both agreement and disagreement between lay midwives and certified midwives in the area of minimal required training

TABLE 2: Future organization that respondents felt the midwife profession should have

Professional dimension	Lay midwives		Certified midwives		
	No.	%	No.	%	p
Professional status*:					
• professionals working under physician's authority	0	0	1	2	
• autonomous professionals required to consult a physician in case of problems	27	100	42	98	0.424
Nature of collaboration*:					
• work independently of current personnel but consult them when needed	9	33	15	35	
• work in close collaboration with current personnel	18	67	27	63	0.839
Professional body regulating midwifery*:					
• midwifery college	26	92	42	98	
• Collège des Médecins du Québec ~	0	0	1	2	0.328
• other	1	8	0	0	
Professional body responsible for quality control in hospitals*:					
• Council of physicians, dentists and pharmacists, to which midwives would be added	2	7	4	9	
• maternity care committee with equal representation by nurses, physicians and midwives	4	15	5	12	
• multidisciplinary committee composed mostly of midwives	18	67	32	74	0.873
• other	3	11	1	2	

*Response choices are mutually exclusive.
~Regulatory body of physicians in Quebec.

TABLE 3: Where respondents felt that future midwives should work

Workplace	Lay midwives		Certified midwives		
	No.	%	No.	%	p
Pre- and postnatal care:					
• private office	26	96	34	79	0.038
• independent birthing centre	27	100	32	74	0.046
• hospital-based birthing centre	24	89	39	91	0.635
• hospital	16	59	24	56	0.747
• community health centre	25	93	39	91	0.755
• client home	26	96	33	77	0.024
Delivery:					
• client home	26	96	18	42	0.000
• independent birthing centre	27	100	27	63	0.002
• hospital-based birthing centre	24	89	41	95	0.299
• hospital	21	78	37	86	0.282

TABLE 4: Level of training that respondents felt future midwives should have

Level of training	Lay midwives		Certified midwives		
	No.	%	No.	%	p
Minimum midwifery training*:					
• practical experience through apprenticeship and passing a certification exam	6	22	0	0	
• college diploma in midwifery	1	4	3	7	
• bachelor's degree	16	56	34	79	0.011
• master's degree	3	11	6	14	
Prerequisite to that training:					
• nursing degree	0	0	12	28	0.001
• human relations training	11	41	19	44	0.752
Special training profiles:					
• certification exam for midwives with degree from outside Quebec	21	78	40	93	0.063
• brief training for nurses experienced in obstetrics	6	22	13	30	0.300

*Response choices are mutually exclusive

(Table 4). The majority agreed that a bachelor's degree was required, but the two groups disagreed on the subject of apprenticeship, which was supported by 22% of lay midwives, but not by certified midwives. Lay midwives rejected nursing as a prerequisite to midwifery training, while a small minority of certified midwives, most of whom are nurses, found that prerequisite adequate, as it corresponded to their profile of training. Compared to certified midwives, lay midwives appeared slightly less in favour of the proposed particular training profiles that would allow a person to practise as a midwife in the short term in Quebec.

Other Factors

It is not just the type of training received that determines the opinions of midwives, but a number of interrelated professional, social, political, and legal factors as well. For example, respondents who were certified midwives, members of the ASFQ and not in current practice in Quebec, were more in favour of the bachelor's level as a minimum training for future midwives. The respondents with these characteristics, as well as being nurses, having practised outside Quebec and having had training for two years or more, were favourable to a nursing prerequisite for midwifery training. Being in favour of home delivery was not only related to the fact of being lay midwives, but also being recently trained as midwives, currently practising in Quebec without having had experience outside Quebec, and being members of the AQSFP.

The study's results confirm certain findings of previous studies.[36] It showed that lay midwives have been trained more recently, and that they are practising as midwives today even if it must be outside a legal framework. Having practised in an unregulated environment, they have struggled to survive and be recognized by the healthcare system. Thus, it follows that they have a greater interest in the legalization of the profession in general.

The lay midwives in Quebec received support from women's groups (e.g. Naissance-Renaissance), who struggled for women to gain control over their bodies and challenged the established medical profession through the natural birth movement that emerged in the 1960s and 1970s.[37] The principal event that marked this movement was the regional conferences organized in 1981 by the *Association pour la Santé Publique du Québec (Quebec Public Health Association)*, with the theme, "Deliver or be delivered." These conferences brought together nearly 10 000 people. The main recommendations of these conferences were the creation of birthing centres and the legalization of the midwifery profession. Due to this support offered by the women's groups, the lay midwives tend to have a closer relationship with their clients and a more client-centred attitude, which is geared towards follow-up and deliveries at home or in the natural environment chosen by their clients.[38] Although some of them are nurses, they preferred that the future training of midwives not require prior training in nursing. As noted by other authors, this may be due to their belief that nursing training could make them lose their autonomy and their philosophy which is oriented towards normality.[39] According to this philosophy, pregnancy and birthing are physiological and natural events in a woman's life which should be respected by health professionals.

A majority of certified midwives are immigrants. Born outside Canada, they moved recently to this country after having completed their midwifery training, and sometimes practising their profession for a number of years in their country of origin. They have an earlier training than their counterpart lay midwives. This profile has had an impact on their current situation in Quebec: they have been distant from clients and full midwifery practice, and they do not seem to be as strong advocates of women's demands for humanized care as lay midwives have been. Moreover, as most of them are nurses, this may explain why they thought that future midwives should first be trained as nurses. In the meantime, they felt that a brief university training in midwifery would qualify nurses experienced in obstetrics to practise as midwives. Since many of them were born and were trained in midwifery outside Canada, they understandably favour having midwives with their background (certified midwives) be recognized as qualified to work in Quebec, on the successful completion of a certification examination.

The differences in the way midwives viewed and practised their profession led them to form two distinct associations. This, in turn, may have accentuated certain divergent points of view (e.g. training required to become midwife, the need for prior training in nursing, the permission of midwives trained outside Canada to practise in Quebec, and the interest in home delivery). However, members of these two associations agree on some key professional dimensions: almost all of them wish to maintain full control over their profession and be recognized as autonomous professionals who would be required to consult a physician only in case of problems.

The tensions that may exist between lay midwives and certified midwives in Quebec are rooted in different forms of prejudice. Lay midwives consider that the renaissance of their profession has been made possible by their militancy over the last two decades. They see immigrant, certified midwives as competitors who arrive the moment midwifery is legalized and then simply threaten to take their place and jobs because of their midwifery diploma. Furthermore, some lay midwives consider that these immigrant, certified midwives are unable to understand and respond to the needs of the women of Quebec because of their different culture; they may also see the approach of certified midwives as too medicalized, since they have received their training under physician supervision in hospital centres. From the certified midwives point of view, a lay midwife may not have a professional approach and may be dangerous to women and children because of some practices already rejected by the medical profession in general (e.g. utilization of herbs). For all these reasons, each group of midwives may consider that the other does not have the legitimacy to practise in Quebec. This situation has been exacerbated by the context of the experimentation of the profession that limited the number of positions available for the midwives who wish to practise in Quebec.

IMPLICATION OF THESE RESULTS: PRESENT AND FUTURE

This is the first study conducted in Quebec which surveyed the opinions of midwives about maternity care, on their role and preferred training and model of practice. This study pinpointed the areas of agreement and disagreement among midwives. Results from the present study, showing that Quebec midwives from different backgrounds share the same philosophy of care, are encouraging. Yet there are also real differences in points of view that should not be overlooked, regarding especially midwife training and home delivery. These issues could become crucial in the definition of the profession of midwife in Quebec.

Workplaces for Midwives: Home Delivery?

Currently in Quebec, in the context of Bill 4, 49 midwives from different backgrounds have been recognized as able to practise, but exclusively in the pilot projects which are established in birthing centres.

Home delivery is not part of the pilot projects. Nevertheless, some lay midwives, who did not pass the accrediting exams recommended by the admission committee, continue to assist home deliveries. Besides, the midwives who were recognized and able to practice in the pilot projects, suggested that the nonaccredited midwives who desire to join in their new corporation should be practising midwifery in Quebec. As the only legal midwifery practice yet in Quebec is taking place through the pilot projects, this suggestion means that the nonaccredited midwives seeking the eventual affiliation to the new corporation must practise 'illegally' at home.

This presents a difficult situation for the certified midwives who have not been accredited to participate in the experimentation of the profession. Because of the immigrant status of most of them, they are unwilling to work in an illegal context, even though they wish to practise one day in the different settings corresponding to women's choice, including client's home, for which their initial midwifery training had prepared them. These certified midwives came from countries where midwifery practice was legal. They were also members of associations affiliated to the International Confederation of Midwives which recognizes 'home' as a normal workplace of midwives. Explaining this contradiction led us to analyze this result in the context where it occurred. At the time this study was conducted, the debate surrounding home births was heated: physicians were against this workplace even if they were not against midwifery practice in Quebec itself. The law adopted in 1990 to experiment with midwifery practice prohibited home births during the experimental period. It was clear that, in such a context, professionals who were generally familiar and respectful of ethics and deontological codes of practice would follow the government recommendations.

Besides, the fact of being immigrants may have reinforced certified midwives' attitudes against illegal practices. In fact, after the disappearance of the profession of midwives in the first half of this century, the lay midwives who dared to practise their art did so despite the opposition of the medical profession. They were considered 'outlaws' practising illegal medicine in a semi-clandestine fashion. The certified midwives, newly arrived in Canada and not yet naturalized, were informed of the nonexistence of their profession in this country prior to their arrival and were thus forbidden to practise their profession. In these conditions, and having practised in the context of a code of ethics in their own country, immigrant, certified midwives preferred not to practise their profession, even if they were willing to do so as soon as they could be given the legal opportunity.

In order to be able to practise their profession in Quebec, certified midwives who do not participate in the pilot projects will either have to wait for the eventual legalization of the profession at the end of the pilot projects in 1998, or hope that the process undertaken by the Quebec College of Physicians, aimed at integrating midwives into hospital settings, will be successful. In fact, the Quebec College of Physicians,[40] which until recently opposed the introduction of midwifery in the province, declared in November 1995 that it will give midwives the opportunity to work in hospitals, granting them autonomy of practice and hospital admitting and discharge privileges. Certified midwives may accept the collaboration offered by the physicians because of the many advantages they can gain from this opportunity. The experience of the other Canadian provinces (British Columbia, Alberta, and Ontario) shows the advantages of the midwifery practice model developed in tertiary care centres.[41] Based on these experiences, the most important advantages for midwifery practice would be to give midwifery care more visibility within academic settings that have national influence, provide medical, nursing and postgraduate students with an opportunity to observe practising midwives, and enhance midwifery skills, as well as foster leadership, political awareness and research skills. Most of these advantages are needed by the re-emerging profession in Quebec.

Quebec has experienced midwifery practice in a hospital setting, in the Hudson Bay region's Puvirnituk birthing centre. This centre was founded in 1986 after consulting with the regional hospital, the Inuit community, the Native Women's Association, the Regional Health Board of Kativik, and the Community Health Department of Laval University Hospital. The objective was to allow Native and Inuit women to give birth safely, in their own community, assisted by competent women speaking their own language. This service may reduce and prevent the disruptive consequences of family separations previously caused by prenatal transfer of women to Moose Factory in Ontario or to Montreal.[42]

Thus far, the Puvirnituk birthing centre has been successful in meeting the needs of the population. Inuit women living in the region served by this birthing centre no longer have to leave their community to give birth to their children, except in the presence of risks or complications. The management of clinical activities in this birthing centre is usually handled by a certified midwife. The members of the team of midwives delivering health care to the women are generally members of the community itself. These midwives receive the training that corresponds to the needs of the women in their communities. They have been able to meet the needs of First Nations women better than any other professionals.

Since it had been favourably evaluated[43] prior to the implementation of the pilot projects under Bill 4, the Puvirnituk birthing centre is no longer considered an experimental project by its staff and the community, and is not subject to the same stringent evaluation as are the other seven pilot projects.

Midwife Training In Quebec

The results of our survey suggest that certified and lay midwives do not agree on all aspects of future training for midwives in Quebec. Their disagreement involves essentially the nursing prerequisite to midwifery training, and particularly, 'apprenticeship' as a model of training. It is clear that the first option is supported by nurse-midwives and the second by lay midwives.

In its review of midwifery training in Europe, Asia, and United States, the Quebec Taskforce on Midwifery[44] noted that England, Finland, Japan, Sweden, and the United States offer nurse-midwife curricula. The Taskforce also stated that the current trends are moving towards midwife training by direct entry, assuming that the curricula would take into consideration the necessity of initiating midwives in the 'nursing care' required for midwifery practice. Regarding the level of training, the same committee indicated that in the consulted countries, the training level is equivalent to a university degree in Quebec. In the province of Ontario, which is ahead of the other Canadian provinces in the implementation of midwifery, the attempt is being made to also train midwives under instructors in an apprenticeship-type model.

> It was agreed, however, that in order to practice autonomously with hospital admitting and discharge privileges in the Ontario health care environment, midwives would need a university degree. In addition, there was a desire to open research to midwives in a way that would not be possible without a university affiliation.[45]

This process is taking place even though the disadvantages may be overprofessionalization and an academically oriented midwife, rather than a 'hands-on' midwife who learns in an apprenticeship model, and values community practice.

Since the apprenticeship model constituted a source of disagreement between the two categories of midwives surveyed in Quebec in the 1991 study, it appears important to consider the Ontario experience. Reflecting on the future training of midwives in their province, some Ontario midwives consider the feasibility of apprenticeship as a model for training to be still uncertain: "How do we remain committed to keeping apprenticeship as the strong core of the relationship between midwives and student midwives?"[46] Quebec, and the other Canadian provinces as well, could learn from Ontario when planning the training of future midwives.

Furthermore, home delivery by midwives poses particular challenges for training. For example, it would take a lot of creativity to manage the program in such a way as to allow for the introduction of student midwives in settings where normal deliveries are assisted (e.g. home settings), and later to the hospital setting, where they can observe and look after complicated deliveries in collaboration with physicians. High-risk mothers would benefit from the midwives' care, along with the adequate care and information related to their specific situation. One of the major concerns of the registered midwife is to remain competent and confident attending births in all settings. There are some constraints in trying to combine the advantages of the apprenticeship and university models of training.

PERSPECTIVES

The implementation of a new profession is always a source of turmoil, and midwifery is no exception. The introduction of midwifery in Quebec has had its way paved by the government, through an experiment (pilot projects) which gives a context for the evaluation of the profession.

The aim of the experimentation has been to determine whether or not to authorize this practice, and should the occasion arise, to determine the professional organization and the mode of integration of midwives in the perinatal system. The evaluation compares midwives' services with the current medical services with reference to humanization and continuity of care, the utilization of obstetrical technologies, mother and child health and safety and costs. Bill 4 charges the Conseil d'évaluation des projets-pilotes (CEPP) to transmit its recommendations of the end of the experiment, to the Minister of Health and Social Services. The CEPP recruited a multi-university research team to conduct the evaluative research and provide it with the information needed for the formulation of its recommendations.[47]

Bill 4 came into force in September 1992 and will expire in September 1998. The report by the research team mandated by the CEPP to do the evaluation is due in the second half of 1997. Based on this report, the CEPP will have to fulfil its mission and make its recommendations to the minister by December 1997. These recommendations will most likely be crucial for the legalization and integration of the midwifery profession in Quebec. But this evaluation does not look at aspects of midwifery training in Quebec. Another study, financed by the Conseil Québécois de la Recherche Sociale, has taken an interest in this area. This research team, concerned with midwifery training in Quebec, seized the opportunity of the experiment in midwifery practice to identify the basics of a professional training program, adapted to Quebec's reality, that can be offered to future midwives. Given the complexity of the study, it adopted the design of a case study where each midwife represents a case. The midwives practising in the pilot projects have been invited to collaborate in this study. Those who agreed to participate are contributing to the development of the midwife profile needed in Quebec and the basic components of a corresponding training model. Based on their personal and professional characteristics, their perception of their training and practice prior to working in pilot projects, and their perception of the context in which the profession is developing in Quebec, the midwives, consulted at different stages of the realisation of the pilot project, contributed to defining models for the re-emerging profession and the training that would be appropriate in the future.

These two studies (evaluation of midwifery practice in pilot projects and study of midwifery training) will go beyond the 1991 survey, showing some disagreement among midwives, on professional issues, related to the workplace and the training of the future midwives. The studies may help find ways to overcome these differences.

CONCLUSION

In many countries, different types of midwives practise their art in their own way and more or less collaborate among themselves. This is particularly true in the United States where certified nurse-midwives and lay midwives have their own field of practice. The bringing together of these different types of midwives in countries where their practice is well established has been difficult, if not impossible.

In Canada, where the process of recognition of midwives is under way, it is possible to observe whether the creation of a 'single' profession is feasible. If midwifery in Canada were starting from scratch — i.e. by first developing a single training program and then granting the title of midwife only to the graduates of this program — things would be simple. However, between now and the time such training programs are standardized, many midwives with different backgrounds want to be recognized and work within the healthcare system. The position currently taken by Canadian healthcare authorities is to recognize the profession of midwife without distinction. The challenge for these midwives with different backgrounds is to develop a unified practice that transcends their differences.

The capacity of the different types of midwives to form a single profession can only be assessed in practice, after midwives have worked for a time together within the same legal framework. The experiment in midwifery practice through pilot projects that is under way in Quebec will provide a unique opportunity in Canada to document how midwives of different origins can succeed in taking up this challenge. Another way to bring midwives together is to involve them in the development and implementation of a training program that take into account the different points of view and benefit from the advantages of their different profiles.

We hope that this chapter has contributed in clarifying some aspects of the context surrounding the process of implementation of midwifery in Quebec.

ACKNOWLEDGEMENTS

A shorter version of this chapter was previously published: Hatem-Asmar, Marie, Régis Blais, Jean Lambert and Brigitte Maheux, "A Survey of Midwives in Quebec: What are Their Similarities and Differences?" *Birth,* vol. 23, no. 2 (1996): 94-100.

This study was supported by grants from the Social Sciences and Humanities Research Council of Canada and the National Health Research and Development Program (Health and Welfare Canada), a National Health Research Scholar Award to Dr. Régis Blais, and a doctoral scholarship to Dr. Marie Hatem-Asmar from the Fonds pour la Formation de Chercheurs et l'Aide à la Recherche. The authors are grateful to the midwives who generously contributed their time to the study.

ENDNOTES

1. Projet de loi 4, Province de Québec, *Loi sur la pratique des sages-femmes dans le cadre de projets-pilotes* (Québec: Gouvernement du Québec, 1990); Bill 56, Province of Ontario, *An Act Respecting the Regulation of The Profession of Midwifery* (Toronto: Government of Ontario, 1991); Bill 50, Province of Alberta, *Professional Statutes Amendment Act* (Edmonton: Government of Alberta, 1992).
2. WHO *Legislation Concerning Nursing/Midwifery Services and Education* (EURO reports and studies, 45), (Copenhagen: Regional office for Europe, World Health Organisation, 1981).
3. Maria De Lourdes Verderese, "La sage-femme," in *La Planification des Personnels de Santé: Principes Directeurs, Méthodes, Problèmes.* Thomas Hall and Alfonso Mejia, eds. (Genève: OMS, 1979).
4. Judith Rooks, "Nurse-Midwifery: The Window Is Wide Open," *American Journal of Nursing*, vol. 90, no. 20 (1990): 30-36; Rose Weitz and Deborah Sullivan, "Licensed Lay-Midwifery and the Medical Model of Childbirth," *Sociology of Health and Illness*, vol. 7, no. 1, (1985): 36-54.
5. Laura-Mae Baldwin, Heidi Hutchinson and Roger Rosenblatt, "Professional Relationship Between Midwives and Physicians: Collaboration or Conflict?" *American Journal of Public Health*, vol. 82, no. 2 (1992): 262-264. Apprenticeship is also discussed in several of the following articles.

6. Nancy Kreinburg and Maryellen McSweeney, "An Attitude Survey of Lay-Midwives and Nurse-Midwives," *Journal of Nurse-Midwifery*, vol. 26, no. 3 (1981): 43-50.
7. Rose Weitz and Deborah Sullivan, "Licensed Lay-Midwifery in Arizona," *Journal of Nurse-Midwifery*, vol. 29, no. 1 (1984): 21-28; J. Rooks, op. cit.; George Giacoia, "Lay-Midwives in Oklahoma," *Journal of Oklahoma State Medical Association*, vol. 84 (1991): 160-162.
8. R. Weitz and D. Sullivan, 1985, op. cit.
9. Carol Hurzeler, "Use of the Certified Nurse-Midwives in the Education of Lay-Midwives," *Journal of Nurse-Midwifery*, vol. 26, no. 3 (1981): 57-59.
10. Carol Sakala, "Content of Care by Independent Midwives: Assistance with Pain in Labor and Birth," *Social Science and Medicine*, vol. 26, no. 11 (1988): 1141-1158.
11. De Lourdes Verderese, op. cit.
12. Irene Butter and Bonnie Kay, "Self Certification in Lay-Midwives Organisations: A Vehicle for Professional Autonomy," *Social Science and Medicine*, vol. 30, no. 12 (1990): 1329-1339.
13. G. Giacoia, op. cit.; R. Weitz and D. Sullivan, 1984, op. cit.; Judith Flanagan, "Speaking Up and Talking Out: Barriers and Obstacles to Nurse-Midwifery Practice," *Journal of Nurse-Midwifery*, vol. 38, no. 4 (1993): 246-251.
14. J. Flanagan, op. cit.
15. G. Giacoia, op. cit.
16. Judith Rooks, "The Context of Nurse-Midwifery in the 1980s: Our Relationships with Medicine, Nursing, Lay-Midwives, Consumers and Health Care Economist," *Journal of Nurse-Midwifery*, vol. 28, no. 5 (1983): 3-8.
17. R. Weitz and D. Sullivan, 1985, op. cit. Melissa Avery, "Advanced Nurse-Midwifery Practice," *Journal of Nurse-Midwifery*, vol. 37, no. 2 (1992): 150-154.
18. Raymond DeVries, "Barrier to Nurse-Midwifery: Is the Enemy Us?" *Journal of Nurse-Midwifery*, vol. 31, no. 6 (1986): 277-278.
19. R. Weitz and D. Sullivan, 1984; 1985, op. cit.
20. Mary Bidgood-Wilson, "The Legislative Status of Nurse-Midwives: Trends and Future Implications," *Journal of Nurse-Midwifery*, vol. 37, no. 3 (1992): 159-160.
21. J. Rooks, 1990, op. cit.; R. Weitz and D. Sullivan, 1985, op. cit.; Laura Mae Baldwin et al, op. cit.
22. R. Weitz and D. Sullivan, 1984; 1985, op. cit.; L. Baldwin et al op. cit.; J. Flanagan, op. cit.
23. Comité de travail sur la pratique des sages-femmes au Québec, *La Périnatalité au Québec: La Pratique des Sages-Femmes* (Québec: Gouvernement du Québec, 1989).
24. J. Rooks, 1990, op. cit.
25. Judith Rooks, Norman Weatherby and Eunice Ernst, "The National Birth Centre Study, Part I — Methodology and Prenatal Care Referrals," *Journal of Nurse-Midwifery*, vol. 37, no. 4 (1992): 222-252; Part II — Intrapartum and Immediate Post-Partum and Neonatal Care," *Journal of Nurse-Midwifery*, vol. 37, no. 5 (1992): 301-330; Part III — Intrapartum and Immediate Post-Partum and Neonatal Complications and Transfers, Post Partum and Neonatal Care, Outcomes, and Client Satisfaction, *Journal of Nurse-Midwifery*, vol. 37, no. 6 (1992): 361-397.
26. N. Kreinberg and M. McSweeney, op. cit.
27. I. Butler and B. Kay, op. cit.; G. Giacoia, op. cit.

28. R. Weitz et al, op. cit.; J. Flanagan, op. cit.
29. J. Rooks, 1983, op. cit.; R. DeVries, op. cit.
30. Linda Baxter, "Cooperation or Competition: The Choice Is Ours," *Journal of Nurse-Midwifery*, vol. 26, no. 6 (1981): 1-2.
31. Shah, Mary Ann, "The Unification of Nurse-Midwives: A Time for Dialogue," *Journal of Nurse-Midwifery*, vol. 27, no. 5 (1982): 1-2.
32. Projet de loi 4, op. cit.
33. Régis Blais, Jean Lambert, Brigitte Maheux, Jacinthe Loiselle, Nathalie Gauthier and Alicia Framarin, "Controversies in Maternity Care: Where Do Physicians, Nurses and Midwives Stand?" *Birth*, vol. 21, no. 2 (1994): 63-70; "Midwifery Defined by Physicians, Nurses and Midwives: The Birth of a Consensus?" *Can Med Assoc. J.*, vol. 150, no. 5 (1994): 691-697.
34. When the survey was conducted, the pilot projects were not yet operating. Midwives who practised did so at home or as 'accompagnantes' for hospital births and without official recognition by the healthcare system.
35. These differences had already been noted in J. Rooks, 1990, op. cit.; I. Butler et al, op. cit.; G. Giacoia, op. cit.
36. N. Kreinberg and M. McSweeney, op. cit.; J. Flanagan, op. cit.
37. Sheila Harvey, Karyn Kaufman and Alison Rice, "Hospital-Based Midwifery Projects in Canada," in *Issues in Midwifery*. Tricia Murphy-Black, ed. (Edinburgh: Churchill Livingstone, 1995).
38. G. Giacoia, op. cit.; C. Sakala, op. cit.; J. Flanagan, op. cit.
39. R. Weitz and D. Sullivan, 1984; 1985, op. cit.
40. Glenn Wanamaker, "Que. Mds and Midwives Test the Water," *Family Practice*, no. 18 (1995): 6.
41. S. Harvey et al, op cit.
42. Comité de travail..., op. cit.
43. André Tourigny, Judy Ross and Pierre Joubert, *Évaluation des Soins et Services en Périnatalité dans la Région de la Baie d'Hudson: Volet Organisation* (Québec: Département de santé communautaire du Centre Hospitalier de l'Université Laval, 1991).
44. Comité de travail..., op. cit.
45. Holliday Tyson, Anne Nixon and Arlene Vandersloot, "The Re-Emergence and Professionalization of Midwifery in Ontario, Canada," in *Issues in Midwifery*, Tricia Murphy-Black, ed. (Edinburgh: Churchill Livingstone, 1995).
46. Ibid.
47. Régis Blais, Pierre Joubert, André-Pierre Contandripoulos, Maria DeKoninck, Andrée Demers, William Fraser, Michael Klein, Deena White, Marie Hatem-Asmar, Louise Bouchard, Claude Gagnon and Isabelle Krauss, "Évaluation des Projets-Pilotes de la Pratique des Sages-Femmes," Devis Présenté au CEPP de la Pratique des Sages-Femmes, Québec, 1993.

REFERENCES

Avery, Melissa. "Advanced Nurse-Midwifery Practice." *Journal of Nurse-Midwifery*, vol. 37, no. 2 (1992): 150-154.
Baldwin, Laura-Mae, Heidi Hutchinson and Roger Rosenblatt. "Professional Relationship Between Midwives and Physicians: Collaboration or Conflict?" *American Journal of Public Health*, vol. 82, no. 2 (1992): 262-264.
Baxter, Linda. "Cooperation or Competition: The Choice Is Ours." *Journal of Nurse-Midwifery*, vol. 26, no. 6 (1981): 1-2.

Bidgood-Wilson, Mary. "The Legislative Status of Nurse-Midwives: Trends and Future Implications." *Journal of Nurse-Midwifery,* vol. 37, no. 3 (1992): 159-160.

Bill 56. Province of Ontario. *An Act Respecting the Regulation of The Profession of Midwifery.* Toronto: Government of Ontario, 1991.

Bill 50. Province of Alberta. *Professional Statutes Amendment Act.* Edmonton: Government of Alberta, 1992.

Blais, Régis, Pierre Joubert, André-Pierre Contandripoulos, Maria DeKoninck, Andrée Demers, William Fraser, Michael Klein, Deena White, Marie Hatem-Asmar, Louise Bouchard, Claude Gagnon and Isabelle Krauss. "Évaluation des Projets-Pilotes de la Pratique des Sages-Femmes." Devis Présenté au CEPP de la Pratique des Sages-Femmes. Québec, 1993.

Blais, Régis, Jean Lambert, Brigitte Maheux, Jacinthe Loiselle, Nathalie Gauthier and Alicia Framarin. "Controversies in Maternity Care: Where Do Physicians, Nurses and Midwives Stand?" *Birth,* vol. 21, no. 2 (1994 a): 63-70.

-----. "Midwifery Defined by Physicians, Nurses and Midwives: The Birth of a Consensus?" *Can Med Assoc. J.* , vol. 150, no. 5 (1994 b): 691-697.

Butter, Irene, and Bonnie Kay. "Self Certification in Lay-Midwives Organisations: A Vehicle for Professional Autonomy." *Social Science and Medicine,* vol. 30, no. 12 (1990): 1329-1339.

Comité de travail sur la pratique des sages-femmes au Québec. *La Périnatalité au Québec: La Pratique des Sages-Femmes.* Québec: Gouvernement du Québec, 1989.

De Lourdes Verderese, Maria. "La sage-femme" in *La Planification des Personnels de Santé: Principes Directeurs, Méthodes, Problèmes.* Thomas Hall and Alfonso Mejia, eds. Genève: OMS, 1979.

DeVries, Raymond. "Barrier to Nurse-Midwifery: Is the Enemy Us?" *Journal of Nurse-Midwifery,* vol. 31, no. 6 (1986): 277-278.

Flanagan, Judith. "Speaking Up and Talking Out: Barriers and Obstacles to Nurse-Midwifery Practice." *Journal of Nurse-Midwifery,* vol. 38, no. 4 (1993): 246-251.

Giacoia, George. "Lay-Midwives in Oklahoma." *Journal of Oklahoma State Medical Association,* vol 84 (1991): 160-162.

Harvey, Sheila, Karyn Kaufman and Alison Rice. "Hospital-Based Midwifery Projects in Canada," in *Issues in Midwifery.* Tricia Murphy-Black, ed. Edinburgh: Churchill Livingstone, 1995.

Hurzeler, Carol. "Use of the Certified Nurse-Midwives in the Education of Lay-Midwives." *Journal of Nurse-Midwifery,* vol. 26, no. 3 (1981): 57-59.

Kreinberg, Nancy, and Maryellen McSweeney. "An Attitude Survey of Lay-Midwives and Nurse-Midwives." *Journal of Nurse-Midwifery,* vol. 26, no. 3 (1981): 43-50.

Projet de loi 4 Province de Québec. *Loi sur la pratique des sages-femmes dans le cadre de projets-pilotes.* Québec: Gouvernement du Québec, 1990.

Rooks, Judith. "The Context of Nurse-Midwifery in the 1980's: Our Relationships with Medicine, Nursing, Lay-Midwives, Consumers and Health Care Economist." *Journal of Nurse-Midwifery,* vol. 28, no. 5 (1983): 3-8.

-----. "Nurse-Midwifery: The Window Is Wide Open." *American Journal of Nursing.,* vol. 90, no. 20 (1990): 30-36.

Sakala, Carol. "Content of Care by Independent Midwives: Assistance with Pain in Labor and Birth." *Social Science and Medicine,* vol. 26, no. 11 (1988): 1141-1158.

Rooks, Judith, Norman Weatherby and Eunice Ernst. "The National Birth Centre Study, Part I — Methodology and Prenatal Care Referrals." *Journal of Nurse-Midwifery*, vol. 37, no. 4 (1992 a): 222-252.

------. "The National Birth Centre Study, Part II — Intrapartum and Immediate Post-Partum and Neonatal Care." *Journal of Nurse-Midwifery*, vol. 37, no. 5 (1992 b): 301-330.

------. The National Birth Centre Study, Part III — Intrapartum and Immediate Post-Partum and Neonatal Complications and Transfers, Postpartum and Neonatal Care, Outcomes, and Client Satisfaction. *Journal of Nurse-Midwifery*, vol. 37, no. 6 (1992 c): 361-397.

Shah, Mary Ann. "The Unification of Nurse-Midwives: A Time for Dialogue." *Journal of Nurse-Midwifery*, vol. 27, no. 5 (1982): 1-2.

Tourigny, André, Judy Ross and Pierre Joubert. *Évaluation des Soins et Services en Périnatalité dans la Région de la Baie d'Hudson: Volet Organisation.* Québec: Département de santé communautaire du Centre hospitalier de l'Université Laval, 1991.

Tyson, Holliday, Anne Nixon and Arlene Vandersloot. "The Re-Emergence and Professionalization of Midwifery in Ontario, Canada," in *Issues in Midwifery.* Tricia Murphy-Black, ed. Edinburgh: Churchill Livingstone, 1995.

Wanamaker, Glenn. Que. Mds and Midwives "Test the Water." *Family Practice*, no. 18 (1995): 6.

Walsh, Linda, and Ann Lynn Jaspan. "Licensed Lay-midwifery in Arizona." *Journal of Nurse-Midwifery*, vol. 29, no. 1 (1984): *21-28.*

Weitz, Rose, and Deborah Sullivan. "Licensed Lay-Midwifery in Arizona." *Journal of Nurse-Midwifery*, vol. 29, no. 1 (1984), Sullivan: 21-28.

-----. "Licensed Lay-Midwifery and the Medical Model of Childbirth." *Sociology of Health and Illness*, vol. 7, no. 1 (1985): 36-54.

WHO *Legislation Concerning Nursing/Midwifery Services and Education* (EURO reports and studies, 45), Regional office for Europe, World Health Organisation, Copenhagen, 1981.

Midwifery in Atlantic Canada

Charlene MacLellan

My philosophy about childbirth, which has matured with experience, is that birth should be shared with other women in order to give experience to women who don't have any, and secondly, to receive wisdom from women who have the experience.

— Suann Morrow

THE HISTORY

It is impossible to think of the tradition and history of midwifery, women who help women in birth, without considering the first people of Atlantic Canada, the Mi-kmaq. While there is little historical documentation by the Mi-kmaq of their childbirth practices, it is known that healers were principal members of the community. The men were responsible for the healing of the mind and spirit and the women focused on the body. The labouring woman was commonly helped by the medicine woman or man who prescribed remedies such as chewing on the root of the Trillium plant to initiate labour. Problems such as malposition of the fetus, haemorrhage, and difficult labours were dealt with by the women healers. The Mi-kmaq believed that expression of the pain of labour should be suppressed in hopes of imparting the mother's stoic courage to her offspring.[1]

The settlers of this region were mainly of British and French origin. Their ideas of birth were based on the European history of midwifery, again, women attending women. However, by the late 1800s, following the witch hunts of the 1500s and 1600s, most European countries regarded doctors as appropriate birth attendants. Many middle- to upper-class women may have been taught to prefer doctors. The reality of life in the new world was that few communities outside Halifax could rely on available physicians for obstetrical services. Community midwives were the primary attendants at births. The vast knowledge and wisdom of their tradition was passed from mothers to daughters.

At the turn of the century and through to the end of World War I, women still attended women in rural areas of the Maritimes. When doctors, who were primarily male, returned from the war, the practice of midwifery was no longer sanctioned through the medical profession. In addition, doctors began to organize and control medical services. However, in rural areas community midwives did continue to help other women living nearby, though these midwives were scarce. In larger towns and cities nurses began to attend births more regularly at home and in maternity homes. The Victorian Order of Nurses (VON) presided at many births in the Halifax region. Physicians viewed this as direct competition to their growing practice and worried that recognition of this work could spell the legitimation of midwifery.[2] The VON's duties in attending births were eventually phased out with pressure from well-organized medical societies.

In rural Nova Scotia, a few doctors continued to employ nurses and women of the community as labour sitters and physician assistants at births. These midwives were often educators to doctors in practice and brought their life-saving skills to countless generations of people. An example of this is evident in the story of Shirley Boates' birth.

Shirley is a grandmother now. She was born at home in 1924, in the small village of Bible Hill, Nova Scotia. Born a twin, her birth weight was 1 1/2 pounds; her twin brother weighed 5 1/2 pounds. The birth was attended by a nurse and a doctor. Because of the demands of his medical practice, the doctor returned to his office after the birth. In the days that followed, Shirley's mother was attended by the midwife whose time-honoured skills and unwavering presence marked the survival of the small baby. Shirley's mother was instructed to bundle her baby in cotton at all times and keep her warm by placing her in a box on the door of the woodstove. At night the tiny baby was to sleep, bundled, on her mother's chest.

By the 1940s, the majority of births in Prince Edward Island, New Brunswick, and Nova Scotia were taking place in hospitals attended by doctors. The threads of midwifery survived in poor urban populations and rural areas of the Maritimes until the arrival of universal health care in the late 1950s. The funding of healthcare services made the difference for poor women who could now afford a hospital birth attended by doctors. Newfoundland and Labrador, however, continued to employ nurse-midwives in cottage hospitals and in regional centres. This was mainly due to the unavailability of physicians in remote areas and the birth culture of arriving immigrants from Britain who were accustomed to hospital-based midwifery.[3] This practice of nurse-midwifery is still present today in Newfoundland and Labrador.

THE RENAISSANCE

The renaissance of midwifery which placed birth back into the hands of women helping women, took place in the 1970s. The resurgence was partly due to the feminist movement and the desire of a rising number of people to take charge of their own health. Women wanted to simplify and de-pathologize the birth process and return to midwifery and home birth.

Due to the unavailability of a practising midwife, women searched out a like-minded healthcare professional and found response in Dr. Winston Makhan. Winston, a physician trained at the Dalhousie Medical School, had moved to the rural Pictou area in 1974. Winston was born at home in his country of origin, Trinidad, as were eight of his siblings. Winston's childhood memories of home births were those of mother and baby always kept together, a happy event shared by the family. Recently I asked Winston how he got started attending home births. Winston remembers: "When back-to-the-landers in the Pictou area wanting to take active roles in their births and resisting the institutionalized medical model of birth, asked me for assistance, I sympathized strongly. For me, the wishes of these people struck a personal chord, an echo of my boyhood." Winston thus became the first physician to regularly attend numbers of home births in Nova Scotia. After several years of attending births on his own, Winston was joined by Joan Richards, a nurse formerly from the New England states, then living in the Pictou area. Joan began to receive requests from women further out of the local area. She travelled alone to a small number of births in the Annapolis Valley of Nova Scotia. By 1980 Joan had moved back to the United States and Winston continued to attend women with a second assistant, Holly Irons.

In the 70s there were also isolated incidents of home births in the urban centres of Halifax and Moncton. These births were attended by foreign-trained nurse-midwives. Fearing the loss of their jobs and scorn from their peers, these midwives who were employed at local hospitals as nurses, kept their attendance at home births secretive.

In Prince Edward Island two lay midwives practised throughout the 1980s. They taught prenatal education, assisted women at home births and accompanied women to hospital where they acted as labour coaches. The midwives eventually ceased their home practice due to declining requests for their services and subsequently were unable to keep up their skills.

In 1980, I completed a midwifery-designed post graduate nursing course, moved to Nova Scotia, and attended my first home birth. To my knowledge, I was the only independent midwife practising in the province, and possibly the Maritimes.

MY STORY

I was born in Prince Edward Island, the fourth in a family of eight children. My ancestors were of Scottish and Irish origin, having settled in Prince Edward Island three generations ago. One of the many gifts passed on to me from my mother, a school teacher, was a keenness to discover knowledge. My father, while keeping a daytime job as a carpenter, was also an entrepreneur. They maintained strong family ties and worked very hard, at home and in the community. I now see the value of these influences.

As a girl of eight or nine years of age, I remember sitting around the kitchen table with four of my brothers doing our school 'lessons.' My mother presided at these weeknight sessions a short distance away in her rocking chair, knitting. Often she would take pleasure in quoting from memory a favourite poem or line from the great poets Longfellow, Shakespeare or Yeats.

When I was 17, I finished high school and entered nurses training at the Halifax Infirmary. As a student on a busy labour and delivery ward, I was to sit with a labouring woman timing her contractions. If she delivered while I was still on shift, then I was allowed to observe the delivery. The first birth I watched was in a small delivery room, with everyone scrubbed and gowned in hospital greens. The birthing woman, draped in layers of sterile cloths and legs up in stirrups, was attended by a doctor, medical student, and a nurse. I stood, observing, along with eight other medical and nursing students at one end of the room, away from the 'sterile field.' The attention of everyone in the room was focused on her perineum and the emerging baby and although the woman cried out, no one paid much attention. That night, I walked back to my student nurses' residence in awe of the woman's enormous efforts in birth and shaken by the fact that she was in pain and alone.

It was seven years later that I was to experience another birth. My travels in nursing took me to Inuvik in the Canadian Arctic where I was employed by the Medical Services Branch of Health Canada at the Inuvik General Hospital. This small hospital served the entire Western Arctic, a circled area of 600 miles in radius. As nurses in a remote region, we worked in a variety of situations, although the majority of my work was on a ward where surgery and maternal/newborn care were housed. Doctors were available on call for births.

During my early days in Inuvik I was very 'green' in my knowledge about birthing women. Native and Inuit women, most of them being multiparous women, often walked the hospital halls in labour. I didn't know that when a woman walked, changing her stoic facial expression from a concentrated look to a deep, furrowed brow, then she was about to push her baby out. Sometimes it was too late for a doctor to arrive and I, with great anxiety, would 'catch' the baby. Shortly after one of these first experiences, I had the fortune to receive first hand instruction from Chipo, a native of Rhodesia and British-trained midwife. I watched as she managed the delivery of a baby that was coming fast. The woman stayed on her labouring bed and a small packet of birth instruments was unwrapped at her feet. With calm and gentle assurance from Chipo the woman eased her baby out without sterile drapes, without bright lights, and, most significantly, without an episiotomy. I immediately knew that I wanted to learn more. I ordered textbooks and searched for routes to midwifery training. The following autumn I left the Arctic to attend the

Advanced Practical Obstetrics (APO) Program at the University of Alberta, in Edmonton, Alberta.

The APO Program was a postgraduate course designed for nurses working in isolated areas of the Canadian North. We were taught both by midwives and by doctors who had themselves worked with midwives in other countries. An integral part of the program included managing the complete care of a woman once admitted to hospital, including the labour, delivery and postpartum; to this end, students were sent to various hospitals across Alberta. While at the University of Alberta, I met Sandy Pullin, my classmate, who at the time practised midwifery and attended home births in the Edmonton area. Sandy became a valuable resource to me and was the midwife for my second child, born at my home in Kingsport, Nova Scotia. In the spring of 1980, I completed my studies in Edmonton and, wanting to live closer to my parents, moved to the Annapolis Valley of Nova Scotia. It was here that my practice as an independent midwife began.

The first birth I attended was the birth of Levon; he will soon be 17 years old. Through mutual friends, Levon's mother had heard about me and my training as a midwife. She had given birth to her first child at home with midwives in British Columbia. She planned to stay at home with this baby, her second, and asked me to assist her. After meeting with her, I sensed that she would stay at home regardless of whether I attended her or not. I felt that with my training and skills, I could help her. After this birth, word spread that there was a midwife in the area and I was asked to attend more and more births. From the beginning days of my practice and through some eight years, I had the good fortune to have Linda Wheeldon as an assistant midwife. Linda, a mother of four children, had a strong intuitive sense and a tender, caring way with people — precious gifts in those days of early practice. Laws surrounding midwifery were nonexistent at the time and therefore midwifery was in a state of legal limbo; it was neither legal nor illegal. We worked with some degree of secrecy: there was always a threat of being found out and charged with practising medicine without a license by a disgruntled doctor. I also worked as a nurse at the time and I knew my colleagues and the nursing profession would not support my involvement in midwifery. Our clients thus came to us through word of mouth. The Annapolis Valley area, where we lived, contained a good-sized counter culture population whose values of birth as a natural process aligned closely with midwifery practice.

Linda and I continued to provide comprehensive prenatal, intrapartum, and postpartum care. In the beginning, we charged nothing for our services. After two years of practice and many dollars spent on travel, childcare, supplies, and phone bills, we set a fee at $200 plus expenses. In those early years, without a senior midwife in the area, I consulted with Sandy Pullin in Edmonton. As well, Winston Makhan was always on call for questions, advice, and kind words of encouragement.

In January of 1983, Linda and I assisted in a birth with another midwife who had just moved to the Halifax area. The baby required resuscitation by us at birth and was transferred to a hospital where she died six months later. Following the birth, all three of us were charged with criminal negligence causing bodily harm, a charge which was later changed to criminal negligence causing death. The charges were instigated by a doctor who worked at the hospital where the baby was taken for medical assistance. We felt devastated for the baby and her family and fearful of what was to come for us and our families. We were requested by our lawyers not to have any contact with the baby's parents. This sudden break in our relationship with the family was very difficult for us. Through a third person, the mother sent a request asking me to meet with her privately. I met her in a small cafe in Halifax. She too, had been told not to have any contact with her midwives. Feeling the bitter effects of the imposed separation and relief of seeing each other again, we cried and hugged each other. This meeting was a significant point of healing for me. Throughout the complex emotional period brought about by the court proceedings, I knew that I had found a place of peace with her.

The case lasted nine months. It went as far as a preliminary hearing and resulted in a decision by the presiding judge that there was not enough evidence to proceed to a trial. Throughout the court proceedings, midwifery supporters in Nova Scotia came forward in large numbers. Hundreds of letters from all over Canada and the U.S.A. offered words of encouragement and monetary contributions. Midwifery support groups were formed in Halifax and the Annapolis Valley. Public events were organized to raise funds for our legal fees. Our legal fund received an anonymous donation of $2500. In all, the legal fees totalled $14,000 — all of it raised by supporters. Today, many of my friends look back to this era as a time that strengthened and built this community.

The media covered the case completely, but not always accurately. The media experience was two-sided. It seemed that the press was using us to make their stories and yet, in the long run, it was their coverage that helped people across the country follow the case and subsequently align themselves with the cause. There was also some sympathy from the press. I remember a woman photographer snapping pictures of Linda and I walking to the court-room with our lawyer and saying, "God bless you midwives." Radio talk shows featured issues surrounding midwifery and home birth. Suddenly everyone was openly discussing their opinions about midwifery in Nova Scotia.

In the spring of 1984, at the end of frantic fundraising activities and with the legal battle behind us, a meeting was called inviting all the midwifery supporters. The meeting, held in Halifax, was organized by Jan Catano of the Women's Health Education Network. The purpose of the meeting was to organize all the midwifery supporters under a single group. The new group,

The Midwifery Coalition of Nova Scotia (MCNS), is still a vital and strong consumer voice for midwifery in this province.

At the same time Linda and I made ties across Canada with midwives and consumer supporters after attending the Creating Unity Conference in Toronto in 1984. We attended the first meeting of the Midwives Association of Canada, now the Canadian Confederation of Midwives/Confederation Canadienne des Sages Femmes (CCM/CCSF). We returned feeling revitalized to continue our midwifery work. The relationships we made at the Toronto conference were important as we worked in isolation — the only midwives practising in Nova Scotia and, most likely, in the Maritimes.

Sometimes I received requests for midwifery services from women in New Brunswick, Prince Edward Island, and Cape Breton. I assisted these women when I was able to go, that is, when I did not have any clients in my area expected to give birth around the same time. Because of the distance, usually six to eight hours of driving to some places, I would stay with the family for several days. Normally I would arrive in the week preceding the expected due date and leave about three days after the birth or when it was clear that the mother and baby were stabilized. Follow-up care would be continued by regular phone calls, the family physician, and when available, a Public Health nurse. Although these long-distance births were a worry to me because I was not able to provide continuous care, the women I attended, living in rural areas and faced with the local hospital fare of shaves, enemas, episiotomies, continuous fetal monitoring, and mother and baby separation, were extremely grateful.

By 1988, Linda had decided to leave midwifery. I continued to practise alone for a time and took breaks from the work to have children myself. Louise McDonald, a previous childbirth educator living in the area, obtained apprenticeship midwifery training in Ontario and Alberta and returned to practise in Nova Scotia. Political work with the consumer group, the MCNS, was ongoing and national ties through the CCM/CCSF were strengthened. Due to the need for an official group representing practising midwives (now there were two practices!), the Association of Nova Scotia Midwives (ANSM) was formed. Standards of practice, protocols, a code of ethics, and membership requirements for midwives were established over the years.

Throughout the 1980s, as hospital births became an increasingly medical event surrounded by the latest technical advancements, more and more women rejected this interventionist approach to care during childbirth and formally expressed their discontent. This was exemplified in the activities surrounding the formation of the Committee of Inquiry into Caesarean Section Rates in Nova Scotia. The impetus for this committee, appointed by the Department of Health, began with complaints registered with the Nova Scotia Advisory Council on The Status of Women. These complaints were received from women in the Yarmouth area who were experiencing Caesarean Section rates at their local hospital of 28 to 30%. Upon investigation, two other areas of the province had similarly high section rates. The Status of Women brought this to the attention of the Minister of Health and hence the Committee of Inquiry was established. In July of 1990, the Report of the Committee of Inquiry into Caesarean Section Rates in Nova Scotia was released publicly. The Report stated: "A nurturing, supportive, less interventionist expert in the process of normal pregnancy and delivery, the midwife concept appears to embody all that is considered lacking in the present day system."[4] The MCNS and the ANSM seized this acknowledgement of midwifery and began actively lobbying for midwifery legislation in this province. The midwifery movement in Nova Scotia was fuelled by political advancements elsewhere in Canada. The implementation process for a midwifery program had commenced in Ontario and a five-year midwifery pilot project had been approved by Quebec's Minister of Health and Social Services. Core members within the MCNS and the ANSM were few but committed to their work. The MCNS printed a newsletter communicating midwifery news and circulated it four times a year to its 300-strong member/contact list. Annual conferences highlighting midwifery and birth were held in Halifax. Guest speakers included Ina May Gaskin and Valerie El Halta who were internationally known midwives. Political parties were lobbied and meetings organized with the Minister of Health. Radio talk shows and breakfast TV programs centred on midwifery and included a midwife and a consumer of midwifery care in their discussions. By the early 1990s the tasks of the midwifery community had rallied an increasing number of supporters.

Throughout the years of growing midwifery support, the Medical Society of Nova Scotia, the official licensing and governing body for physicians in the province, continued with attempts to strengthen their monopoly on birth. In November of 1986, the Medical Society released a "Policy Summary on Homebirth." The policy strongly supported the principle that all births occur in the hospital setting. The policy stated that the hospital setting should include:

> a pleasant home-like environment for the expectant mother. Hospital policies must be altered to reflect the concept of family-centered maternity care so that in all hospitals in N.S., companions of the mother's choice may be present with her during labour and delivery.[5]

Following this statement, peer pressure towards doctors attending home births escalated. As a doctor, Winston Makhan recalls feeling "like being out on a branch, alone, in the wind." Local physicians who sympathized with, and supported Winston were intimidated by obstetricians in the area. To this day, most doctors in Nova Scotia refuse to provide prenatal care or backup in case of hospital transfer for mothers planning home births with midwives.

Another incident of appropriating birth and placing it within the domain of doctors occurred in December of 1995 when the Medical Society of Nova Scotia attempted to change the *Medical Act*. Until this time, the *Act* had included birth in the practice of obstetrics. Changes to that section of the *Act* as proposed by the Medical Society were stated as:

> The practice of medicine includes but is not restricted to: offering or undertaking to prevent or to diagnose, correct, or treat in any means, methods, devices, or instrumentalities any disease, illness, pain, wound, fracture, infirmity, defect, or abnormal physical or mental condition of any person, including the management of pregnancy and parturition.[6]

By the time news of the proposed changes reached the ANSM and the MCNS, the *Act* was about to have it's third and final reading before it was passed. Members of the ANSM and the MCNS met with the Law Amendments Committee, a government-based committee which is a vehicle for public comment regarding proposed changes to legislation. Midwifery supporters requested that the management of pregnancy and parturition, which we considered a normal state, not be included in the practice of medicine, and secondly, that the profession of midwifery be regulated under a separate health services and disciplines act. A victory for the midwifery movement followed when the Law Amendments Committee deleted the Medical Society's phrasing.

Meanwhile the Association of Nova Scotia Midwives were in the throes of planning a large meeting of Canadian midwives in Halifax. In April of 1996 the ANSM hosted the Annual General Meeting of the Canadian Confederation of Midwives/Confederation Canadienne des Sages Femmes. The political effects surrounding this event were pivotal in the lobbying focus towards midwifery regulation. Planning well in advance of the forthcoming national assembly of midwives, the ANSM and the Midwifery Coalition arranged meetings with the Minister of Health, asking him to create a working group on the implementation of midwifery. "What better time to announce such a working group than in April when the Canadian midwives are gathered in Halifax?" we petitioned. The Minister promised a working group. The day before the CCM/CCSF meeting, Mr. Stewart, the Minister of Health, announced that the Department of Health had commissioned the Reproductive Care Program (RCP) of Nova Scotia to look into the issues surrounding midwifery, including it's potential need, scope of practice, education and remuneration. The RCP is described as a multi-disciplinary group of professionals including representatives from the Medical Society of Nova Scotia, Dalhousie University, the Registered Nurses Association of Nova Scotia and hospital staff.

The ANSM and the Midwifery Coalition publicly expressed immediate disappointment with this decision to involve the RCP. We questioned the

RCP's ability to provide an impartial view respecting midwifery. The newly formed committee, The Midwifery Review Group, consisted of five doctors and nurses of the RCP, a Department of Health Representative, a project assistant, one member of the Association of Nova Scotia Midwives, and one member of the Midwifery Coalition of Nova Scotia. Throughout the year, public opinion was solicited through voice mail, written submissions and focus groups held in a number of communities across the province. The process of the Midwifery Review Group, however, was again very disappointing for the midwifery community. The representing consumer and midwife were relieved of their involvement before the third and final draft of the Group's report was written.

Three months later, on September 16, 1997, the report entitled "The Potential for Midwifery in Nova Scotia" was publicly released. The main recommendations of the report state that midwifery should be implemented as a regulated healthcare profession separate from medicine and nursing. It advises the establishment of a working group coordinating the implementation and integration of regulated midwifery in Nova Scotia. Future action upon these recommendations and the timetable for achieving legislation hinges on public demand, the medical profession's agenda, political will and financial restraints.

THE FUTURE

Earlier in this chapter I told the story of Shirley Boates. Suann is Shirley's daughter. I attended the births of three of Suann's children at home, including the birth of her daughter, Hannah Morrow, now five years old. What will the future hold for midwifery and how it will be for little Hannah if she has children? The regulation of midwifery is inevitable. The losses and gains for women need to be scrutinized.

Perhaps the most beneficial effect of regulation will be that more women will receive midwifery care. The foundations of midwifery care embody woman-centered care, choice of birthplace and continuity of care. These key concepts will provide increased satisfaction with the birth experience for women and their families. Highly personalized care lends more parental attachment to the birth process and strengthens the family unit. Some midwives believe that family support is a key ingredient toward excellent birth outcomes.

Funded midwifery opens care to all classes of people. Currently in Nova Scotia, clients must pay the fees for a midwife, thereby rendering the service unattainable for women likely to benefit most — poor women and teens. With funded midwifery, childbirth will take on a new social concept as unnecessary medicalized routines are avoided. Women will return to the idea that birth can be an empowering event in their lives. Child health will improve as babies are born into a gentle environment and nourished with supported breastfeeding. A healthcare system for birthing that is based on midwifery will be less expensive than the status quo once the initial provisions for midwifery training sites are recovered.

With regulation, however, comes concessions. Midwives, consumers and babies will clearly be affected by legislation. Concessions will mostly be made by clients of 'free midwifery' before regulation. Women may have fewer choices around birthing because of the regulating laws; home birth, for example, is threatened, at least in the preliminary stages of regulated midwifery practice, until backup systems are in place. The possibility of less appointment time and less personalized care exists as midwives are placed in high demand and practice loads increase. Potential clients may experience disappointment when accessing a midwife only to find the midwife completely booked and unable to take on new clients.

Certainly the midwife will gain more independence with the ability to order tests and prescribe medications. The midwife's services will be complete in its delivery to clients. Midwives will acquire more skills as competent caregivers with the expansion of duties provided for under a midwifery act. The midwifery profession as a whole will reach greater public profile with more acceptance from health professionals and the general public. The number of practising midwives will increase. In Nova Scotia, midwives will have more centralized work regions. At the moment, three practising midwives in Nova Scotia cover all the Atlantic provinces. Training sites will be available for those seeking to become a midwife. Educational faculties will provide more opportunities for continuing education of midwives. Midwives will be paid for their work. To charge appropriately for the many hours involved in caring for a woman at the present time would make the price of midwifery services too high for most. Midwives have worked too many years without full compensation. The practice of a midwife will include more support staff. A secretary will be available for office duties and midwifery students will assist the midwife.

Again, there will be downfalls to legislated practice for midwives. The initial costs for licensing will need to be paid. Thus far, these costs have come from the midwife's pocket. In Alberta, each midwife candidate paid $2750 to complete the first stage, a comprehensive assessment process. One midwife told me that it will cost her about $10,000 to do what she has already been doing for the last fifteen years.

As midwifery services become a standard care, midwives may be overworked initially with an increased number of clients combined with various committee obligations. As well, the restrictions on practice will affect midwives who previously practised in a free environment.

Midwives at work will be watched with a critical eye by other health professionals initially. There will be increased pressure on the midwife to always do the right thing. At the same time, more high-risk clients will access midwives, creating more stress for the midwife. The midwife's personal life will be affected with increased work stress. She will need to balance all of these factors as she continues her professional work.

Midwifery legislation is something I have strived for over many years despite some personal reservations. Women have the right to midwifery care. In my heart I keep coming back to the fact that more women and babies will receive better care with midwives. That thought keeps me on track with the sometimes discouraging political work. At the same time, I want to protect midwifery from domination by government and the medical community. I have a role in deciding the fate of midwifery for midwives and for birthing families. I respect and honour this role. I trust that those who have guided me thus far will remain my truth.

ENDNOTES

1. Margot Jean Ferguson-Parker. "Feminism and Midwifery," (Master's thesis, Acadia University, 1990).
2. Ibid.
3. Ibid.
4. "Report of the Committee of Inquiry into Cesarean Section Rates in Nova Scotia," (Department of Health, Halifax, Nova Scotia, July 1990).
5. Medical Society of Nova Scotia, "Policy Summary on Homebirth." (November 1986), 1.
6. Bill 59, Section 2 (WIII) *The Medical Act of Nova Scotia* (December 1995).

REFERENCES

Department of Health, Halifax, Nova Scotia. "Report of the Committee of Inquiry into Cesarean Section Rates in Nova Scotia." July 1990.
The Medical Act of Nova Scotia. December 1995.
Ferguson-Parker, Margot Jean. "Feminism and Midwifery." Master's thesis, Acadia University, 1990.
Medical Society of Nova Scotia. "Policy Summary on Homebirth." November 1986.

Community Birthing Project:
Northwest Territories

Maureen Morewood-Northrop

PREAMBLE

In this paper I examine factors and forces in the establishment of a pilot community birthing project at the central Arctic community of Rankin Inlet, in the Northwest Territories. Until the 1950s, birthing was in the hands of Aboriginal women, but the high mortality rates prompted the federal government to intervene in the delivery of northern health services. As a result, birth was redefined from a community event to a medical problem, requiring the intervention of nonaboriginal medical workers. Initially, women birthed in Nursing Stations in their home communities; however by the 1970s, many women were being transferred to southern hospitals. This had a dramatic impact on the isolated communities, leading to social, economic and political problems both for the family members left behind and the pressure on local political leaders. Aboriginal women and their communities were particularly concerned about the potential loss of Aboriginal status to children who were not born in their home community in the Northwest Territories; they were also concerned about the loss of Aboriginal traditional midwifery knowledge. The community birthing project was established in this context. The goals of the project are many: to improve maternal and perinatal outcomes, to reduce the economic and social costs of transferring women out of the community, to revitalize Aboriginal traditional midwifery knowledge and more generally, to empower the community by giving it control over birthing. The following description of this project points to the need for community-controlled birthing practices which reflect and empower indigenous culture.

INTRODUCTION

Childbirth, in the scattered isolated areas of the Northwest Territories (NWT), has undergone a dramatic change in the past forty years. In the years prior to the 1950s, it was seen as a natural and normal event for the nomadic and family Aboriginal group. Health care for the Northwest Territories population was provided from within this group or from the missionaries, RCMP or

Hudson Bay personnel. Aboriginal traditional lay midwives were women with varying areas of expertise. No one midwife had all the prenatal and delivery experience. One woman would spend time with the prenatal mother talking about the nutritional foods to eat, and how to exercise and prepare for a healthy pregnancy. Another woman may do the delivery, assisted by her sister, friend or the husband. The postnatal care to the mother and baby was provided by another woman who would visit frequently in the tent or home. Local herbs and berries were used to ease discomfort, arrest bleeding and encourage the stimulation of breast milk.

Depending where the nomadic group or community would be, the women always gave birth in their own home. If the husband was out hunting or trapping, other families in the group or community would care for any children in need of attention or care. If an infant or mother died during childbirth, although the people mourned the loss, it was accepted as a part of life. Today, childbirth has become a medical event, away from the home community and removed from the everyday life of families; it is treated as potentially abnormal, until proven otherwise.

This change, initiated by government and medical personnel, has been brought about in the hope, that with increasing medical care of the reproductive process, improvements in maternal and infant mortality and morbidity rates will occur. The changes are also meant to reflect the goal of rendering healthcare services available to all, as well as providing women with access to well-equipped medical facilities and physicians.

As the Northwest Territories population is widely dispersed across many hundreds of square miles, it is not possible to have a hospital based in each isolated community. Therefore, rather than taking the health facility to the pregnant woman, the woman is taken out of her home community to a hospital. This can occur anywhere from two to four weeks prior to the expected date of delivery. It is important for this discussion, to be aware of the scattered remoteness of the majority of the NWT's communities.

BACKGROUND

The Northwest Territories includes an enormous geographic area of 1.3 million square miles: one-third the total area of Canada. It stretches across almost the entire width of the country, yet the population is just 60,000 distributed amongst 68 communities. Interestingly, 63 of the communities are home to fewer than 1,500 people. Forty-four of these communities are completely isolated, and community health programs and emergency and treatment services are delivered from local community health centres (formerly known as nursing stations). These are staffed by primary healthcare nurses recruited from the southern provinces. The six larger and urban communities have hospitals of various sizes, depending on the population served. The remaining communities, with populations under 100, receive emergency services from an individual from the community who has some basic first aid training.

Transportation is limited, but has improved dramatically over the past twenty years. The majority of travel between communities is by aeroplane, which is expensive, and regularity varies from one community to another. Other modes of transport include snowmobiles, all-terrain vehicles and boats. Dog teams used to be a regular mode of travel, but these have been replaced by the faster, but not quite so reliable, snow machine.

In 1954, the Federal Government of Canada, undertook the responsibility for the provision of health care to Aboriginal and nonaboriginal residents of the Northwest Territories. This new area of responsibility introduced the building of nursing stations staffed by southern Canada and overseas nurses (usually with midwifery training) into the isolated scattered communities. This initiated the introduction of Western medicine.

In the 1960s, the very high infant mortality rate was seen to accompany the marginal economic conditions of the Aboriginal people. This was redefined as a medical problem, and the solution at that time was to provide nonaboriginal medical workers to perform the childbirth activities. Low-risk births took place in the community nursing station with nonaboriginal nurse-midwives, with some assistance from an Aboriginal lay midwife. Women who were seen to have a moderate to high-risk pregnancy, were flown to the nearest hospital facility. It was felt a 'medicated' delivery by physicians may reduce the complications to the mother and newborn infant. An example of a risk pregnancy was seen to be previous complicated deliveries, i.e. forceps delivery, Caesarian section, haemorrhage, or retained placenta. Twin and breech pregnancies were also seen as a risk for the mother and infant.

Dr. Otto Schaefer (one of the first doctors in the Northwest Territories), was not initially convinced of the need for more hospital deliveries, as the Aboriginal lay midwives seemed to handle deliveries just as well as the 'trained nurses.' There were very limited efforts in the 60s and 70s to evaluate mortality and morbidity rates, prior to the introduction of an evacuation policy for pregnant women, since it was believed that any move in the direction of medicalized birth would be a move towards better health. The move towards referral for *all* prenatal women therefore, was not based on an evaluation of mortality data, but on a belief in the superior safety of hospital births. So, gradually, in most areas, all prenatal women were electively evacuated to a hospital setting for delivery of their infants. In some regions of the Territories, this also meant an 'out of territory' birth. A factor which may have enhanced this process was a substantial lack of Canadian nurse-midwives to work in the isolated nursing stations. Up until the mid-70s the majority of northern nurses were recruited from Britain, and were registered nurses with midwifery qualifications. As the immigration laws tightened it was soon no longer easy to recruit overseas midwives into Canada. Another factor was the shortage of Canadian nurses willing to work in the remote northern communities. As a British trained nurse and midwife, I have worked in northern Canada for 17 years. My experiences range from that of a community health nurse in a remote community, a nursing officer overseeing Health Units in a specific region, to a nursing consultant at the ministry level of the government of the NWT's Department of Health. During this time, I have had the opportunity to practice and consult on all aspects of childbirth, both with professionals and community members. I have seen discussions on community-based birthing take a complete 'U- turn.' Government policy used to dictate mothers transfer out of the community, away from the practice of lay and nurse-midwives performing the deliveries, to medicalized birthing in a hospital setting by physicians. This was followed by the reintroduction of community birthing with nurse midwives delivering the infants and an attempt to reorient to traditional midwifery practices. However, this has been for low-risk pregnant women only, thus a 'U-turn' and not a complete circle, to a past when all women were delivered in their home communities by traditional lay midwives. My early years working alongside Aboriginal lay midwives was a wonderful experience, as they supported my professional role with their traditional ways and beliefs.

CURRENT PRACTICE

In some parts of Inuit society today, childbirth is seen as a medical event and each pregnant woman is encouraged to attend a prenatal clinic at the newly named local community health centre. These centres are normally staffed by registered nurses who are recruited from the southern provinces of Canada. The majority of the nurses who work in the isolated communities have little obstetrical training and even fewer have midwifery training. Legislation has restricted the practice of midwifery in most provinces. This has led to a situation where mothers are no longer delivered in their home community, and the natural reproductive process they have known has become medicalized. Childbirth itself is seen as a medical process outside the realm of 'normal family life.'

The current practice is one where the pregnant mother is assessed and followed throughout the pregnancy by the community health nurse and visiting community physician. Prenatal teaching is done either through group sessions, or on an individual basis by the community health nurse. A local, Aboriginal person, called a Community Health Representative (CHR), with some training in health promotion and health educational activities, will assist in this teaching. An example would be teaching nutrition and exercise, promoting a healthy pregnancy to produce a healthy infant. Local foods would be encouraged in this teaching, i.e. wild meats such as caribou or moose, arctic char or other fish, and berries. Participation in community activities would also be encouraged. At approximately two to four weeks before the expected date of delivery, the pregnant mother is 'referred out' from her home community to a southern community, which has either a secondary or tertiary hospital facility (depending on the risk factor of the pregnancy). This entails the mother leaving her family and friends and going to another community, which in most instances has a different culture and a different first language.

Many people believe that such absences create social, economic and political problems for First Nations families and communities. Evacuation for birthing without family support, attended by people of differing cultures with differing first languages, creates psychological and physiological stress.[1] This absence from home is seen to result in social, economic and health consequences, both for the mother and the family she leaves behind.

Some of the social consequences voiced include loss of control of the birthing process and the knowledge associated with it. The diminishing role of respected community elders in assisting with pregnancy care and delivery, resulting in a generation gap. Without the father's involvement in the birthing event, mothers feel they lose some of their partner's respect. Siblings tend to show resentment towards the baby who has taken the mother away from them for awhile.

The economic consequences include the increased cost of phone bills, due to the number of long distance phone calls between the pregnant mother and her family. There is also the cost of using babysitters for the children left behind, when fathers are working or hunting and trapping out on the land. As a substitute for her absent family, out of loneliness, the pregnant mother sometimes spends money on entertainment and clothing in the urban setting, which increases the strain on the family budget.

The health consequences identified in the research by Kaufert, O'Neil and Postl,[2] are a result of mothers being isolated from their families in an unfamiliar environment. They worry about the family they have left at home and being in an unknown urban environment can be very stressful, resulting in an increased temptation by alcohol and drugs. Seeing a differing culture serving unfamiliar foods may result in a decrease in nutritional foods for the pregnant mother and her unborn infant. A lack of exercise, from being away from their own home environment, i.e. no housework, meal preparation, laundry, etc., results in boredom and watching more television. There is also the added risk of having the pregnancy medically induced if the mother is past her expected date of delivery, stressing the need to return to her family. Induced labour can often result in a poor progression of labour and a forceps delivery, or even a Caesarien section having to be performed.

The medical model deals only with narrow individual factors, here narrowed to issues of safety. However, aspects of health are influenced by not only the individual factors, but also by aspects of sociocultural background and economic status.[3]

Since the early 1980s, the number of deliveries conducted in isolated communities in the Northwest Territories has dramatically reduced, from a situation where most births occurred in the community, to the present day practice of routine medical evacuation of all prenatal women, irrespective of their risk category. With routine evacuation of all prenatal women, women have expressed their concerns about the resulting social, economic and health problems, which are more far reaching than purely the issue of safety. It appears, in the Aboriginal community these issues have more impact on their daily lives and family relationships, than the risk of a problem pregnancy.

The (Central Arctic) Keewatin Region of the Northwest Territories has seen much work focused on birthing. In 1980, there was a report on the health needs assessment of the Keewatin and this identified the issue of birthing (at this time 'low-risk' deliveries were still the normal practice in the nursing stations), as an important one. Most recently O'Neil et al[4] have undertaken a five-year study looking at the various birthing concerns within the Keewatin. These papers have demonstrated that the issues surrounding birthing are multiple and complex, and have changed — with the transition of community birthing for all prenatal women, prior to the intervention of southern medical care — to today's policy of hospital birthing for all. Many Aboriginal women believe strongly that the evaluation of maternal-child healthcare services by the use of maternal and perinatal mortality rates alone, is inappropriate. They express the belief that instances of family violence, incest and marriage breakdowns should be used as additional evaluation indicators.[5] It is felt these social problems within the family are consequences of a mother being separated from her husband and children for several weeks. Husbands left behind with the stress of childcare and homemaker duties are tempted to abuse alcohol and 'stray' from their family responsibilities. The new mother returns home and has to deal with a new situation which very often results in marital disharmony.

In the North, the issues of midwifery and birthing, although intricately interwoven, are separate issues. Midwifery is an issue that is very broad in scope and deals with many more aspects of the care of the pregnant woman and family than just the actual delivery. Today, especially in the more developed countries, including Canada (and its remote areas), birthing has become increasingly medicalized, from a normal life event that carried with it certain inherent risks, to an event where many of these risks have supposedly been reduced. This has been done by removing the event from the everyday life of the community to a hospital setting, and, as in the case of the Northwest Territories, this is often in a community hundreds of miles away from the mother's home. Over the past decade perinatal and mortality rates have been seen to decrease, which supports the government's prenatal transfer policy and their reluctance to change it.

During the summer of 1989 a comprehensive literature review, including extensive interviews to access provincial activity concerning midwifery, the legalization of midwifery and traditional Aboriginal midwifery practice, was undertaken by a nursing consultant for the Northwest Territories' Department of Health. In developing countries and elsewhere (Holland and Scandinavia), midwifery had emerged as a means of lowering maternal and infant mortality, as local women were trained in prenatal education, birthing techniques and postnatal care. Here, in the Northwest Territories, midwifery appeared to offer a solution to dissatisfaction with the Northwest Territories birthing practice of evacuation from one's home community several weeks prior to the delivery date.

The urge to enhance Aboriginal traditional midwifery and reintroduce nurse midwifery, was supported by the Keewatin Inuit Association, Inuit Women's Association, Native Women's Association, the Dene National Organization, Northwest Territories Women's Secretariat, and nationally by the Ontario Midwives Association, and the Canadian Confederation of Midwives.

COMMUNITY BIRTHING PROJECT

Dissatisfaction from families and communities in the Northwest Territories was being recognized by many Native organizations and women's groups. Concern was being voiced that birthing outside of the Northwest Territories would lead to nonrecognition of the child within tribal funding, which could effect future land settlement claims. Social, cultural and economic concerns were being expressed, as discussed earlier, associated with the separation of the mother from her family and home community. Also, women were expressing their concerns that Aboriginal knowledge around childbearing was being lost, due to the medicalization of pregnancy and birthing. The political pressure from all these groups, led to the announcement from the Minister of Health, in October 1990,[6] "that a pilot birthing project should be developed for low risk deliveries only, in a community in the Central Arctic Region of Keewatin, keeping in mind the safety of the mother and newborn." A two-year project was developed collaboratively with the Department of Health, Government of the Northwest Territories, and the Keewatin Regional Health Board. The community of Rankin Inlet was chosen by the Health Board because it had an airstrip, and a medical evacuation plane based there, a resident regional physician, and the largest prenatal population in the Keewatin Region.

It was felt, that, by having a community-based midwifery/birthing team in place, it could significantly affect the health and well-being of the mother and her new infant, thus reducing the perinatal and infant mortality and morbidity rates. A reduction in the incidence of low-birth-weight infants, through increased nutrition counselling, could reduce anaemia. Involvement of local elders and/or Aboriginal lay midwives could improve the physical and psychological supports to the prenatal women through community members involvement. Avoiding family disruption, by keeping the mother at home, could reduce the problems associated with alcohol abuse, i.e. child neglect, and marital or partner disharmony. Prenatal women have voiced their concern that alcohol consumption, by their partners left behind and by some of them in their strange environment away from home, increases during long family separation. There would be a reduction in travel and boarding costs to the government's Department of Health. There would be a revitalization of skills, experience and knowledge of community Aboriginal lay midwives, by having them involved in prenatal education — thus also providing a cultural support system for new mothers. The rate of medical intervention in childbirth, i.e. forceps delivery, induced labour, and Caesarian sections, may be minimized, when the mother is in a nonmedicated (hospital) setting for her delivery care. The uncertainty and risk of Aboriginal rights or identity would be removed, by having prenatal women give birth in the Northwest Territories (instead of Manitoba hospitals), and thus giving their children territorial status for future land claims. A significant contribution could be made to the contraceptive and childrearing knowledge of members of the community's childbearing and rearing age group.

To help achieve the above improvements, the combined principles of health promotion, community support and seeing the birthing process as a normal life event, formed the basis of thorough perinatal care, education, screening and follow-up — which in turn would allow for the provision of effective and safe midwifery practices. Through application of these principles, the community birthing project attempts to realize the following objectives: to bring low-risk birthing back to the community, and to provide high quality services to all childbearing families through the perinatal period. These services would include education and care extending to areas of: family planning, sexuality, gynaecological health, familial violence, newborn and child development, care and feeding — all focused at both the individual and community level. This would also foster the progressive autonomy of women and the community in self-health care, particularly related to childbirth and pregnancy.

This new initiative established a community-based birthing project steering committee, which included Health Board staff (two), board trustees (two), one of which must be a traditional (Aboriginal) midwife, a regional physician, an interested Aboriginal community resident, and a nurse/midwife consultant from the NWT's Department of Health. The terms of reference of this committee were to design and develop the scope of the project, from the principles and objectives which had been agreed to by both the Department of Health and the Keewatin Health Board.

Once in place and approved by both parties, funding was sought through the government of the NWT's Financial Management Board, as this was a new program which required salaries for new personnel and funding for renovations to the existing Community Health Centre structure. Due to the territorial 'financial climate' at the time, which included a monetary freeze on all new initiatives, the funding proposal was reviewed by the Department of Health's senior financial personnel with the Regional Health Board. It was decided to omit the budget for the evaluation of the project and apply for a research grant for the evaluating component once the project was underway.

Funding was approved in June 1992, and a Project Coordinator, Northern Nurse-Midwife (nonaboriginal) was hired in January 1993. The coordinator worked on job descriptions for the project staff, and the project's policies and procedures, in consultation with several professional and community members. The steering committee met frequently to review the progress of the development of the project. Renovations to the local Health Centre commenced early in the spring of 1993, with some delay due to an extension to the Rankin Inlet airstrip. Project staff were hired in August of 1993. Two nurse-midwives (nonaboriginal) were recruited from Ontario, with current midwifery experience from birthing centres around the Toronto area.

The Inuit Maternity worker, a well-respected individual with no midwifery experience, was recruited from the Rankin Inlet community. Being a mother with a keen interest in the project and a willingness to share community knowledge and learn from the nurse-midwives and local Aboriginal lay midwives, it was felt she was an appropriate choice. It should be noted here that the local elder lay midwives did not wish to actively participate in the project themselves, but were very willing to pass on their skills to a younger woman and teach the nurse-midwives also. They were on the advisory committee that selected the maternity worker.

The official opening of the project was November 22, 1993, which happened to be the day the first two babies were born, therefore tours of the birthing rooms had to be postponed to a later date! The project is being delivered out of the local Community Health Centre, where currently, community health nurses provide primary healthcare programs. The project staff provide prenatal care to all prenatal women in the Rankin Inlet community, and select, through a local Peri-Natal Committee, those of low or no risk, for delivery in the community. Given the complete isolation of the Rankin Inlet community, moderate and high-risk prenatal women are still transferred out of the community for delivery in a medicalized setting, to either Churchill or Winnipeg in Manitoba, or Yellowknife in the western Northwest Territories.

The mothers, who deliver in their home community, stay in the health centre up to eight hours following delivery and are then visited daily for three days in their own homes by one of the nurse-midwives or the maternity worker. All postnatal women are monitored up to six weeks postpartum, regardless of their location of delivery. It is hoped, with the concentrated focus on preconceptual and prenatal education, that many 'at risk' pregnancies can be reduced, thus allowing more prenatal women to have the opportunity to remain in their home community.

Traditional Aboriginal lay midwives in Rankin Inlet, who have not practised for over 20 years act, as 'consultants' to the project and as a resource for the maternity worker. They assist in incorporating some of the old Inuit traditions into the current midwifery birthing practices, i.e. position of the woman for delivery, local herbs to stop heavy bleeding, immediate infant care following delivery, and the encouragement of breastfeeding.

With establishment of the program, project staff are also focusing on other areas of reproductive health. For example, prevention and reduction of sexually transmitted diseases. Establishing well women and well men clinics, and introducing HIV pre- and post-test counselling. These activities are done in collaboration with the community health nurses in the Health Centre. Funding for evaluation of the project has been provided through the federally funded National Health Research Demonstration Project. North of 60 and the Keewatin Regional Health Board have contracted a credible evaluator to conduct the evaluation. The project will be evaluated in many areas, including quality of care, individual, family and community satisfaction, overall funding (savings for the NWT health system), staffing mix, and future training requirements to encourage more Aboriginal workers.

The evaluation will attempt to examine all prenatal care provided by the nurse midwives and maternity work and approximately 40 low-risk deliveries in Rankin Inlet. This will occur over a period not exceeding two years, and determine whether the current contingencies are well integrated within the existing health services. A control group, prenatal women from another Keewatin community receiving their prenatal care from nurses (none midwives), will also be included in the evaluation. This group will continue to be evacuated out of their community for birthing in a southern hospital as is the current Northwest Territories practice. Some pre- and post-interviews will be done, to determine their satisfaction or dissatisfaction with this practice and compared with the mothers delivered in their Rankin Inlet community.

The Rankin Inlet Community Birthing Project is a major step taken toward community wellness. To date, the benefits of the establishment of the birthing project have been many and varied. It has seen 31 percent of the total prenatal services and costs of confinement of the Rankin Inlet prenatal population, repatriated to the community. Travel, boarding and hospital costs have been saved by not sending women south for their deliveries. These costs contribute to the costs associated with additional staffing (nurse-midwives and maternity worker) for this new program in the Rankin Inlet Health Centre. The project has successfully reintroduced the expertise of traditional Aboriginal and nurse midwifery to the Central Arctic Region of Keewatin.

Midwives are providing holistic care, by not only caring for the prenatal and newborn infant, but involving the whole family in the 'special event.'

On average, every prenatal woman, during her pregnancy, receives two hours of health promotion information, which is expected to assist families to make informed decisions concerning their care. The community health nurses say that mothers appear happier and more confident in their parenting role. Members of the community have noted that prenatal teens are better prepared for birth and childcare, and the demand for escorts to accompany them for their confinement has lessened. Babies born in the community are immediately and strongly bonded to the father and family, as well as with the community. In addition, the mother gains respect from her attending partner. The partner, having participated in some of the prenatal education and experienced for the first time the stages of labour with his wife and the birth of their baby, appears to have created a new dimension to their relationship. Being involved in this special event in their lives and observing the strength of his wife, releases a personal sense of pride in him for her.

The midwives are introducing more natural and traditional methods of caring for mothers and babies. The maternity worker not only supports the nurse-midwives, but also gives advice to other health centre staff on incorporating a cultural approach to care. Within the project the difficult issues of childhood sexual abuse and family violence have been brought forward through the maternity worker. This was quite a revelation for the nurse-midwives and other nurses in the Health Centre. It appears much of this abuse does take place during pregnancy and had never been revealed in past prenatal clinics. Staff have advocated successfully for more family counselling services within the community to assist those families with victims of abuse and violence.

The successful lobby by the Aboriginal groups and Northwest Territories women, to bring birthing back to the community, is an indication of Aboriginal self-determination. One can empathize with women who are separated from home and family during childbirth. However, personally, as a nurse-midwife and professional, I feel there is an obligation to communities and to the unborn, to ensure safe births and the best possible start to life. This can only be achieved with careful attention to the legal issues.

To date (1996), the Northwest Territories government has not pursued midwifery legislation before this project has been formally evaluated. However, in my role as the Department of Health's consultant for this project and the Territorial contact on issues pertaining to midwifery, I have been able to keep the Department up to date on the progress of legislation in other provincial jurisdictions. Lessons learned from other lobbying groups would be an asset to assisting the Northwest Territories with development of their own legislation.

It would appear that the success rate thus far of this birthing project is forming the basis for legislation, given the uniqueness of the geographically scattered population of the Northwest Territories. The policies and procedures developed by the Keewatin Regional Health Board have provided the parameters for safe, quality birthing practices in a remote Northern community, with back-up support systems should an obstetrical emergency occur.

It is interesting to note that, to date, a physician has only been present in Rankin Inlet for two births, both of which, attended by the midwives, had normal outcomes. When the Keewatin Health Board were choosing one of their eight communities in which to reintroduce community birthing, Rankin Inlet was chosen because there is usually a physician based in the community a minimum of one week per month. The second year of the project has seen several high-risk prenatal women, going into premature labour, who have been successfully delivered in the community by the midwives. Minimal postpartum haemorrhages occurred, which were controlled by the midwives, an unexpected still birth and a premature twin delivery also happened. In the latter instance, the mother and infants were evacuated by air in a medically equipped plane to a Manitoba hospital, which resulted in a healthy outcome. It will be interesting to see in the Health Board's evaluation, if the on-site physician criteria remains, given the above outcomes. Community health nurses in other health centres within the Keewatin region have consulted and utilized the project's midwives when premature deliveries were imminent and no physician was available on site.

If midwifery is to be legislated in the Northwest Territories, high- and extreme-risk women (should their home community be isolated), will continue to be delivered in a hospital setting. However, with the increase of focused preconceptual and prenatal education, these risks may be seen to be reduced over time, thus increasing low-risk community births. Unlike the days of the nomadic groups and the 'lay' Aboriginal midwives, when infants and occasionally mothers would die during childbirth, there appears today to be an expectation that for every pregnancy there will be a healthy mother and baby, and that any problems that do arise can be dealt with in an appropriate manner with the appropriately trained staff.

The recruitment of southern trained midwives may hinder the practice of midwifery NWT-wide, given that there is currently only one training program in place in Canada (in Ontario). The Northwest Territories may need to look at a training program for Aboriginal community members, given the intricate role of the local maternity worker in this project. The formative evaluation of the project should identify these concerns with possible recommendations.

It is hoped that after a complete evaluation of this project, the integration of modern and traditional Aboriginal midwifery practices can be successfully added to the current primary healthcare programs offered in an isolated community, without risk to a new mother and her infant. Combining the skills of nurse-midwives with the cultural practices of traditional lay midwives, brings hope for the future that more local Aboriginal women can be trained in midwifery, for a revitalization of past practices!

ENDNOTES

1. See P. Kaufert, L. Paulette and J. Stonier's articles in *Childbirth in the Canadian North: Epidemiological, Clinical and Cultural Perspectives*, J. O'Neil and P. Gilbert, eds. (Winnipeg: Northern Health Research Unit, University of Manitoba, 1990).
2. P. Kaufert, J. O'Neil and B. Postl, *The Impact of Obstetric Evacuation Policy on Inuit Women and their Families in the Keewatin Region, NWT* (Winnipeg: University of Manitoba, proposal, 1986).
3. G.C. Helman, *Culture, Health and Illness* (Bristol: Wright, 1985).
4. J. O'Neil, et al, *A study of the impact of Obstetric Policy on Inuit women and their families in the Keewatin region* (NWT: unpublished, 1990).
5. L. Paulette, "The Changing Experience of Childbirth in the Western NWT," in *Childbirth in the Canadian North*, J. O'Neil and P. Gilbert, eds. (Winnipeg: Northern Health Research Unit, University of Manitoba, 1990).
6. Minister of Health, Ms. Nellie Cournoyea, Legislative Transcript (GNWT, Yellowknife, October 1990).

REFERENCES

Government of the Northwest Territories, Nursing Services Division. *Report of the Midwifery Issues as it Pertains to the Northwest Territories*. Yellowknife: 1989.

Government of the Northwest Territories. Legislative Transcript. Yellowknife: October 1990.

Government of the Northwest Territories. *NWT Data Book.* Yellowknife: 1991.

Helman, G.C. *Culture, Health and Illness.* Bristol: Wright, 1985.

Kaufert, P., J. O'Neil and B. Postl. *The Impact of Obstetric Evacuation Policy on Inuit Women and their Families in the Keewatin Region, NWT* (proposal). Winnipeg: University of Manitoba, 1986.

Kaufert, P. "The Epidemiology of Obstetric Care in the Keewatin District: Methodological Issues." In *Childbirth in the Canadian North: Epidemiological, Clinical and Cultural Perspectives.* J. O'Neil and P. Gilvert, eds. Winnipeg: Northern Health Research Unit, University of Manitoba, 1990.

Keewatin Regional Health Board. *First Annual Report of Rankin Inlet Birthing Project.* 1995.

Lessard, Pierre, and David Kinloch. "Nothern Obstetrics: A Five Year Review of Inuit Deliveries." *Canadian Medical Association Journal*, vol. 137, no. 11 (1987): 1017-1021.

Mason, J. "Midwifery in Canada." In *The Midwife Challenge.* S. Kitzinger ed. London: Pandora, 1988.

O'Neil, John, and Patricia Kaufert. "The Politics of Obstetric Care." In *The Inuit Experience in Birth Power, Social Change and the Politics of Reproduction.* Boulder/San Francisco: Westview Press.

O'Neil, John, Patrick Brown, Eva Voisey, Michael M. Moffatt, Brian Postl, Rosemary Brown and Bernard Binnis. *Inuit Concerns about Obstetrics Policy in the Keewatin Region, NWT.* Paper presented at the 7th International Congress on Circumpolar Health, Umea, Sweden, 1987.

O'Neil, John. et al. *A Study of the Impact of Obstetric Policy on Inuit Women and their Families in the Keewatin Region.* Unpublished, NWT, 1990.

Pauktuutit. "The Inuit Way." In *A Guide to Inuit Culture.* Updated.

Paulette, Lesley. "The Changing Experience of Childbirth in the Western NWT." In *Childbirth in the Canadian North: Epidemiological, Clinical and Cultural Perspectives.* J. O'Neil and P. Gilbert, eds. Winnipeg: Northern Health Research Unit, University of Manitoba, 1990.

Stonier, Jennifer. "Innulitsivik Maternity." In *Childbirth in the Canadian North: Epidemiological, Clinical and Cultural Perspectives.* J. O'Neil and P. Gilbert, eds. Winnipeg: Northern Health Research Unit, University of Manitoba, 1990.

Smith, Shirley. *Perceptions of Parents and Health Workers Regarding Childbirth in the Inuit Community of Rankin Inlet, NWT.* A discussion paper for NWT Department of Health and Keewatin Regional Health Board, 1991.

Closing Questions

As this book goes to print, more changes to midwifery and its regulation will be occurring, particularly in Alberta, British Columbia, Nova Scotia, Manitoba, Quebec and Saskatchewan. This book thus has no conclusions because the landscape is continually transforming. The 'new' midwifery — regulated and legalized — is still in its first trimester all over the country.

Midwifery has been nurtured in Canada by practitioners who have been willing to take legal risks to give women choices in childbirth. Midwifery gives women an opportunity to feel strong and powerful during pregnancy, labour and postpartum. Clients attest to the emotional/mental/social connections they develop with their midwives and how their births marked transitions in their lives which they will always remember. Midwives hold very special roles in the families of their clients, so much so that many practices have yearly gatherings for their former clients for the babies to meet their midwives as they grow older and for the clients to reconnect with their midwives. Clients often seek to have the same midwife for each of their births, so midwives often have a long-term role in clients' lives. Many clients feel a loss when the official period of their midwives' scope of practice is over (six weeks postpartum). They miss their midwives and continue to contact them for advice and support. Many midwives have maintained long-term relationships with clients, as friends, and provide advice for free. Most midwives are not motivated by monetary concerns and genuinely care for their clients. Being with clients at a (usually) joyous time — new life — midwives are associated with positive memories, excitement, growth and transitions.

The proven safety of midwifery, coupled with this kind of bonding between midwives and their clients, and other factors, have been viewed as a threat by the entrenched system of medicine in this country. Under the care of this system of medicine, many women experience further oppression when they are recipients of medically-managed childbirth services. Some women have likened their hospital birth experiences to rape; they have felt degraded, humiliated and violated by disrespectful personnel and invasive technology.

They have felt that their bodies were literally taken away from them and 'owned' for a time by hospital workers. Working-class women, women of colour, lesbians, new immigrant and refugee women, teen women, women with disabilities and others who experience exploitation, have often felt furthered punished by medical staff for being pregnant. Dominant Canadian society does not value groups of women outside the status quo, so when these groups choose to reproduce, some of the most damaging weapons of the medical profession are brought to bear on them.

In contrast, midwives strive to be caring and compassionate to all their clients. Midwifery has been marginalized for over one hundred years largely because physicians wanted to maintain their position as the most legitimate providers of perinatal care. Territoriality, professional jealousy and power struggles have characterized much of the relations between midwifery and medicine. In Canada today, this is slowly changing. While tensions still exist, midwifery has moved from the margins to the centre.

IS STATE REGULATION OF MIDWIFERY A GOOD IDEA?

The answer depends on many factors, perhaps most importantly on the perspective of the questioner. Some people will probably never be convinced that midwifery — especially home birth — is safe; they will continue to be against the inclusion of midwifery on state-covered medical insurance plans and for them, state sanctioning of midwifery has brought peril for consumers. Others will see the 1990s as heralding in the 21st century's new era of financially-covered birthing services; for them, the new midwifery has brought hope and the promise of empowered women/families giving birth to healthy babies. Still others will be in between these two extremes, seeing the indignities that occurred as a result of state sanctioning of midwifery, but not being willing to write off the entire profession because of the unsavouriness of some members in its leadership. Some of those who sit in this middle category ask if working-class women, new immigrants, women of colour, women for whom English is not a first tongue, or women with disabilities have been trained as midwives or have become midwifery consumers. If diversity has not been achieved in both the practitioner and client base, many critics will claim that state regulation maintained the privileges and access of elite Canadian women who could have afforded to pay for midwifery anyway. It is possibly too early to fully evaluate these issues but they are worthy of examination if only to remind those at the helm of midwifery that embracing diversity is a central need for Canadian birthing women.

The controversies over state regulation of this ancient women's calling continue to rage. For those who support the idea, being enfranchised by the state has brought many benefits. Midwives and consumers who have worked and/or are working for state regulation view legalization as: provision of funded choices for birthing women; protection of the public through the establishment of safety and professional standards for midwifery; better emergency care for birthing women as midwives gain hospital privileges; entrenchment in law and institutions of a genuinely woman-centred model of care; an opportunity to influence the broader healthcare system with social justice ideals; the possibility to have state-funded and therefore highly subsidized midwifery education, training and assessment; a victory for feminist organizing and years of hard work; a promise that midwifery will grow and continue (the numbers of midwives appeared to be declining in most parts of the country before movements for legitimation/regulation emerged, due to the risky legal status of midwifery and its poor remuneration); steady and adequate income for midwives; enhanced interprofessional relationships; an opportunity for midwives to practise openly; and the only logical choice in an untenable quasi-legal situation.

Those who do not support midwifery's regulation and enfranchisement are largely concerned with the compromises to midwifery care that this could bring. The practitioners among them want to be able to continue working in intimate and caring ways with women and decide how to operate their practices. Some are concerned that an elite group of midwives has been supported by the state and are helping their friends and shutting out their enemies. In-fighting amongst midwives continues, particularly for those midwives who lost their livelihoods and are legally barred from claiming the title "Midwife" and especially "Registered Midwife." This group is relegated to practice as labour coaches if they wish to continue legally working with birthing women. A few have gone 'underground' and practised illegally. The homogeneity of practice that state-regulated standardization enforces could take away from individual midwives' professional strengths and force them to work on their professional weaknesses. Making it compulsory for all registered midwives to practise in hospitals is intensely unappealing to midwives who want to do only home births. Others preferred being entrepreneurial private practitioners in the quasi-legal environment because they set their own rules and answered only to their clients — unless legal issues arose.

For some labour and delivery nurses, midwifery has been a threat, for it could take away some of their work. Other medical professionals, including some physicians, are also threatened by midwifery. These 'turf' battles will continue for many years. On a large scale, however, midwives will not be 'taking over' birthing in Canada. After almost four years of regulation in Ontario, for example, less than 3% of births are being managed by midwives. In Saskatchewan, those shaping the regulation of the profession are hoping that 4% of the births will be midwifery-assisted. The small numbers of midwives and the number of women they serve will thus not have a major impact on the healthcare scene in this country in the foreseeable future.

DOES THE IDEOLOGY OF THE PARTY IN POWER INFLUENCE DECISIONS REGARDING MIDWIFERY?

We have seen that the ideology of the party in power does not necessarily shape their views on midwifery. Both the left and the right may be in favour (or against) it. While much of the woman-centred philosophy resonates with the left, the potential cost-savings attract the right. In (extreme right-wing) Premier Klein's Alberta, midwifery is being regulated largely because it is perceived to be cheaper and it may be funded only in certain regions of the province. In (centre/left-wing) Premier Rae's Ontario, midwifery was welcomed for its woman-centred model and promise of support, education and caring for birthing women. In (extreme right-wing) Premier Harris' Ontario, midwifery continues to be funded at the same level as it was funded by Premier Rae's New Democratic Party (NDP) administration (although this could have been due to bureaucratic — as opposed to political — decision-making processes, i.e. it was simply easier to continue to fund midwifery than to evaluate it). In British Columbia, the NDP is behaving very differently than their counterparts did in Ontario; the B.C. College of Midwives has received much lower levels of funding than that in Ontario (even when the smaller population in British Columbia is accounted for). There is very little chance that a fully funded, separate and direct-entry midwifery education program will be started in British Columbia this decade (whereas three universities in Ontario received funding even before the official and final declaration of the act to regulate midwifery occurred), and midwives refused the first salary/income offer made by the B.C. government. Saskatchewan, on the other hand, under an NDP leadership, will probably adopt midwifery in a similar manner to the whole-hearted support that the NDP gave it in Ontario.

The *way* in which the left has implemented midwifery has thus been more supportive of the social justice/feminist ideals of midwifery. The right may legislate/regulate/implement it but not necessarily support a woman-centred mode of practice.

Generally, however, it is not possible to look into the crystal ball of midwifery's future by examining the ideology of governing parties. Sociologically, this could partly be due to the relatively similar agendas of various political parties in this country, given the capitalist system in which we live. Pleasing their electorate and saving money are prime aims of both the left and the right.

LOOKING INTO THE CRYSTAL BALL OF MIDWIFERY'S FUTURE

Midwifery will continue to be the choice of a relatively low percentage of Canadian women. Why? Partly because most Canadians consider hospital births to be the safest and most scientifically proven means of birthing. And partly because most Canadian women are not taught to learn about our bodies

(especially their reproductive organs), to understand the physiological processes that go on during childbirth, and to trust in the body's ability to undergo
the enormous changes which are normal and healthy during pregnancy and
childbirth. From many sources, women are taught to fear the pain of childbirth at such a deep level that the thought of 'natural childbirth' is unfathom-
able.

Canadian women are bombarded with media, peer and family messages
regarding their bodies; these messages have a profound impact on ideas
regarding pregnancy, childbirth and mothering. Messages that women:

- are definitely overweight (no matter what their size);
- need cosmetic surgery (to lift their breasts, make their noses smaller,
  or in the case of Asian women, to slit their eyelids so as to appear more
  European);
- must bleach their facial hair and shave/wax their legs and their arms;
- must straighten their hair, in the case of African women;
- smell awful and need to wear perfume;
- are hysterical and need to take drugs to calm down OR are too lifeless
  and need to take drugs to perk up;
- must spend most of their energies as caregivers for children and
  families;
- should always put their own needs after those of others;
- ought to accept poorly paid work which replicates nurturing work in
  the household (cleaning, food service/preparation, clerical, childcare
  etc);
- deserve emotional, economic and physical violence in their everyday
  lives;
- should be subservient and obedient to males, even boys, at every level
  of their lives;
- should acquiesce to the 'expertise' of the medical profession.

After a lifetime of these — and many other — oppressive messages, it
is no wonder that most women do not feel comfortable with the thought of
midwifery-assisted pregnancy and natural childbirth. The thought of giving
birth at home is even more frightening for many women. And even if women
are not afraid of trying to birth naturally, peer and family pressure is often
very strong and convinces us not to 'risk' the life of our children and
ourselves. Yet taking risks may be encouraged in many other situations;
statistically the most dangerous thing that Canadians (under the age of 35
years) do every day is to get into a car, but minimal discourse about this
everyday risk exists in mainstream culture. Risk is indeed a relative concept.

Canadian mainstream culture is profoundly mother-blaming. Mothers are
blamed for virtually everything that is 'wrong' with their children. Mothers
are blamed for not contributing to household income if they take time away

from the workforce in order to raise their children. Mothers are equally blamed for neglect if they put their children in daycare. This catch-22 situation prevents many women from making autonomous decisions about their lives which may be viewed as dangerous to the newborn. Mothers are told that it is normal and natural for them to be the sole caregivers of children. The lived reality of isolation of many young mothers who receive minimal support from others is drowned out by this message. And malestream messages indicate that the fetus/newborn's life is more valuable than that of the mother, so it's okay if the mother suffers. To some extent, many Canadian mothers have become resigned to this mother-blaming reality and turn to medical practitioners who uphold and are part of this status quo.

For these and other reasons, Canadian women will not be flocking to midwives in droves (at least not this century). Even in countries where midwifery is widely accepted, such as many nations of the South, midwifery is considered second-rate care. Most midwives are women. Since women are taught to undervalue ourselves, it is difficult to respect the knowledge of other women and to trust them as caregivers. Women who can afford obstetrical fees choose medically-managed births in most parts of the world where two-tiered medical systems exist.

Canada's tax payers will possibly save money in the long term with the introduction of midwifery services but more importantly, the small percentage of Canadian babies born in the presence of midwives will likely enter the world in a positive environment, with their mothers feeling empowered and connected to their bodies. This is the greatest potential of the new midwifery.

Contributors

IMAN AL-JAZAIRI was born in Basra in southern Iraq, and grew up in Kuwait. She came to Canada in 1981. She is a community activist, feminist and writer. She participated in coalition-building between the various Arab groups, between Arab people and other communities, and Canadian mainstream society. Iman has worked extensively with Arab women who are survivors of abuse. She was part of the organizing committees for Arab Heritage Day. In 1995, she was elected the Executive Secretary of the Canadian Arab Federation for a two-year term.

CECILIA BENOIT is an associate professor in the Department of Sociology and Assistant International Liaison Officer at the University of Victoria. Dr. Benoit's primary teaching and research interests are in work, occupations and professions, women's work and social rights, comparative healthcare systems, gender and health. She is author of *Midwives in Passage*, and has published journal articles and book chapters on mothering, midwifery and comparative healthcare systems. Her current writings are on changing reproductive care systems in Canada, Sweden and Finland, and a forthcoming book, *Women, Work and Social Rights: A Comparative Study*. She is a core-partner in a national Centre of Excellence on Women's Health.

RÉGIS BLAIS holds a PhD in psychology from the University of Quebec at Montreal. He is an associate professor in the Department of Health Administration and member of the Interdisciplinary Health Research Group at the University of Montreal. His research interests include the analysis of health services utilization, the evaluation of midwifery practice in Quebec, and the training of future midwives.

BRIAN BURTCH is an associate professor in the School of Criminology, Simon Fraser University, and also associate member with the Women's Studies Department, S.F.U. He has published articles, chapters, and books addressing issues of gender and legal regulation. His books are *The Sociology of Law* (Harcourt Brace Canada, 1992) and *Trials of Labour: The Re-emergence of Midwifery* (McGill-Queen's University Press, 1994). He also co-authored (with Kerri Reid and Paul Woodward) a government report, *Discovering Barriers to Legal Information* (Department of Justice Canada, 1994), which addressed problems identified by first-generation immigrants in accessing legal information and services in the lower mainland of B.C. He is now working on a co-authored book about the work of the late prison abolitionist, Claire Culhane.

CAROL COUCHIE was born and raised in Niagara Falls, Ontario and moved to Toronto as a young mother. She began her academic life at age 30 through the Transitional Year Program at the University of Toronto. At U of T, Carol studied psychology and was involved in the Aboriginal Health Professions Program. She eventually transferred to Toronto's Ryerson Polytechnic University upon being accepted into the Midwifery Education programme. Carol will be the first of many Aboriginal women to practice midwifery under the new legislation and looks forward to a time when she will be free to offer more midwifery services to women in the North. Currently she is practising midwifery in Toronto, where she lives with her two teenage daughters, Sarah and Rachel.

MARIE HATEM-ASMAR holds a PhD in Public Health from the University of Montreal. The subject of her thesis was the future education of midwives in Quebec. She has a Master's degree in Obstetrics and Community Health Care from Lebanon and a Master's degree in Health Administration from the University of Montreal. She is a certified nurse-midwife who was trained in Lebanon and France. In Lebanon, she taught in a school of midwives which she also directed for several years. Apart from this, she developed several programs in primary health care, particularly in the area of mother and child care in extraordinary war circumstances. Since she moved to Quebec a few years ago, she has given short training sessions for midwives. Her domains of specialization correspond to mother and child's care, education of health professionals, particularly midwives and nurses, and healthcare organization.

CAROL HIRD qualified as a midwife in 1969 in the United Kingdom. After immigration to Canada in 1973, she became active in the movement to legalize midwifery in British Columbia. A founding member of the Midwives Association of B.C., she helped to establish the B.C. School of Midwifery, and was its academic director from 1984-88. Her commitment to the aims of Safe Motherhood developed while she was a board member of the International Confederation of Midwives (ICM) for nine years. Carol was ICM President from 1990-93, during which time the Midwives Association of B.C. hosted the 23rd Triennial Congress of the ICM in Vancouver in May 1993. In fall 1993, she began an MA degree in Midwifery Practice at the Queen Charlotte's Hospital, London, in collaboration with Thames Valley University. Her thesis was accepted in 1996. She is now participating in the registration process to become a midwife in B.C.

AMY HLAING, RN, worked as a Research and Teaching Assistant within the Ontario Midwifery Education Programme and was a consumer of midwifery services. Currently she is working in Toronto at the York Public Health Department and Mount Sinai Hospital.

PAT ISRAEL is a disabled feminist who has worked in both the disability rights movement and the women's movement for the last 25 years. She is a consultant on disability issues and continues to be involved in presenting workshops on women with disabilities and their issues. Health, sexuality and mothers with disabilities are just some of the topics that Pat lectures on. Pat lives in Toronto with her partner John and four wonderful cats.

SUSAN JAMES is a practising midwife in Edmonton, Alberta. She is politically active in the Alberta Association of Midwives and the Canadian Confederation of Midwives, as well as a member of the Alberta Midwifery Regulation Advisory Committee. She serves as an assessment consultant for the British Columbia and Ontario Colleges of Midwives. Her doctoral research was a phenomenological study of the relations between women and their midwives.

CHARLENE MacLELLAN has been a practising midwife in rural Nova Scotia for 17 years. She is a graduate of the Halifax Infirmary School of Nursing, and the University of Alberta. She is co-founder of the Association of Nova Scotia Midwives and founding member of the Midwifery Coalition of Nova Scotia. She has been the Nova Scotia representative to the Canadian Confederation of Midwives/Confederation Canadiennes des Sages Femmes since 1988. She resides with her husband and two children in Kingsport, Nova Scotia.

MAUREEN MOREWOOD-NORTHROP, BScN, RN, SCM, trained as a Registered Nurse and Certified Midwife in England and Scotland. She has worked in many areas of nursing in the British Isles, Bermuda and Canada. From 1979-96 she worked in several of Canada's northern communities in various positions at the community, regional and government levels. She has participated in pre- and postnatal care and well-baby clinics as a community health nurse, also assisted in some emergency home births with community lay midwives. Maureen was the consultant for the Department of Health in 1989 when discussions on midwifery in the NWT began with political groups, and Native and professional organizations. She was a member of the NWT's maternal and perinatal committee 1990-95 and the NWT representative for the Canadian Confederation of Midwives 1991-95. She also participated in national conferences on midwifery and northern health issues. Maureen now resides on Texada Island, one of B.C.'s northern Gulf Islands, where she works part-time at the local medical clinic and is an ardent gardener.

HERBERT NABIGON (*Maangiins* — Little Loon), MSW, is assistant professor and coordinator of the Native Human Service Program at Laurentian University. He is a pipe carrier and traditional teacher who was taught Cree healing methods by several elders from western Canada. He has written chapters for *Rebirth: Political, Economic and Social Development in First Nations* and *Schooling and Employment in Canada*.

SAPNA PATEL is a feminist writer, editor, and community activist. She taught ESL in a Latin American women's community centre, and has been active in various grassroots organizations in Toronto. In the aftermath of the Gulf War, she edited and co-produced *Middle Eastern Times*. Sapna has been published in *Fireweed, Diva, Middle Eastern Times,* and *Elixir.* She is currently working on a poetry manuscript. For this paper, her interest is in the personal and global politics of midwifery. She would like to hear what other Ontario women of colour have to say about midwifery.

J. ALISON RICE, RN, BSN, MS, SCM(UK) is a midwife and a nurse currently teaching at the University of British Columbia School of Nursing and practising at B.C. Women's Hospital with the Midwifery Practice. At the time of writing this article she was in the process of applying for registration as a midwife with the College of Midwives of British Columbia. She has been actively involved with the evolution of midwifery in B.C. for many years. She has held the position of President of the Midwives Association of British Columbia from 1995 to the present and served on the Midwifery Implementation Advisory Committee from 1993-97. She received a BSc in Nursing from the University of British Columbia and a MSc in Nursing (Maternal Child) from the University of California, San Francisco. She earned her midwifery qualification at the Birmingham Maternity Hospital in the U.K. in 1981 and was a founding member of the first hospital-based midwifery practice in Canada, at the Grace Hospital in Vancouver, B.C.

MARY SHARPE, Registered Midwife (RM), BA, MEd. Over the last thirty years, Mary has worked as a teacher, childbirth educator, lactation consultant and midwife. She began attending home births in 1976 and since 1979 has been practising as a midwife in Ontario. In addition to her current practice with Riverdale Community Midwives in Toronto, she is working towards a doctoral degree in Adult Education at the Ontario Institute for Studies in Education at the University of Toronto and is a faculty member in the Ontario Midwifery Education Programme at Ryerson Polytechnic University in Toronto. Over the past two years she has served as a midwifery assessor for the Alberta government and the British Columbia College of Midwives. She has six children and recently had the privilege of being her eldest daughter's midwife.

FARAH MAHRUKH SHROFF, BSc, MEd (Primary Health Care), PhD, works in the areas of health, social justice, and holism. As an activist, educator and health professional, she had worked in many parts of the South, in Europe, and all over Canada. She sees her biggest challenge as bringing together structural analyses/action of race/class/gender struggles with analyses/action of spirit and ecology. She has taught in Canada's only university program to educate midwives for over four years. Her research areas include holistic health, policy, HIV/AIDS, women's health, and community development and health.

BETTY WU-LAWRENCE, RN MED, is a public member who was appointed by the Minister of Health in 1993 to sit on, first the Transitional Council, and then the Council for the College of Midwives of Ontario (1993-1996). She has chaired the Registration committee for the Council for a year.

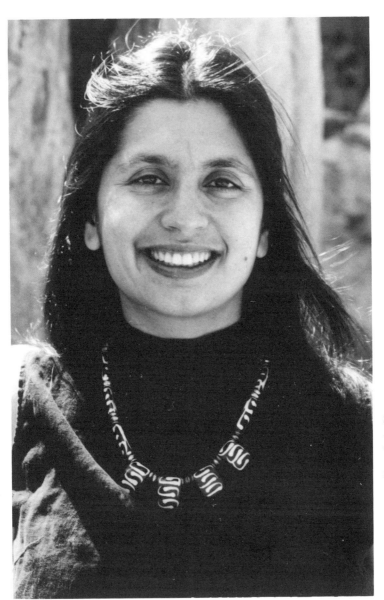

Photo: Janice Pinto

Farah M. Shroff, PhD, works in the area of public health as a researcher, educator/
professor and activist. She has worked all over the world for community
organizations, universities and governments. Her current research focuses on holistic health, health policy, and social justice issues.